Composite Materials

Luigi Nicolais · Michele Meo
Eva Milella
Editors

Composite Materials

A Vision for the Future

Springer

Editors
Prof. Luigi Nicolais
IMAST Scarl
Piazzale Enrico Fermi 1
Località Granatello
80055 Portici Napoli
Italy

Dr. Eva Milella
IMAST Scarl
Piazzale Enrico Fermi 1
Località Granatello
80055 Portici Napoli
Italy

Dr. Michele Meo
Department of Mechanical Engineering
University of Bath
Bath BA2 7AY
UK
e-mail: m.meo@bath.ac.uk

ISBN 978-0-85729-165-3 e-ISBN 978-0-85729-166-0

DOI 10.1007/978-0-85729-166-0

Springer London Dordrecht Heidelberg New York

British Library Cataloguing in Publication Data.
A catalogue record for this book is available from the British Library.

Cover design: eStudio Calamar S.L.

Printed on acid-free paper

Springer is part of Springer Science+Business Media (www.springer.com)

Contents

List of Contributors

L. Ambrosio, Institute of Composite and Biomedical Materials (IMCB-CNR), National Council of Research, Piazzale Tecchio, Naples, 80125, Italy

A. Beukers, Delft University of Technology, Kluyverweg 1, Delft, GB, 2600, The Netherlands

H. Bersee, Delft University of Technology, Kluyverweg 1, Delft, GB, 2600, The Netherlands

J. I. R. Blake, School of Engineering Sciences, University of Southampton, Southampton, SO17 1BJ, UK

S. W. Boyd, School of Engineering Sciences, University of Southampton, Southampton, SO17 1BJ, UK

L. Chang, King Saud University, Riyadh, Saudi Arabia

O. Choi, Mechanical and Aerospace Engineering Department, University of California, Los Angeles, CA, 90095, USA

J. M. Dulieu-Barton, School of Engineering Sciences, University of Southampton, Southampton, SO17 1BJ, UK

S. Feih, School of Aerospace, Mechanical and Manufacturing Engineering, RMIT University, GPO Box 2476V, Melbourne, 3001, Australia

K. Friedrich, Technical University Kaiserslautern, 67663, Kaiserslautern, Germany

A. G. Gibson, Centre for Composite Materials Engineering, University of Newcastle upon Tyne, Stephenson Building, Newcastle upon Tyne, NE1 7RU, UK

H. T. Hahn, Mechanical and Aerospace Engineering Department, University of California, Los Angeles, CA, 90095, USA

J. C. Halpin, JCH Consultants Inc., 7143 Hunters Crk., Dayton, OH, 45459, USA

F. Haupert, School of Aerospace, Mechanical and Mechatronic Engineering, University of Sydney, Sydney, 2006, Australia

S. Koussios, Delft University of Technology, Kluyverweg 1, Delft, GB, 2600, The Netherlands

A. P. Mouritz, School of Aerospace, Mechanical and Manufacturing Engineering, RMIT University, GPO Box 2476V, Melbourne, 3001, Australia

P. A. Netti, Department of Material and Production Engineering (DIMP) and Interdisciplinary Research Centre on Biomaterials (CRIB), University of Naples Federico II, Piazzale Tecchio, Naples, 80125, Italy

S. Quinn, School of Engineering Sciences, University of Southampton, Southampton, SO17 1BJ, UK

R. A. Shenoi, School of Engineering Sciences, University of Southampton, Southampton, SO17 1BJ, UK

T. Triantafillou, Department of Civil Engineering, University of Patras, Patras, GR-26500, Greece

Chapter 1
Future Aircraft Structures: From Metal to Composite Structures

A. Beukers, H. Bersee and S. Koussios

1.1 Introduction

During just 5 years after the 2003 centennial celebration of the Wright brother's first motorised flight, the price of a barrel of oil more than quintupled, to over US $100. In the first half of the year 2008 more than 25 air carriers went bankrupt and in January more than 35 regional airports in the United States had a 100% decline in flights. Imagine 35 cities, like Wilmington Delaware, hometown of polymer materials giant DuPont de Nemours, lost all connecting flights to main airports. Main airports in their turn had flight declines of more than 10%. Chicago O'Hare, for instance, had to deal with a decrease of over 3,000 flights in January.

In the middle of that same year, some time before the opening ceremony of the Olympic games, the Chinese HVT, a modified Siemens Velaro, set a new speed record of 394.3 km/h between Beijing and Tianjin, a 115 km track, thereby reducing travelling time to 30 min, centre to centre.

Together with the centennial of manned motorised flight, which was dominated by aluminium and pressurised fuselage structures for almost 70 years, there was yet another centennial to celebrate: oil supremacy as a prime energy carrier. From this fossil liquid derive various fuels with an unsurpassed energy content per kg, a property that is crucial for the success of transport in general and for aircraft in particular. In this age of transport by air, on the road and on water, the western hemisphere underwent an enormous technological boost followed by economical prosperity (Fig. 1.1).

Abundant availability of cheap energy carriers such as oil derivates is an essential stimulant for economic growth, like other precious resources,[1] but

[1] Cheap labour, commodities and precious materials.

A. Beukers (✉), H. Bersee and S. Koussios
Delft University of Technology, Kluyverweg 1, 2600 GB, Delft, The Netherlands
e-mail: A.Beukers@tudelft.nl

L. Nicolais et al. (eds.), *Composite Materials*,
DOI: 10.1007/978-0-85729-166-0_1, © Springer-Verlag London Limited 2011

exploitation is based on a classical approach: short term profits and slash and burn. For the first time this happened on a global scale.

As a consequence in the years to come cheap exploitable oil will become scarce and enforce a shift to other energy carriers for transportation and industrial use. Scarcity of cheap energy will also become a stimulus for new technological developments like miniaturisation of "systems" and dematerialisation of "structures". The cost of energy and the cost of pollution, particularly of water and air,

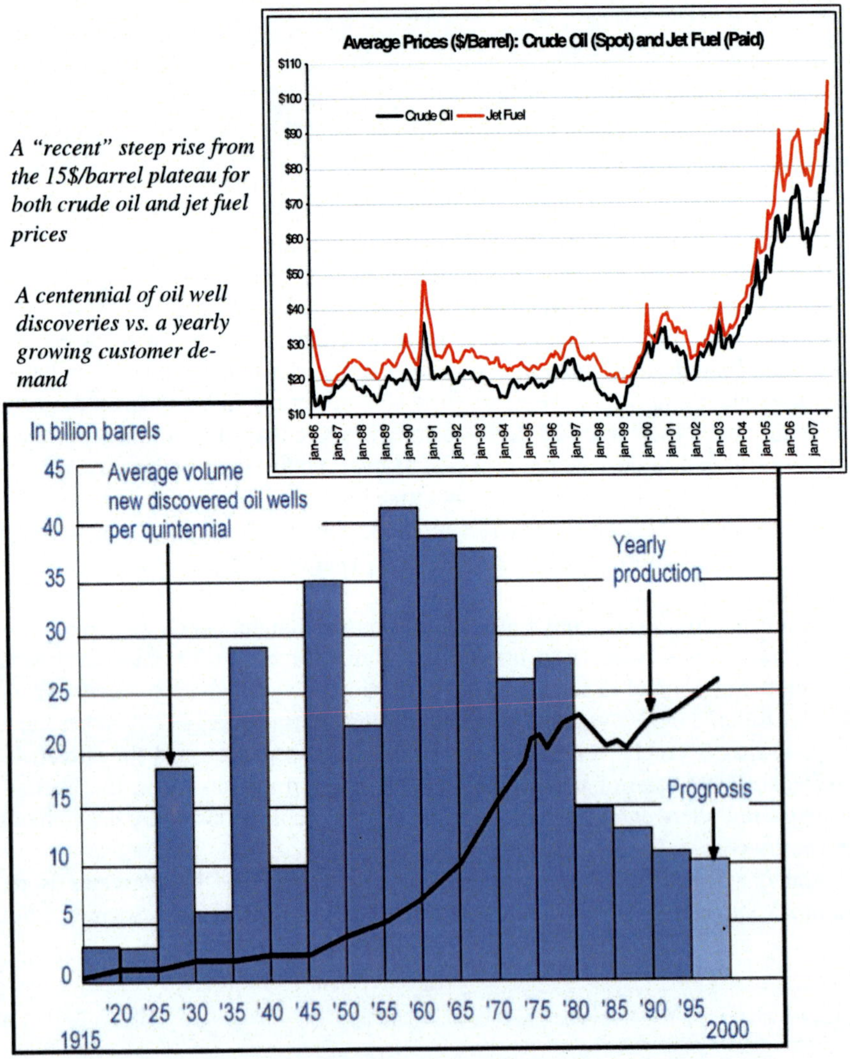

Fig. 1.1 Cheap oil and new economies 1998–2008 a decade of rising consciousness that burning oil is a cheap activity

are becoming essential economical parameters and will have a direct impact on yet another important parameter: quality of life.

So for all goods moving or being moved (transport and packaging) a reduction of mass is one of the major drivers to develop new concepts, materials and manufacturing processes without affecting the intrinsic system qualities (safety, comfort, reliability and durability). Most building blocks to design and build reliable metallic aircraft, the best long distance transport for busy people, were developed in the 1930s. From then on industrially produced all-aluminium aircraft appeared on the market, such as the Boeing 247 (1932) and the extremely successful Douglas DC 3 (1935). Especially the ability to build airtight pressurised cabin structures, as in the Boeing 307 "Stratoliner" (1937), became the start of a 70-year evolution into today's very efficient high velocity air transport systems, equipped with high bypass jet engine aircraft configurations. Since the 1960s most aircraft efficiency improvements came from technological development outside the realm of aircraft materials, structures and manufacturing. The biggest share consists of the reduction of specific fuel consumption (SFC) by advanced turbofan propulsion technology (40%) and improved aerodynamic efficiency Lift/Drag (15%). However, the structure efficiency of the aluminium aircraft concept did not change all that much. For about 90% of their weight, from the B707 until the B777 aluminium aircraft, structure development hardly contributed to aircraft efficiency improvement. Structural efficiency, the ratio of empty operating weight (EOW) versus maximum takeoff weight (MTOW) tended to shift to numbers higher than 0.50. For modern aircraft the EOW/MTOW is ranging from 0.50 to 0.66 and improvement by weight reduction was mainly annulled by other technological improvements: reliability, durability, passenger comfort and safety [1].

Fortunately, science in aeronautics and lightweight structure engineering is at the brink of the next revolution: the change from all-metal technologies to hybrid structure technologies, based on textile-reinforced polymers that are locally "blended" with metal elements.

In the near future a tremendous leap in material morphologies will take place: from intermediates such as solid plates and slender beams that are assembled and jointed mechanically, to flexible bundles of fibres (yarns), which are materialised into integral three-dimensional structures through both traditional textile manufacturing techniques and modern fibre placement machinery.

These textile structures are impregnated ("pre", "in situ" or "post"—before, during or after moulding) and finally "frozen"[2] or "solidified" into ultra modern integral multipart and multifunctional solid lightweight composite structures.

In the following chapters the authors present a personal view on ways to transform "state of the art" aircraft concepts into more efficient (more pay-load per unit weight and per dollar) transport, both by increasing structure simplicity and efficiency, and by a more straightforward use of modern materials and processes.

---

[2] The word "frozen" is used in this "essay" as a metaphor for the controlled polymerisation or solidification of polymeric media (both thermosetting and thermoplastic).

1.2 Carrying Load, Carrying Energy

By evaluating the forces that could transform new aircraft materials and structural concepts into a next generation of aircraft (and vice versa), classic and new morphologies of aircraft materials and structures will be presented and discussed, but first there are two essential questions to answer: (1) what is the future of transport, especially aviation, and (2) do innovations in materials and structures really matter?

1.2.1 Introduction, Future Transport and Energy

Recent price increases in fuel and the first attempts to tax CO_2 emission show that the future use of aircraft is no longer bound by creating low cost accessibility of transport for an unlimited number of people. Neither is the aircraft the sole solution to meet all transport and mobility demands in an increasingly urbanised world. Future continental air transport has to compete with high velocity trains that don't depend on liquid fossil energy carriers. What surely most limits transport, flying included, is that it will have to account for air pollution, which damages health, blights the environment and threatens vital natural systems. Technology cycles in aircraft technology of the past and the European goals for future developments are listed in Fig. 1.2.

For future ambitions, like EC 2020, a new technology aircraft technology cycle (S-curve) is essential to replace earlier aircraft technologies. Typical for successful transport system cycles is a maximum lifetime of 70 years. Seventy years of rise and seventy for decline: the change from animal traction to steam, from steam to electricity, from low velocity to high velocity trains are typical examples of that phenomena.

1.2.2 Energy Carriers

A very important "external" parameter for the development of new and more efficient transport is the world's general future demand for new energy technologies, based on gases (Table 1.1). Several energy system innovations,[3] beginning with the introduction of steam engines in the nineteenth century, have shown a fundamental change in dominant energy source from solid fuels to liquid ones, and in the near future to gases (natural gas CH_4 and hydrogen H_2). It is striking that the principal driving force for energy innovations, which we could regard as

[3] Energy system is fuel source plus the energy transformer (like coal, steam engine/electric dynamo).

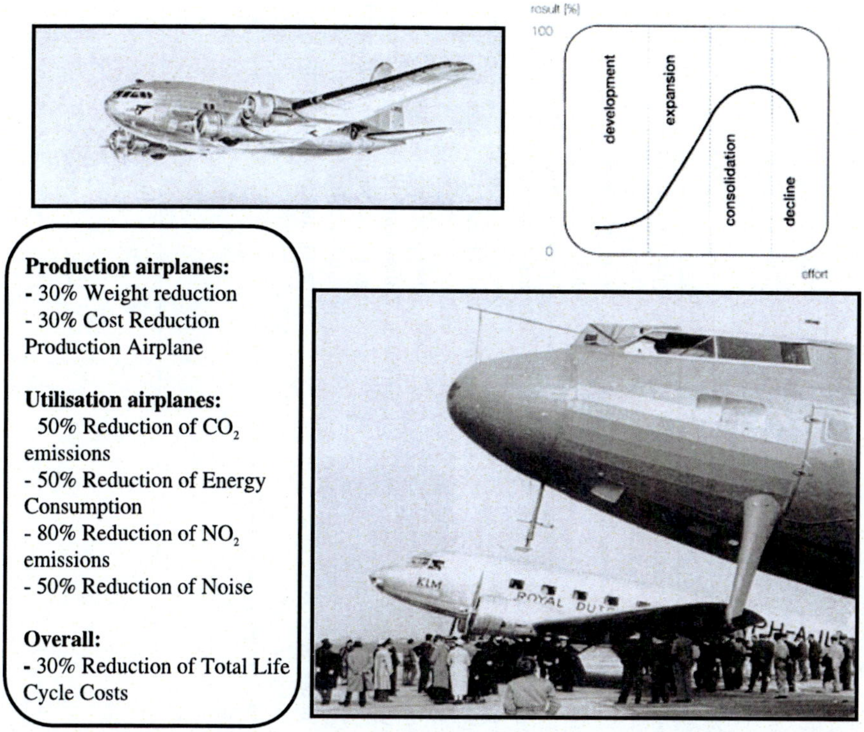

Fig. 1.2 Aircraft technology cycles and ambitions for 2020 wood linen and steel, 1880–1940 light alloy "tubes", 1930–2000 composites, "tubes", 1998–2060

discontinuities in energy technologies, is not so much the availability of fuel, but rather a market pull effect caused by end-use equipment development, which allow new superior services.

Future discontinuities in energy source exploitation could seriously affect future aircraft configurations. If hydrogen-powered fuel cells would cause a transition in road transport for reasons of improved performance, efficiency or sustainability, then oil production would decline, despite the availability of oil. This could have a serious negative effect on the availability of liquid fuels for air transport.

Therefore, although impractical in terms of energy content per mass and volume, the leap from liquid fossil fuels to hydrogen[4] is a possible future discontinuity in energy technology.

The critical problem for hydrogen, which is an energy transformer rather than an energy carrier, is how to store it, particularly in aircraft. For storage solid, liquid, gas or in situ production are the four basic options.

---

[4] The Peoples Republic of China is heavily investing to become a hydrogen based economy.

Table 1.1 Discontinuities in energy technologies, related types of transport and applied material families

Period	Energy carrier/transformer		Transport system	Materials
Up to 1830	Direct	Wood, wind, water, animals, man	Walking, horses, barges, coaches	Wood, linen, copper, brass and iron
1830–1900	Coal	Steam engines	Coaches, ships, trains	Wood, linen, iron, steel
1900–1940	Coal	Electric dynamo	Trains, cars, buses	Wood, linen, plywood, iron, steel
1903–2003	Oil	Internal combustion engines, piston and turbine engines	Cars, buses, flying machines, all aluminium aircraft with pressurised fuselages	Wood, plywood, linen, iron, steel, aluminium, polymers
1960–2025?	Oil	High efficient by-pass turbine engines	Supersonic aircraft Classical subsonic aircraft	Iron, steel, aluminium, polymers, titanium, composites
1970–1990	Nuclear	Centralised electricity distribution	High velocity trains	Steel, aluminium, composites
1990–2025?	Gas	Clean and efficient energy supply, CH_4 and H_2	City transport	Steel, aluminium, titanium, advanced composites, advanced alloys, ceramics
2025–future?	Hydrogen?	Fuel cell? Gas? Bio-fuels? Direct electricity Direct elektrocutie Highest caloric value Per unit volume and mass	Sustainable transport: smart cars, buses, new train concepts, high velocity trains Composite aircraft/BWB	New polymers, ceramics, fibres, new reinforcing materials and improved metals

For future aircraft only liquid storage of hydrogen seems to be realistic. If air transport cannot follow the discontinuity it is likely to become a niche market for the traditional organic or fossil fuel suppliers.[5]

On the other hand, if hydrogen will become the fuel for future aircraft then we will have to enter the era of cryogenic storage. Relatively heavy and bulky pressure vessels would considerably affect aircraft configuration and structural layout.

1.2.3 Vehicles Velocity and Vehicles Efficiency

In economical prosperous areas the different major public transport systems will evolve to optimal efficiency, each in a characteristic velocity domain. The optimal transport velocity results from the travelling distance and from the desire and ability of people to invest in time reduction.

Every moving vehicle has to overcome different forms of resistance or drag. The required effort, energy, and therefore fuel consumption depend directly on this resistance. Its nature varies from rolling resistance to aerodynamically induced friction and wave drag. In order to compare the efficiency of different transport systems in various velocity domains a specific drag (D_{spec}) is introduced. It is defined as drag per unit total vehicle weight.[6]

Because specific drag depends on speed, various characteristic velocity domains can be defined. But if transport systems for low, intermediate and high velocity, are selected on the basis of optimal fuel efficiency (as a function of the specific drag value), only three systems are likely to survive for the local, regional and (inter-) continental markets:

- "Smart" road transport systems[7]
- "High" velocity trains and
- "Subsonic" air transport[8]

Improving transport vehicle efficiency not only challenges innovative aerodynamicists and developers of active vehicle systems, but also structure designers, not as independent designers, but as actors in a multi-disciplinary approach.

---

5 Like Aviation Gasoline (AVGAS) for general aviation.

6 $D_{spec} = 0.30$ (equal to 30%) means: for 1 kg in transport about 3 N is needed to overcome resistance.

7 Smart could mean: (1) speed and separation controlled, (2) satellite navigation/control, when necessary manual control is overruled, (3) active, instead of heavy passive safety precautions (an enormous reduction of weight).

8 Increasing the cruising altitude reduces the specific drag of aircraft. The result is increased travelling speed.

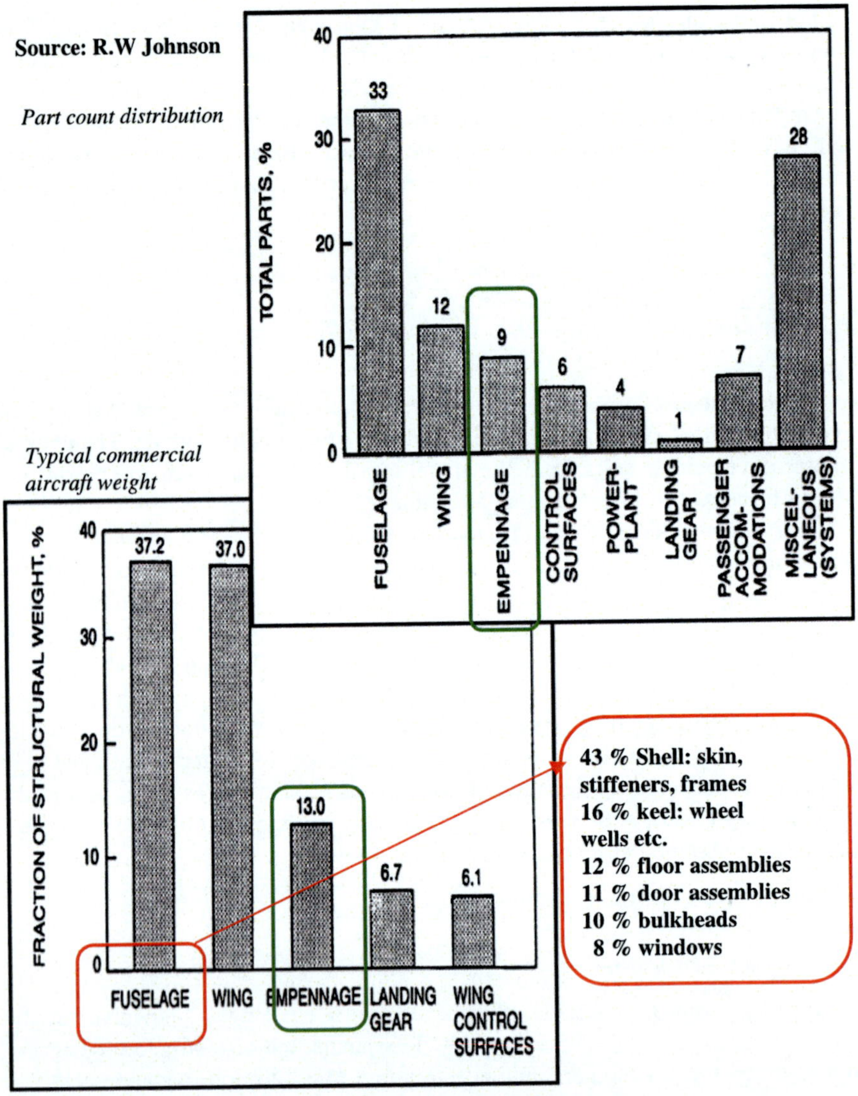

Fig. 1.3 AC structures in fractions 1985 fractions of weight and parts

To give an example: the empennage for passive stability and control used in traditional aircraft is a rudimentary drag and weight increasing leftover. It is "dead" weight in optima forma, 13% of structural weight, 9% of parts (Fig. 1.3).

Apart from weight reduction through a change in configuration, weight reduction of the system itself is a major challenge. When considering the vehicle efficiency $W_{system}/W_{payload}$ of conventional "state of the art" transport vehicles, the structure as a "small" part of the system (=structure, fuel and propulsion) itself still offers a considerable weight reducing potential, especially on the system level where acoustic and thermal insulation are important requirements.

In terms of their fuel efficiency, aircraft are performing well for continental transport and they have no real competition on intercontinental operation (Fig. 1.4). Since 1960, however, there is a continuous tendency to a rise in airplane cost per seat and to a decline in profit per passenger [2]. The question is how this can be reversed?

For traditional, well optimised, aluminium aircraft concepts no revolutionary breakthroughs are to be expected in the future. The same appears to be true in the

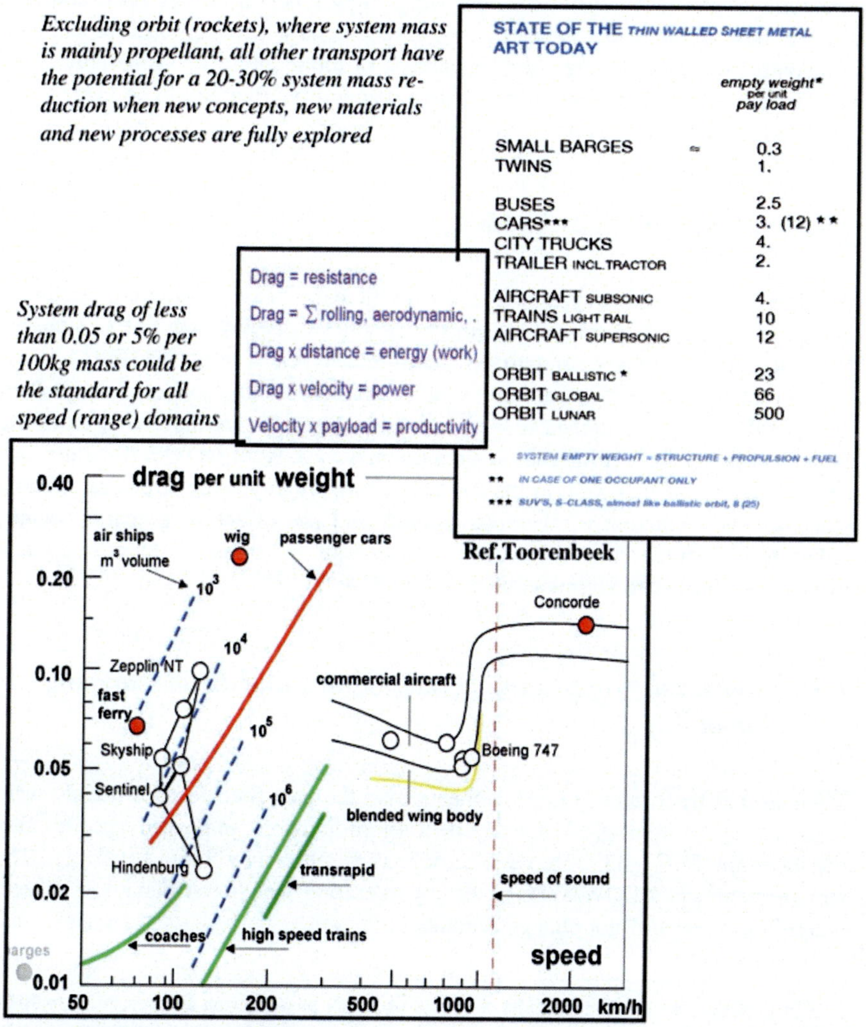

Fig. 1.4 Vehicle efficiencies 1932–2003—resistance to overcome per unit (total) mass—system mass required for carrying pay load

field of traditional aerodynamics and systems for stability and control. In addition, cost of personnel, taxes, insurance and fuel will probably keep on rising. Profits per passenger seat[9] will decline due to fierce competition in "open skies" markets. Therefore, only new aircraft with improved performance and durability per unit cost could create positive and more competitive perspectives and when international environmental regulations are tightened, these new aircraft even are the sole solution. Overall system weight reduction, improved aerodynamic efficiency or the aircraft lift versus drag ratio L/D, should lead to better performance per unit weight. In addition, improvement of L/D can be achieved through a change from passive to active (smart) stability and control in combination with advanced boundary layer control systems in the wing. New types of energy provision and storage, new aerodynamic aircraft configurations and a new approach to stability and control will have to affect the appearance of future aircraft considerably. This will be reflected in future structures. To be competitive they are to be made from more durable and sustainable lightweight materials.

1.3 Structural Weight Counts

An aircraft is a complex system. Transport efficiency between different aircraft is not a simple matter of comparing empty weight versus payload, not as straightforward as the efficiency comparison of different types of transport (Fig. 1.4). At take-off the mass of fuel, necessary to fulfil the aircraft's mission, especially when it's long distance, is dominant to the point that it becomes an important part of the "load" to be carried, from 18% for continental to 37% of MTOW for intercontinental flights (Sect. 1.3.2). In the following subparagraphs the structural mass is identified as a fraction of the total system and the effect of potential weight reductions is expressed in the reduction of energy and emission over an aircraft lifetime (according to Helms et al. and Lee et al. [1, 3])

1.3.1 Improved Propulsion, Aerodynamics and Load Carrying Capability

Most aircraft performance improvements over the past four decades mainly were achieved by technological development in propulsion, improved specific fuel consumption SFC and improved aerodynamic efficiency ratio Lift/Drag. The structure efficiency EOW/MTOW (empty operating weight vs. maximum takeoff weight) however did not change dramatically.

[9] In 2003 major airlines claimed to have a profit of $5 per passenger on average, equal to $0.05 per kg including luggage. The same profit per kg is claimed for competitive international road transport. Low fare airliners claim profits of $1.2 per passenger, which is equal to the profit of one sold cup of tea.

The improvement of the SFC with 1.5% per year, measured at cruise speed, resulted in a more than 40% reduction from 1959 until 1995 [1]. This mainly happened in the years before 1970 and was achieved through the increase of by-pass ratios (turbo-fans), the increase of peak temperatures (better materials and cooling) and increased pressure ratio (higher aerodynamic and component efficiencies). Due to the interdependency of changes, the SFC improvement also had negative by-effects, such as an increase in drag and weight (increased fan diameter and engine "ex-centricity"). The aerodynamic efficiency L/D has been improved with 0.4% per year on average for the same period of time, adding up to approximately 15%.

In comparison the improvements in structure efficiency EOW/MTOW are less evident, since materials, structural concepts and manufacturing technologies have not changed much since WW2. From the onset aircraft designers skilled in metallic structure design did very well in distributing aluminium (90%) to carry all loads over the aircraft lifetime. In the course of time most fuselages became in fact heavier due to safety and passenger comfort improvements and the ratio EOW versus MTOW decreased from 0.53 (B737) to 0.56 (A320-200) with extremes for down sized aircraft (A318) ranging from 0.60 to 0.66.

If we want to improve the average structure efficiency of mid sized aircraft to 0.50, as claimed for the B787–8 (and already a standard in the 1960s), we will have to reduce the total empty weight by 6–12%.

Let us take the typical singe aisle aircraft (A320–200 or the B737–700/900) as an example. Then we can identify how and where structure weight reduction can be achieved, for instance with carbon-epoxy composites that are considered 20–25% lighter in similar structures designed in aluminium (Sect. 1.5).

To identify the structure mass reduction impact on an aircraft system as a whole, the most common typical single aisle aircraft data are taken as a starting point:

$$\mathrm{EOW/MTOW} = 42\ /74\,\mathrm{ton} = 0.56 \tag{1.1}$$

In this type of aircraft the Operational Empty Weight is distributed as follows (Fig. 1.5):

50% = 21 ton, for systems, crew and power plants
50% = 21 ton for the structure in total.

If the aim is to reduce structure weight with 2.5 ton ([3], Fig. 1.5), this signifies on a "system level":

~25% weight reduction of either the wing or fuselage, or
~12% weight reduction of the total structure, or

for the total aircraft weight of an Airbus A320 type aircraft this only represents:

~6% weight reduction of the total empty operational weight.

For the structure efficiency (empty vs. maximum takeoff weight) this reduction of 2.5 tons (6% EOW), however, implies an improvement of EOW/MTOW from 0.56 to 0.53. When a old fashioned structure efficiency ratio equal to or less than

	Weight (kg)		Weight reduction	
OWE	40'925kg		- 2'500kg (-6.1%)	
Load	13'607kg		-	
	Short-distance		Long-distance	
	Weight	Weight reduction	Weight	Weight reduction
Fuel	8'823kg	- 319kg (- 3.6%)	19'144kg	- 664kg (-3.5%)
Fuel consumption	5'569kg	- 226kg (- **4.1%**)	15'399kg	- 563kg (- **3.7%**)
Total take off weight	63'355kg	- 2'819kg (- **4.4%**)	73'676kg	- 3164kg (- **4.3%**)
Relative energy savings	9.3%		8.6%	
Source: [FZKA 2003]				IFEU 2004

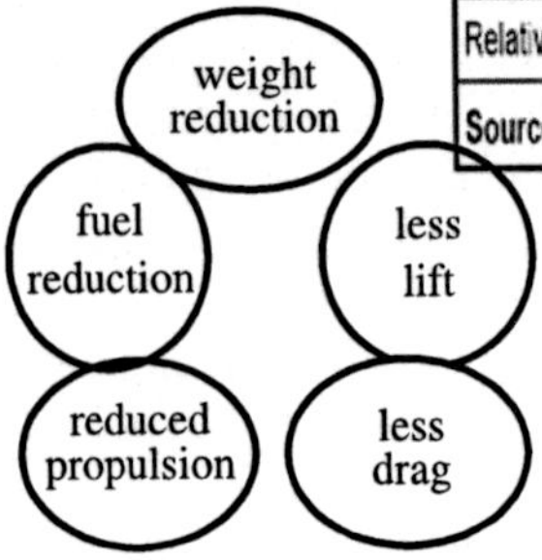

Snowball effect of a 2.5t operational empty weight reduction. Via 'fuel' reduction, the total take off weight is reduced 3.0t on average

A320, thirty year life time

Airbus A320	Short-distance	Long-distance
Take of weight (t)	63t	74t
Relative energy savings (%)	9.3%	8.6%
Life-time fuel consumption (t)	200'000t	222'000t
Life-time fuel savings (t/100kg)	295	258
Life-time final energy savings (GJ/100kg))	12'683	11'084
Life-time primary energy savings (GJ/100kg)	14,579	12,740
Source: [FZKA 2003]		IFEU 2004

Energy savings per 100 kg weight reduction for various aircraft types ("weight manager" tool, Lufthansa AG)

Aircraft type	Flight pattern	Annual fuel savings (t/100kg/a)	Life-time final energy savings (GJ/100kg)
A319-100		13.2	17,012
A320-200		12.3	15,852
A321-100/200		11.7	15,079
737-300	Short distance	13.4	17,270
747-400	Long distance	21.2	27,323
A340-300		17.2	22,167
Source: [Lufthansa AG 2003]			IFEU 2004

Fig. 1.5 Weight reduction counts *A320 short and long haul—2.5 ton ≈ 12% structure—* different aircraft types—100 kg lifetime reductions

Table 1.2 Weight percentages for "system" elements

Weight or mass "fractions"	Single aisle %		Long range %	
Pay-load		24		18
Fuel		18		37
Systems, crew, etc.	18		12	
Power plant(s)	11	29	10	22
Structure		29		23

0.5 is required to meet future environmental and economical demands, then the total weight reduction must be doubled to 12% of the EOW and in the case of this type of aircraft a structure weight reduction of 25% over the total structure, which is 50% of the total EOW.

1.3.2 Fuel Reduction by Empty Weight Reduction

For modern single aisle and long-range aircraft, designed in the 1980s, the following weight percentages for "system" elements can be determined in relation to maximum take-off weight as listed in Table 1.2.

Weight reduction of structures in traditional aircraft (tube, wings, empennage), and its effect on fuel consumption and CO_2 reduction was not really an issue in the past decades. Programs to diminish mass generally were executed to meet the specifications of the initial design, since traditionally, apart from being delayed, new aircraft when launched on the market are more expensive and heavier than originally proposed.

The traditional after launch weight reduction programs, often worth thousands of dollars per reduced kilogram, were meant to reach or increase the prototype's proposed payload or flying range (fuel). Recent growing societal and political interest, however, were the incentive to start studies to determine a broader impact of mass reduction [1, 3].

According to the most recent study by Helms et al., a 100 kg weight reduction for a long distance aircraft results on average in the following energy and fuel savings per year:

Energy saving:	667 GJ/year·100 kg
Specific energy content:	35 MJ/litre
So fuel saving per year per 100 kg:	19,000 litres

Because aircraft do have an operational life of at least 30 years, an initial 100 kg weight saving here has more impact than in any other form of transport.

We can use the estimated fuel saving as a crude indication for the consequence of weight decrease in a large passenger carrier. According to Boeing data a B747-400 navigates on average 1.9 million miles per year. A 747's fuel consumption is about 19 l/mile[10](5 gallon/mile), so the annual (365 flight days) fuel consumption equals 36 million litres.

For a 1% weight saving, 1,810 kg of the B747 empty weight of 181 tons, the result in a fuel consumption is a reduction of 190 l/kg × 1,810 = 0.344 million litres (2,177 barrels, 25 kerosene transport trucks), which is a slight reduction of 0.96% fuel consumption per year.

Although for 1% of weight saving (~4% structural weight saving required) the percentage of <1% fuel saved is low, but the absolute values saved per year are not.

For a B747–400, 1% mass reduction is equivalent to 0.344 million litres of kerosene per year and the cost saving, at the price level of $100/158 litres, is at least $218,000 per year with a CO_2 emission reduction of about 160 tons, tax free, per year.

1.4 Aircraft Structures: the Past, the Present and the Future

The choice of materials in relation to structural concepts is usually based on designer skills and the company's manufacturing traditions. Materials are selected accordingly. When emerging materials and technologies provide opportunities to improve products or even develop distinguished new ones, local customs and interests generally frustrate that. In the case of international collaboration programs, local interests and politics often feed emotional and irrational decisions. Change based on realism usually is hard to swallow for all stakeholders from worker to shareholder, who are active in obsolescent technologies. Aerospace business was and still is a rich source of examples of this phenomenon. In airplane history, however, several technologies have been overruled by new emerging opportunities.

Fuel cost per passenger

For modern long-range aircraft the next average jet fuel consumption per passenger per 100 km can be determined [4]:
Boeing 747: 3.5 litre/passenger × 100 km
Airbus 380: 3.0 litre/passenger × 100 km
The flying distance between Amsterdam and New York is about 6,000 km.
Both aircraft for this flight need per passenger, respectively:
B747: 210 litre = 1.32 barrel,
A380: 180 litre = 1.13 barrel,
since 1 barrel equals 158 litres.
For the "old fashioned" barrel price of $100 ($0.633/litre), the fuel cost per passenger for a trip Amsterdam–New York will be US $132 and $113, respectively.
The difference of $19 is for "successful" main carriers, which is about four times the average profit of $5 per passenger and 16 times a $1.2 profit per passenger in the case of the best performing price fighters.

The first attempt to build flying machines was based on the use of natural materials like silk or flax that was woven to dense square fabrics (taffeta), supported and pre-stressed by "fingers" of young birch or ash sprouts. This shaped the lightest

[10] Expressed in a standard for cars: ~11 litre per km (11/400 = 0.03 litre per passenger km).

possible bird and bat inspired wing structures, similar to the sketches of Leonardo da Vinci. Artisans from guilds of weavers, upholsterers and furniture and shrine workers thus became the first builders of bird mimicking contraptions. This kind of artisan technology was applied to build Otto Lilienthal's glider, the first successful attempt to mimic soaring birds.

Later on coach and bike manufactures, using primitive industrial means, enabled the evolution from floppy surrogate bat wings to frames and truss structures made out of steel wires (tendons), spruce for compression rods (bones) and beams loaded with bending forces (stems).

Firmly pre-tensioned linen was used to upholster spruce ribs, spars and girders to form aerodynamic airfoils. The development of plywood laminates allowed the creation of stressed skin wings and fuselages (Lockheed Vega, Fokker wings). Industrially manufactured wooden plate and shell structures were glued together with natural starch adhesives. In the 1930s the change was made to synthetic glues of phenol resins in order to overcome temperature and moisture sensibility.

Although the Fokker passenger aircraft, the Lockheed Vega and the fast and stealthy Mosquito of De Havilland outperformed most metal aircraft in their days, plywood was soon to be replaced by aluminium. Sheets of this metal were assembled into riveted plate structures, basically following iron shipbuilding methods.

Stressed skins, supported and reinforced by stiffeners and frames, allowed unforeseen improvements and developments. The introduction of aluminium, however, was purely ideological and political. A similar phenomenon hampered the introduction of new composite structures, in today's civil transport aircraft.[11]

The arguments against composites used by current metal designers are almost the same as those in favour of replacing wood with metals. They include: poor understanding of mechanical behaviour, hard to predict, anisotropy, large scatter in properties, lack of fire resistance and fast degradation. But these arguments are no longer valid for modern synthetic composites. Composites, fibre reinforced polymer plies, stacked and cured to laminated structures nowadays are well-understood and predictable with respect to mechanical and physical behaviour. In addition several composites are fire resistant and very durable (Fig. 1.6).

Aircraft structure history revisited

The successful replacement of wood by aluminium in the 1930s was based on four presumed improvements [5]:

fire safety

- weight reduction
- production cost reduction
- improved durability

[11] This has been different for sailplanes, helicopters, including rotor and propeller blades, military fighters and stealth bombers. Here rationalism is prevailing and composites have largely replaced metals in shell structures. It is likely that geopolitical arguments were overruled by value for money criteria.

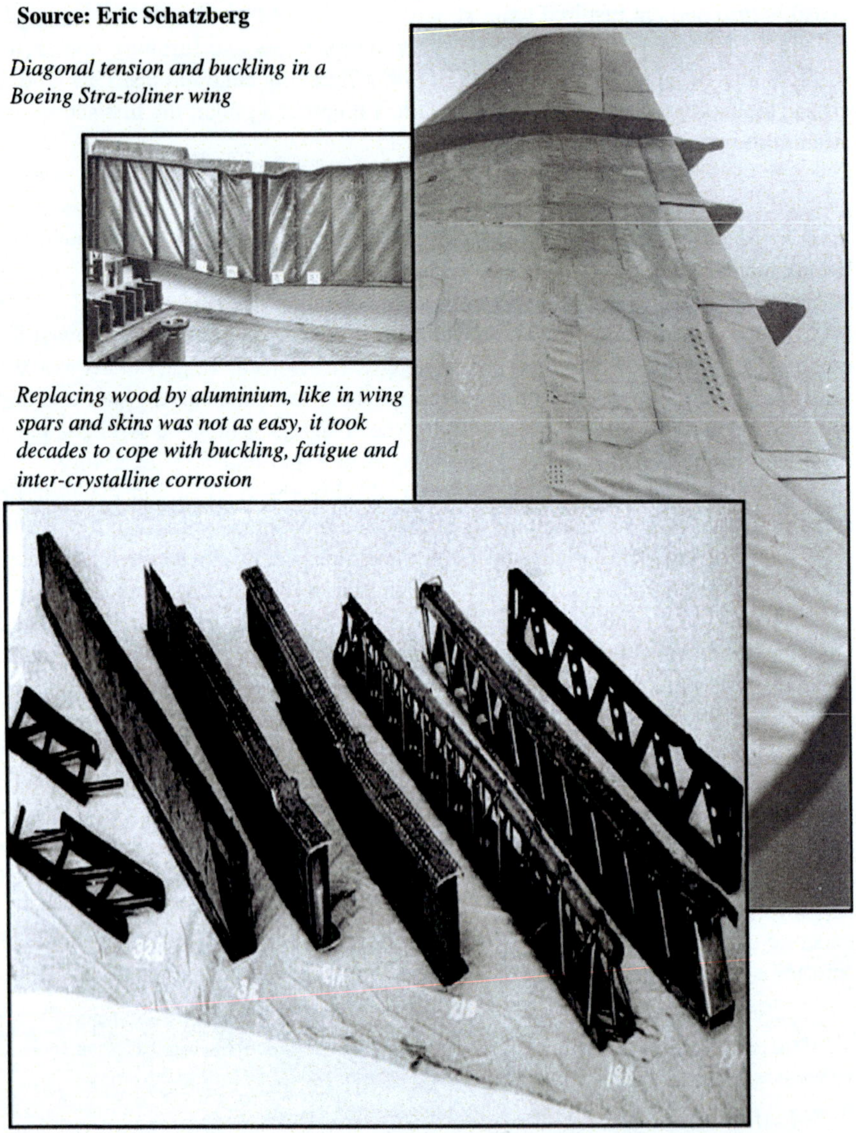

Fig. 1.6 Aircraft structures history revisited 1932–2003 aluminium structures the latest standard

This belief and the predictability of mechanical properties linked metals to "science" and "progress" and made wood "old-fashioned", even artisan. It was purely rhetorical and not based on research, let alone experience. The idea that metal airplanes were "incombustible" proved to be naïve. Weight appears to be an even more complicated issue as it depends, by nature, on structural efficiency, which in its turn varies with the nature of the loads that structural components have to bear. It took enormous effort to build lighter planes in metal. Buckling, a failure mode based on structural instability in compression, became a new phenomenon and appeared to be a dominant design criterion. Stressed skin concepts could handle shear by diagonal tension. However, diagonals loaded in compression were not weight competitive: thin skin would become unstable and susceptible to buckling. Control of the buckling phenomenon in aircraft resulted in complex locally stiffened aircraft structures with the accompanying high parts count and abundant riveting.

Problems of buckling and durability of aluminium structures like inter-crystalline corrosion and fatigue were scientifically investigated and either solved or made controllable. When these structural problems were under control, the metal airplane proved to be much more expensive to produce than wooden ones. The reason that the production of metal airplanes was not stopped, originated from the firm belief that mass production of intermediate parts and well organised assembly would reduce the production costs in due time, like in the automotive industry.

The wrong initial arguments in favour of the change from wood to aluminium were rapidly overtaken by other, more substantial but rather unexpected advantages such as the pressurisation of the fuselage necessary for high altitude, high-speed, flight combined with aerodynamic smoothness. The capability of the metal airframe in this respect changed large-scale transport by aircraft into a success. Now, after 70 years of improvement and optimisation of aluminium alloys, parts manufacturing and assembly, the traditional metal semi-monocoque structure has reached the stage of consolidation and even decline of the technological life cycle.

The same four arguments that were falsely used to advocate the change from wood to metal aircraft can now be truly used to promote the change from metals to composites for future aircraft structures. To these arguments can be added the crash energy absorbing capability (formula I racing) and the durability and sustainability of composite structures.

1.4.1 Modern Aircraft Structures, Light and Efficient

All modern aircraft structures are assemblies of thin skins lengthwise reinforced by stringers, which in their turn are supported by either frames in a fuselage, or ribs in a wing. In fact this is a "semi-monocoque" structure, whereas a pure monocoque—a shell without reinforcements similar to a sandwich structure, is rarely found in primary structures. The all aluminium sandwich structure of the Breguet Atlantic suffered extremely from its operational environment, with difficult repairable corrosion spots and de-bonds as a result. When in the near future well designed and processed polymer sandwich structures will have proven their reliability (Extra 500, Raytheon Premier business jets), this structural concept might offer specific advantages for fuselage structures, such as integration of both mechanical, and thermal and acoustic insulating properties with a minimum of frames and stiffeners.

One of the reasons for stressed skin structures to become the standard in lightweight structure design is the fact that in thin-walled, slender aircraft structures multiple load conditions (magnitude and orientation) occur and that individual structure elements can be dimensioned for specific roles. In plane tension and compression loads are always combined with out-of-plane loads. The material volume that is necessary to sustain tension loads has to be distributed in the out of plane direction as well, in order to create stabilizing bending stiffness that will resist buckling, which is caused by in-plane compression or shear loads (tension–compression).

Through this mechanism stringers prevent skin buckling, but also contribute to the load carrying capacity of a structure as a whole and offer a (once unexpected) advantage: they act as crack-stoppers to restrict the growth of through thickness cracks in metal skins under tensile loads.

In addition the stringers, together with ribs or frames, provide rigidity for loads perpendicular to the skin, and crushing loads, and they redistribute local loads over the entire cross-section as well. These individual elements apparently enable designers to orchestrate multi-functional behaviour of structural elements responsible for the efficiency of the structure as a whole ([6], Fig. 1.7).

1.4.2 Structural Efficiency a Matter of Geometry and Continuity

It is known that, without taking the engineering constants of materials into consideration, structures critical for compression or bending vary in their effectiveness to sustain these loads by the way material is distributed over the cross-section. Well-designed cross-sectional dimensions, plate thickness, stringer pitch, stringer height and of course the stringer cross-section design itself are major parameters to improve the load carrying capacity per unit weight. However, many applied stringer configurations were not selected for their efficiency, but for reasons of manufacturing and assembly cost reduction. In future structure design a rethink of stringer concepts is necessary to establish whether metal design solutions that are attractive for numerical machining, bonding or riveting are the appropriate solutions for lighter laminated composite structures.

Examples of structure efficiency improvement for buckling critical wing panels are presented by comparing the panel efficiency coefficient (Fig. 1.8).

This value of η depends on the various ratios that define the shape of the cross-section, such as the stringer height to pitch ratio. If the equivalent thickness $\bar{t} = t + A_s/b$ and the skin thickness t have a fixed relation, in other words the ratio $\bar{t}/t$ is kept constant, the efficiencies of different stringer/skin cross-sections can be determined, of course in relation to both global- and different forms of local-buckling, for major parameters to improve the load carrying capacity per unit weight. However, many applied stringer configurations were not selected for their efficiency, but for reasons of manufacturing and assembly cost reduction. In future structure design a rethink of stringer concepts is necessary to establish whether metal design solutions that are attractive for numerical machining, bonding or riveting, are the appropriate solutions for lighter laminated composite structures. For example, the Z-stringer, having a fixed characteristic web/flange dimension ratio, d/h = 0.3, the maximum efficiency value $\eta = 0.955$ is reached at about a ratio $\bar{t}/t = 2.5$. In general reasonably efficient panels are obtained at $\bar{t}/t$ values above 1.5 with the advantage that more cross-section material is part of the skin itself. A "robust" skin has many advantages and allows a larger stringer pitch. In

Sources: Schatzberg, UniDelft

Douglas DC3, riveted aluminium plates and (extruded) girders

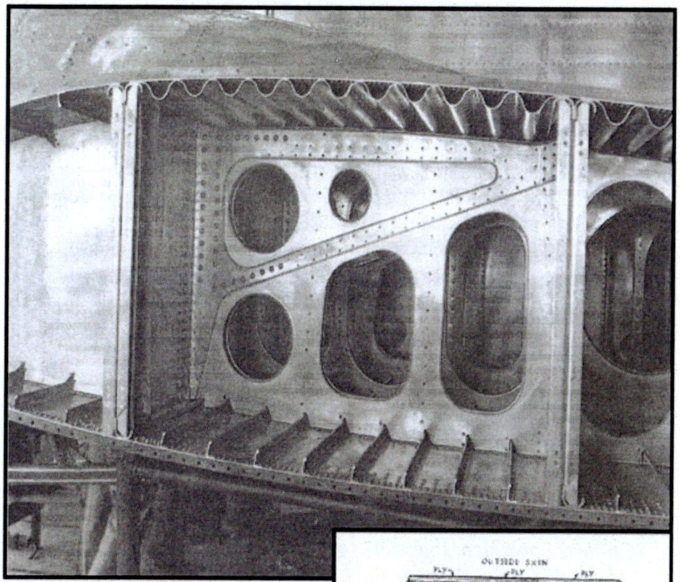

DH Mosquito, laminated and bonded ply-wood wing structure, and a sandwich mono-cocque fuselage

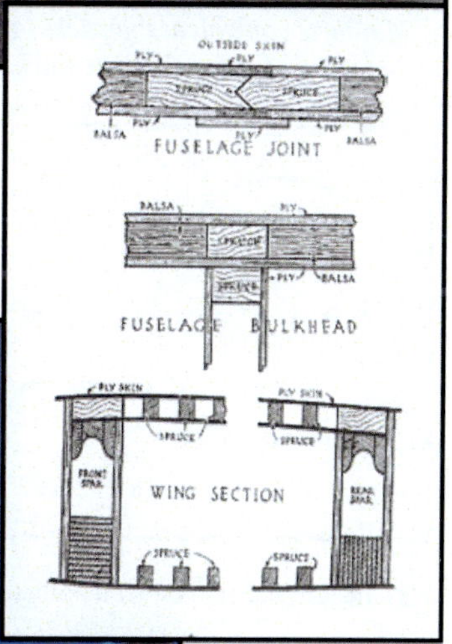

Fokker F28, laminated and bonded aluminium plates and (rolled) girders

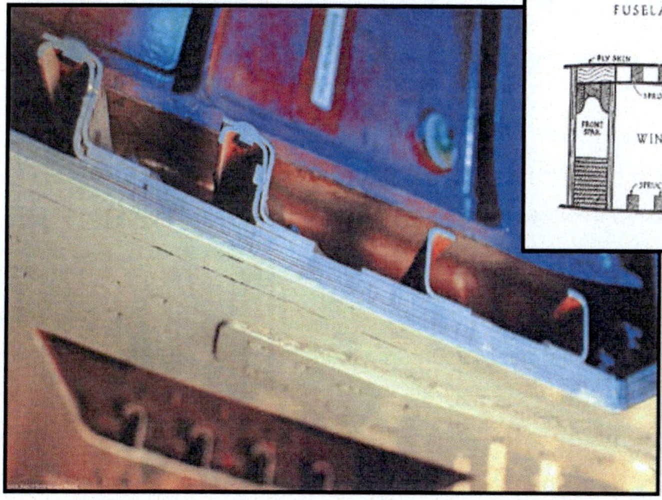

Fig. 1.7 Aircraft structures designed for manufacturing 1930th, 40th and 50th

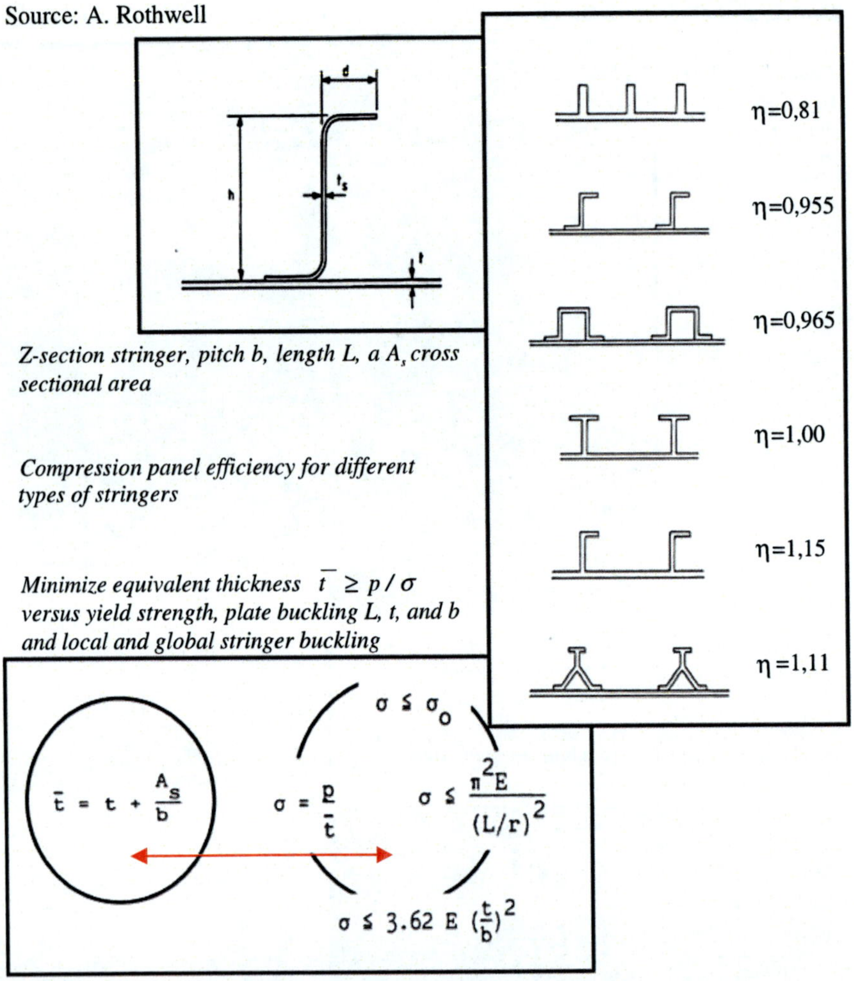

Fig. 1.8 Stiffed skin structure efficiency 1932- buckling or compression critical wing panels

the same reference [6] the mass per unit area $\bar{t}.b$ is determined,[12] showing that the only variable of the panel efficiency is the material efficiency $E^{1/2}/\rho$ (Fig. 1.8) in case all other parameters (loading and geometry) are fixed, which mostly is the case in comparison studies of existing structures.

This efficiency comparison of slender structural panels loaded in compression, which is exclusively based on cross-sectional material distribution optimisation, shows the enormous potential of weight saving by stringer design. The popular

[12] $W/\bar{t}.b = (\sqrt{E}/\rho) - 1.\sqrt{(\sigma.\,\bar{t}.L)}.\eta - 1$

Diagonal tension fields around windows, during complete fuselage static tests

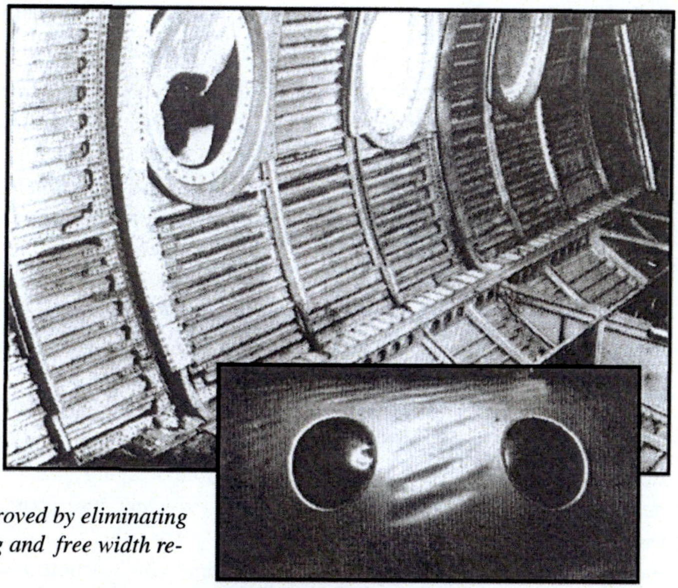

Static strength improved by eliminating inter-rivet buckling and free width reduction by bonding

STRENGTH OF SHEAR PANELS

Panel	Sheet thickn. (in)	Stiffnr. thickn. (in)	Stiffnr. spacing (in)	Height of web (in)	Ult. shear stress (lb/sq in) riveted	Ult. shear stress (lb/sq in) bonded	Mat.
I	.032	.040	5	10.5	20,700	23,900	24 ST
II	.040	.032	3	18.0	12,400	15,100	24 ST
III	.060	.048	3	18.0	25,400	29,800	75 ST
IV	.032	.032	6	18.0	8,500	9,100	24 ST

Fig. 1.9 Continuity counts 1955 F27 fuselage, "Redux", phenol formaldehyde adhesive lquid + powder, 150oC, 14–100 psi

blade stiffener is only attractive because milling is cheap. So if new materials and processes enter the picture, it is worthwhile to re-optimise the total cross-section and to replace rivets by adhesives or integral designs. The Fokker F27 fuselage tests in the 1950s, showed the benefits of bonded structures: metal laminates without fibres. Static strength was about 10% higher compared to the riveted versions, and the improved fatigue resistance gave the structure a (pilot equivalent) life of 90,000 flights.

Composite materials may not only improve these achievements of metal laminates, but they will reduce the maintenance costs to fight corrosion as well.

Of course in the impact-sensitive areas special protective measures have had to be taken. Amazingly in the F27 these include the application of glass-fibre-reinforced composites in all leading edges, and in door edge- and propeller ice-protection plates (Fig. 1.9).

1.5 Laminated Structures: from Metal to Composites

The greatest benefit for future “frozen” textile structures is the sustainable way of manufacturing large structures. Starting with simple intermediates, like bobbins of yarns, tapes and fabrics, the textile pre-form representing the “core of the structure” can be transformed into a “cloth”. This is then impregnated with a resin after or during fibre placement in a mould. A final cure in an oven (no size limitations) and the application of atmospheric over pressure (vacuum bagging) is all that remains. This procedure, in which various fibre/textile placement machines can play a role, is the ultimate form of “downstream manufacturing”. It implies a maximum reduction of intermediate steps between basic material selection (the “ingredients”) and product realisation (the “cooking”).

When fibre reinforcing materials extend beyond glass- and carbon fibres and include yarns of metal fibres that can be shaped in the same way through available textile fibre placement techniques (weaving, tape laying, filament winding, etc.), a new range of applications should emerge. If steel and aluminium mills could produce appropriate steel and aluminium yarns, the unprecedented textile-like formability affords complex three-dimensional shell structures, unlimited in size. Any mechanical, physical and electric magnetic property can be realised by blending. Expressed in textile terms, by inter-mingling, co-mingling and laminating with fibres and yarns of metals, minerals and polymers the number of applications will become infinite.

If we compare two existing fibres for application in shell structures, carbon and glass, in terms of mechanical performance per unit weight (the structure efficiency) we can compile the following list for differently loaded structural solutions. Starting point for comparison to aluminium 2024 sheet is a simple cross-ply laminate (50% 90°@50% 0°) of plain fabrics, a 50% fibre volume content and equal cure cycles (120°C) see Table 1.3.

The comparison is based on ideal materials, without defects, but sensitive to higher temperatures and humidity (80°C/wet).

For the time being the determined allowable strain levels,[13] at least the carbon-epoxy laminate design thresholds, are too ambitious for strength comparison studies, even for hot/wet conditions (Table 1.3, Limit Load Strain = 4,200 $\mu\varepsilon$). In recent composite aircraft designs the allowable values of contemporary carbon-epoxy laminates, being rather brittle and notch sensitive, the values for fibre-dominated[14] designs are in the following range in Table 1.4:

[13] No matter the built up of the laminate: different to stress distributions, strain distributions over the plate thickness are uniform in pure tension/compression and linear in the case of bending.

[14] Mechanical properties of resin sensitive or matrix dominated laminates may be harmful affected by temperature and humidity.

Table 1.3 Structure efficiency or performance per unit weight, for different existing materials, virtually materialised into a few typically loaded structural members

Structure efficiency or static performance per unit weight		Engineering constants	Carbon fibre yarns (T300, 1581)	Glass fibre yarns, e-type (181)	Alu 2024 plate values (e.g. cladding)
Fibre properties	Density	$(\rho)\ 10^3\ \mathrm{kg/m^3}$	1.76	2.58	
	Young's moduli	$(E)\ 10^9\ \mathrm{N/m^2}$	230	73	
	Yield stress	$(\sigma_y)\ 10^6\ \mathrm{N/m^2}$	3530	3450	
Cross-ply laminates, plain weaves, styles 1581, 181, $V_f \approx 50\%$, 120°C, "B" values, RT/dry, "compression"	Sheet values	$(\rho)\ 10^3\ \mathrm{kg/m^3}$	1.5	1.9	2.7
	For composites	$(E)\ 10^9\ \mathrm{N/m^2}$	50	23	72
		$(\sigma_f)\ 10^6\ \mathrm{N/m^2}$	420	260	–
	$\sigma_y = \sigma_f/1.5$, to have a limit load reference	$(\sigma_y)\ 10^6\ \mathrm{N/m^2}$	280	173	320
		$\sigma_f/E\ (\%\varepsilon)$	0.84	1.1	–
		$\sigma_y/E\ (\%\varepsilon)$	0.56	0.75	0.4
	Hot and wet	$\sigma_y/E\ (\mu\varepsilon)$	5,600	7,500	4,000
	Knock down factor	$\sigma_y^{h,w}\ 10^6\ \mathrm{N/m^2}$	211	130	320
	<1.33 For strength values	$\sigma_y^{h,w}/E\ (\mu\varepsilon)$	4,200	5,600	4,000
Cross-ply, hot, wet	Material coefficient	$(E^{1/3}/\rho) \times 10^3$	2.46	1.43	1.54
		$(E^{1/2}/\rho) \times 10^3$	149	79.8	99.4
		$(E/\rho) \times 10^6$	35.4	10.4	26.7
Cross-ply, hot, wet	Load	$(\sigma_y/\rho) \times 10^3$	141	68	118
	Coefficient	$(\sigma_y^{1/2}/\rho)$	9.7	6.0	6.6
	Limit load	$(\sigma_y^{2/3}/\rho) \times 10$	23.6	13.5	17.3

Table 1.3 (continued)

Efficiencies	Structure elements	Dominant parameter			
Cross-ply relative to aluminium 2024					
Solid shells					
Compression	Buckling critical	$(E^{1/3}/\rho)$ vs. $(E^{1/3}/\rho)_{alu}$	~1.6	~0.9	1
Bending	Strength critical	$(\sigma_y^{1/2}/\rho)$ vs. $(\sigma_y^{1/2}/\rho)_{alu}$	~1.5	~0.9	
Tension	Strength critical	(σ_y/ρ) vs. $(\sigma_y/\rho)_{alu}$	~1.2	~0.6	
Beams					
Compression	Buckling critical	$(E^{1/2}/\rho)$ vs. $(E^{1/2}/\rho)_{alu}$	~1.5	~0.8	1
Bending	Stiffness critical	$(\sigma_y^{2/3}/\rho)$ vs. $(\sigma_y^{2/3}/\rho)_{alu}$	~1.4	~0.8	
	Strength critical				
Sandwich shells					
Bending	Stiffness critical	(E/ρ) vs. $(E/\rho)_{alu}$	~1.3	~0.4	1

The relative values are related to aluminium 2024. The yield stress is the lowest stress at which a material undergoes plastic deformation or failure

Table 1.4 The allowable values for fibre-dominated carbon-epoxy laminate designs

μStrain	Limit	Ultimate "B" basis	Factor(s): SF × knock down
Tension ε_t	3,500/4,000	9,000	2.6 = 1.5 × 1.7
Compression ε_c	2,700/3,000	7,200	2.7 = 1.5 × 1.8

Source: Airbus

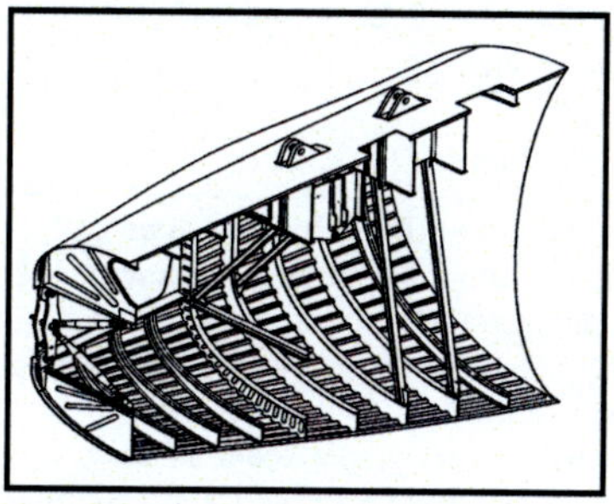

Fig. 1.10 Classical laminated skins stringers and frames accomplished redesign A300⟹A330 tail section, 1 to 1 metal to composite replacement >455 kg saving

The applied static maximum "B"-values[15] are being reduced by a standard safety factor 1.5 and knockdown factors of 1.7 in tension and 1.8 in compression (Boeing). The bold printed LL strains are values used by Airbus (Fig. 1.10). The knock down values used by Boeing are almost the square of 1.33, which is a factor to cover hot/wet conditions alone. It seems that these critical static strain data are determined by tests on specimens containing a "saw cut". Therefore they are severely affected by "standard deviations" and "stress raisers". When in structure design these maximum strains are used they will largely cover fatigue spectrum loads as well. This explains the statement: "Composites must be considered as materials exhibiting poor static properties rather than good fatigue ones" [7], which means that compared to aluminium, composites are rather more critical for static strength than for fatigue.[16] So what the efficiency ratios in Table 1.3 show is that for the loaded structural elements presented, which are those known to be critical for buckling and fatigue, a change to carbon fibre composites give most weight reduction profit. For static strength dominated structures (fittings, joints) the structure efficiency data presented must be corrected for stress raising effects (factor above the environmental knockdown factor 1.33). The most important lesson to be learned for future design is that the best strategy to reduce weight and to improve durability is a maximum elimination of stress concentrations or raisers,

15 "B" value: the value above which at least 90% of the population of test results is expected to fall with a confidence of 95%.

16 Endurance strain limits for different structural details, S–N curves, have values at 105 cycles of about 4,000 με for composites, 3,000 με or less for aluminium.

Table 1.5 Preliminary estimated savings per structural group, CFRP versus AL

Structure	Design allowables[a]		Saving potential of CFRP (%)		Weight (kg)		
	AL (MPa)	CFRP (με)	Optimistic	Pessimistic	AL	CFRP Optimistic	CFRP Pessimistic
Shells	300	3,000[b]	35[c]	20	650	420[d]	520
Frames	200	4000	65[e]	40	230	80	140
Fittings	200	4000	50[f]	30	150	75	105
Total of selected groups			44	26	1,030	575	765
Total of section					1,750	980	1,295

Aluminium: 100 MPa ≈ 1,400 μstrain
[a] Maximum allowable values: stiffness, instability and fatigue
[b] Maximum strain: stiffness, instability
[c] Saving potential: higher in stability critical areas
[d] Weight estimation: 435 kg CATIA
[e] Optimistic value: simple beam bending
[f] Saving potential: experience stabiliser fitting

imposed by discontinuities,[17] notches, open and riveted holes, resin dominated areas: reduce the local reduction factors. In local areas it also saves the "beef-up" or local thickness increase to house the counter sunk rivet heads and additional local factors, such as the bearing factor (1.15) (Fig. 1.10).

On the material level a better match of fibres and resins (stiffness, adhesion and toughness) and better hot/wet properties is another strategy to follow: reduce the global reduction factor < 1.33 for hot/wet conditions. The reduction of global factors affects the total structure. The reduction of local factors by part integration is smaller, but creates simpler and more durable structures, with savings of fastener weight, cost and assembly.

By comparing the respective efficiencies of different structural members (same load, same geometry) in Table 1.5, even for the "simple" laminate selected, carbon-fibre reinforced composites offer the best mechanical performance per unit weight in large shell structures. For buckling and stiffness critical parts, the improvement compared to aluminium varies from 1.6, 1.5 to 1.3 or, inverted to weight reduction per unit load, from 0.63 and 0.67 to 0.76, which on average entails a potential 30% weight reduction. In the case of structural members that are critical for static strength at limit load, but have no (expensive) stress raisers (a future scenario!) improvements are in a range from 1.5, 1.4 to 1.3. After inversion weight reduction per unit load ranges from 0.6 and 0.71 to 0.83 when compared to

[17] The original steep thickness and stiffness variation in the A320 vertical tail fittings suffered from de-bonding by shear and peel stresses during fatigue tests. Reduction of the thickness, thus gradient, and increase of the number of fittings in later fin designs solved this problem.

the unit aluminium. For members critical for bending a maximum reduction promises to be 30% on average and about 15% for tension critical members.

If we consider glass-reinforced polymer structures, like extensively applied in aircraft interiors (floors, sidewalls, ceilings, bins, etc.), Table 1.3 shows that a change to carbon fibres can achieve an easy weight reduction of let us say 20%, without any drawback regarding Fire, Smoke and Toxicity regulations. An educated guess: in this respect for an F27 weight saving potential would amount to about 200 kg, and for an A320 about 600 kg. By today's standards these are attractive savings (Fig. 1.1).

1.6 Composites and Multidisciplinary Aircraft Design

For aircraft structures dominated by stiffness or strength, the potential of aluminium alloys to improve the mechanical performance has been explored exhaustively. A change to new morphologies, from solid plates and profiles to fibre metal laminates or even wires and fabrics, offers the potential for new hybrids with improved specific mechanical and fatigue properties. Companies make huge investments to consolidate proven technologies on the threshold of obsolescence and try to stay ahead of potentially stronger emerging technologies. However, it is a known phenomenon that in the stage of decline in any given technology life cycle, "optimization" only leads to minor improvements (on top of S-curve). Every advance in, for instance, metal yield or failure stress is at the expense of a decrease in fatigue or corrosion resistance. All modifications and new formulations within one material family mostly leave Young's modulus of elasticity unaffected, but that is the key to stiff lightweight structures (deflection, vibration or buckling critical). So in general, major improvements can only be achieved by the introduction of more potent material families, with better specific properties and more attractive manufacturing possibilities to build structures with higher added value.

This latter argument is also important because newly developed materials and their technology are almost by definition more expensive than their traditional rivals. Therefore adding maximum value for money becomes the leading principle. Replacing just a material in order to save weight, for instance aluminium by carbon fibre reinforced epoxy on a one to one basis (black metal structures), is the most convenient, but also most inattentive approach imaginable. It ignores extreme risks due to differences in material response to local overload or to design failures (friendly and slow cracking vs. nasty and explosive de-bonding or de-integration).

If we have to select the most challenging and for innovation most attractive part for multidisciplinary design, then the pressurised fuselage in conventional aircraft, or the passenger compartment in a flying wing, is the ultimate candidate. It is the heaviest, the most expensive and by number of parts and assembly time the most complex structure of all (Figs. 1.4 and 1.6).

1.6.1 Multi-disciplinary Fuselage Design, Integration of Mechanics and Acoustics

Starting point for the choice of new combinations of materials, structural concepts and manufacturing technologies should be efficiency improvement by integration of functions. Fig. 1.11 shows schematically which requirements have to be fulfilled for development and design of aircraft fuselage structures.

The most important structural design and material requirement categories are distributed along the horizontal axis. The level of function integration during manufacturing as realised through the structural design concept is plotted along the vertical axis. The wave-like envelopes moving away from the origin represent materials, structures and technologies, with increasing potential for the integration

Sources: [8]

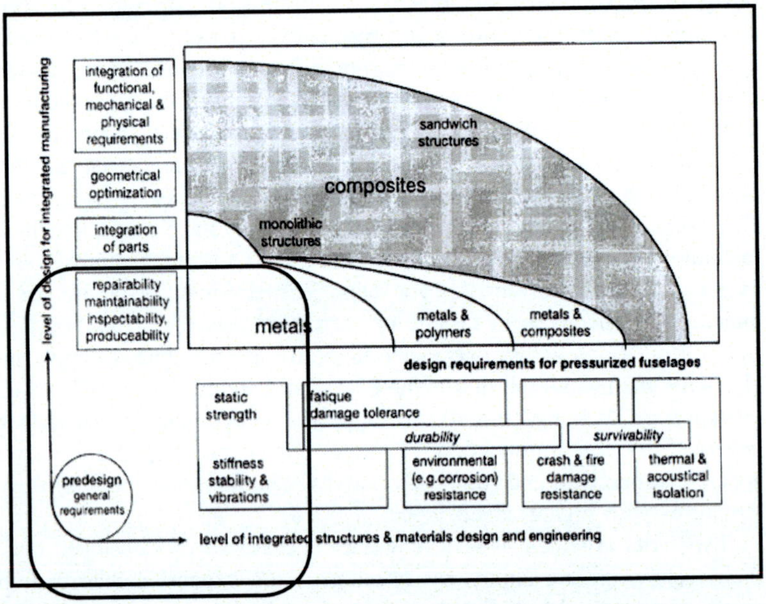

Fuselage & Empennage:
41 % of total number airframe parts

50.2 % of structural weight

1.25 average cost for airframe

Fuselage design requirements in a nut shell:a change to composite structures opens the door for integration of parts and functionalities (manufacturing) and the integration of static and dynamic structure integrity with durability and survivability requirements (design & engineering)

Fig. 1.11 Fuselage design in fractions 2000 integration–segregations. Integration–segregation integrated design material and structure design for manufacturing of functions further to the right. When properly executed the result for a company is a more competitive product (compare with the electronics trade). In practice, however, structure design is characterised by sequential activities with poor interaction. For the major part optimisation is limited to stiffness and strength. Towards the end of the manufacturing process, adding insulating and vibration reducing elements, at the cost of labour, weight and money, meet physical requirements such as thermal and acoustical insulation.

Applying the philosophy of renewed segregation and integration allows exploration of a very basic potential of composite fuselage design. First the influence of a very elementary design parameter, the frame pitch, on the metal and composite fuselage weight is now investigated.

The structural efficiency of a stiffened fuselage panel can be judged by the panel weight required for sufficient strength and stability, presented in "design graphs", see Fig. 1.12. All the design curves have the same characteristic shape. Below a certain frame pitch the fuselage weight is constant (in reality it is rising again) and governed by the maximum allowable material stress. Above this frame pitch stability of the skin panels governs the fuselage weight. In the stability critical region, an increase in frame pitch is only possible with increasing skin thickness. As a result the stress level in the fuselage diminishes. The lightest possible fuselages are those with the thinnest skins (not including physical requirements). It is clear that the lightest aluminium fuselage is about 30% heavier than the lightest carbon-epoxy fuselage [9].

The diagram also shows that a design window for frame pitch selection appears when we change from metal to carbon/epoxy composites. This allows us to create structures that are in weight equal to or lower than metal ones with the opportunity to apply renewed segregation and integration to fulfil other fuselage requirements.

In the next section we will explore the potential of the integration of fuselages.

1.6.2 Sound Insulation in Aircraft Fuselages

The sound insulation of a fuselage depends on many parameters, for instance the noise source spectrum incident on the fuselage, the resonance frequencies of the fuselage structure and the pressure difference between the in- and outside of the fuselage. To get an impression of the effect of structural parameters on sound insulation, it is sufficient to consider a flat stiffened panel with identical air conditions on both sides.

The reduction in noise transmission is characterised by the so-called transmission loss (TL). Sacrificing some of the weight savings achieved by exchanging aluminium with composites can improve the acoustical insulation of a stiffened shell fuselage. As shown in the diagram this can lead to an increase in transmission loss of 1.4 dB. The acoustical insulation can be improved by increasing frame pitch and skin thickness. These adjustments also lead to a reduction in the number of parts, lower stress levels, better fatigue behaviour and better impact resistance.

Source: [10]

Increased composite skin thickness and 50% reduction of frames and 1.4dB extra sound transmission loss as a result

Boeing commissioned several design studies for novel composite fuselage solutions, but firmly established the frame pitch at 20 inches!

Weight tendency by varying stability critical plate thickness versus frame pitch width

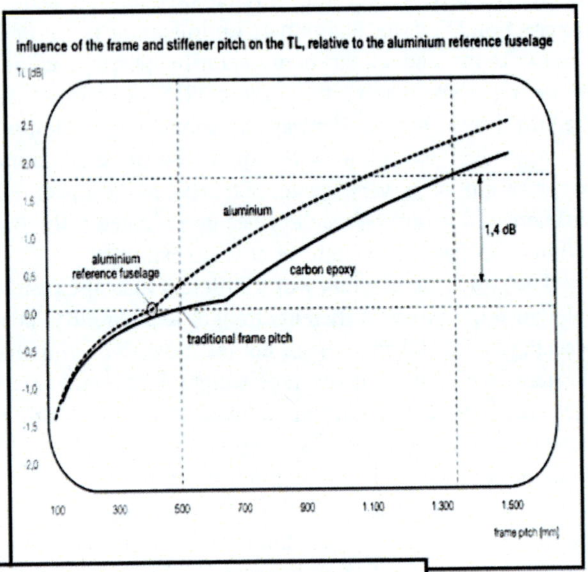

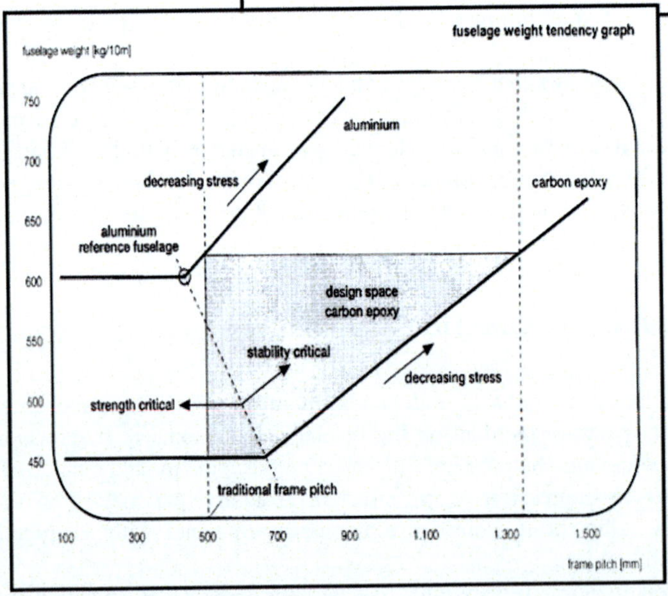

Fig. 1.12 Fuselage structures pitch the frame pitch 1998 bendings stiffness increase by carbon-epoxy offers a new design envelope

If we neglect the new measures necessary to support systems and interior parts, it becomes clear that the weight, and the costs of production and maintenance of an aircraft with such a fuselage all decrease, e.g. due to a 50% reduction of stiffening

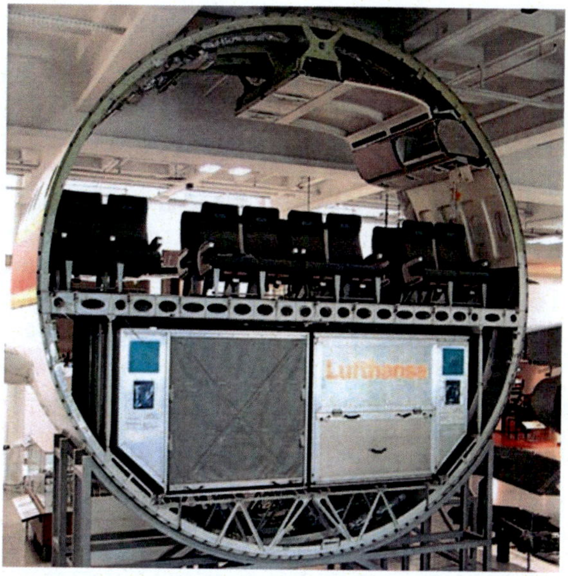

Fig. 1.13 The sandwich concept

elements. Apparently the design window's exploitation can make this aircraft more competitive with the conventional aluminium aircraft than if it were just designed to be the lightest possible composite solution.

Until now we discussed the structural concept with a stiffened skin. A different option is the sandwich concept see Fig. 1.13.

Sandwich panels hardly need stiffeners. Therefore no mass will be lost in those, resulting in a relatively high value of mass per unit skin area, which, according to the mass law, results in a better TL. In addition, the core can be made of a material with high acoustic and thermal insulating properties. The number of discrete stiffeners can then be minimised, since they are only required at places where concentrated high forces are introduced (wing, landing gear, etc.) or diverted (from cutouts). This can reduce the production and maintenance costs. The potential of the sandwich concept for integrated design is part of an ongoing Delft University research program [9] and will not be discussed in this article.

1.7 Safe and Saving Laminates

The classical laminate theory (CLT) was formulated in the 1950s after the translation in English of Russian books that were published in the first decennia of the previous century. They treated the mechanics of anisotropic plate materials. Anisotropy in its most generic form express the relation of all possible stress (six) and deformation components (six) in macroscopic homogeneous and elastic anisotropic materials. The compliance or stiffness [6 $\times$ 6] matrix is symmetric and contains 21 independent elastic constants. By building up plates out of thin anisotropic lamina, all having their own orientation, the CLT, for loaded plates in a state of plain stress, links all possible plate loads to possible deformations. The symmetric matrix consist of three domains A, B en D of elastic constants and in each domain the elastic constants are determined by different "laws of mixture" (Fig. 1.14). The mixture law equations to determine the A, B and D constants possess respectively a linear, a quadric and a cubic character. For material and structure designers coupling of in- and out- of plane deformations and stresses via the elastic B constants is complicating. By sticking on an orthogonal system of coordinates, both for loads and elasticity, the orthotropic structure still rely on nine independent elasticity constants, provided that the laminate is symmetric and balanced. Symmetry means that every layer has a counter part relative to the mid-plane of the laminate (stiffness, thickness and relative position are equal). Balanced means counter parting each off-axis orientated layer by a nephew in the other direction (+ angle by a − angle). In the case of a generalised state of plane stress (no out of plane stress) and a balanced symmetric laminate the A en D matrix are independent, like the independence of the in-plane loads and shear load in the A matrix, with the consequence that dimensioning and analysing of orthogonal structures become a clear activity for structural engineers. Most important effect of the "de-coupling" is that areas for fixation and support (of finite plates) are not loaded by off-plane loads. Loads caused by parasitic bending and torque, in the case of non-symmetric and unbalanced laminates generated by in-plane loads (Fig. 1.14, [11, 12]).

So simple laminates do not surprise or embarrass designers and users, and when just one type of fibre and resin is used, it reduces certification tests and makes production and repair procedures straightforward, the latter is a matter of restoring the original continuous lay-up after being damaged with a minimum of discontinuities and ex-centricities, distortions who in general affects strength, not stiffness.

By excluding exotic laminates and lay-ups the CLT is brought back to its most rudimentary form and become an access-able "tool" for creativity not just on plate level, but on assembled structure level. For example the negative coupling of bending and torsion deformations, which can be attractive for wind turbine blades and forward swept wings, is not a matter of laminate design, a-symmetric and unbalanced, but a matter of coupling wing-cells in possess of non-orthotropic behaviour [13].

For symmetric and balanced laminates, the A_{11}, A_{22}, A_{12} and A_{66} are elastic constants and based on linear relations between the familiar engineering constants[18] in x and y-direction E_x, E_y, ν_{xy}, etc. For all families of laminates tapestry plots or nomo-graphs of equivalent average engineering constants can be plotted (Fig. 1.15).

For dimensioning structures, like beams assembled of girders and webs, like plates and stringers supported by frames, the external loads must be brought in compliance with the global and local extensional and bending properties (EA, EI and strain). By using allowable strains, for static and dynamic loads, notched and

[18] 1 Msi = 6.89×10^3 MPa.

A-symmetric unbalanced laminates generate, loaded in plane, out of plane deformations or when hindered reaction loads, moments and torque loads

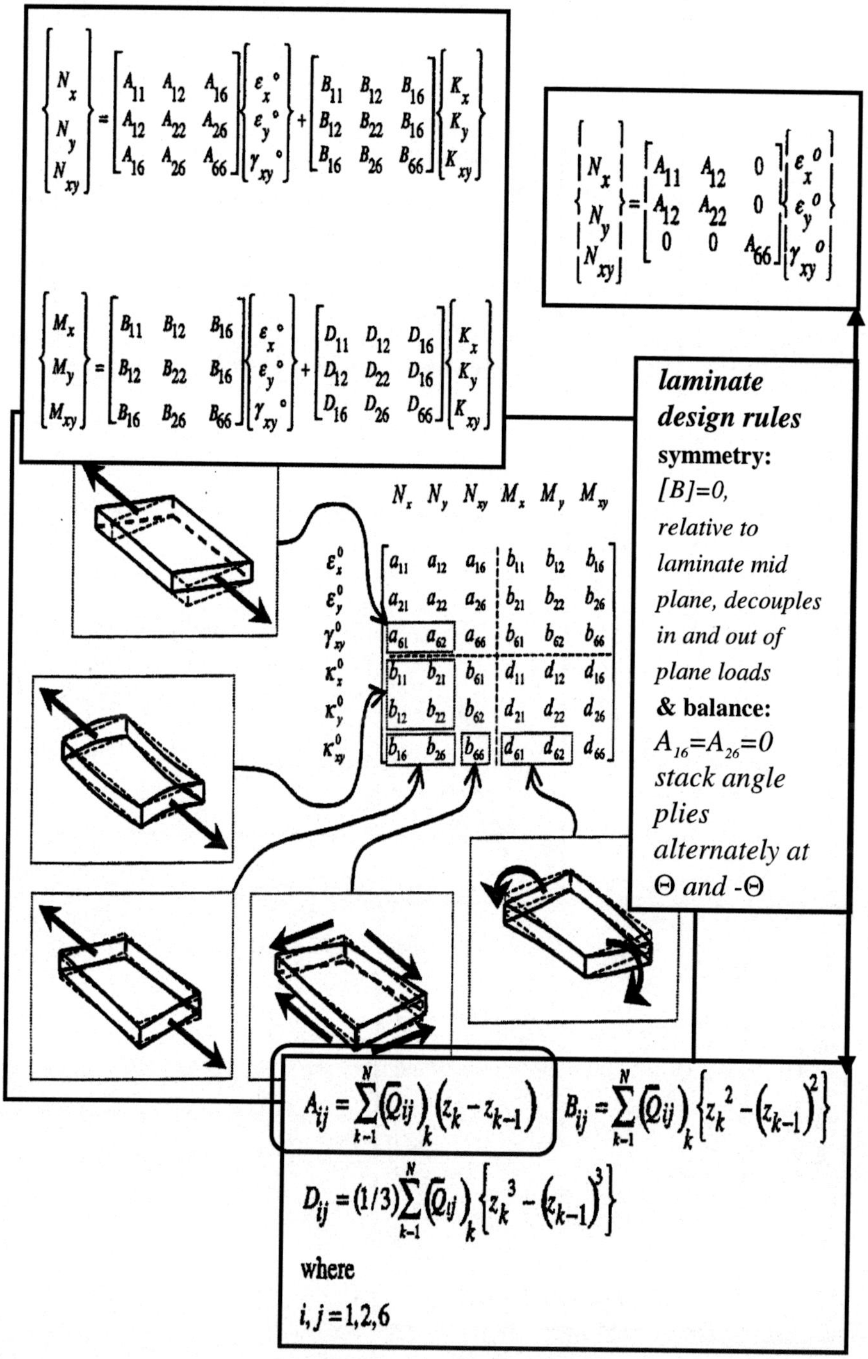

Fig. 1.14 Simple laminates are safer and saving over a lifetime design for simplicity: "balance, symmetry and continuity"

Sources: Boeing, Northrop

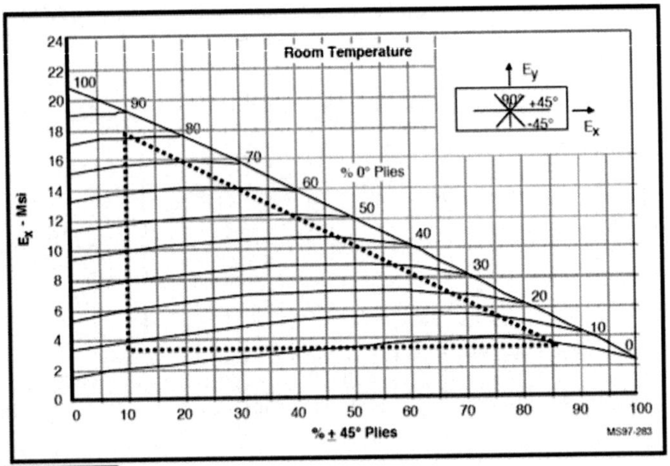

Classical laminates balanced & symmetric

$$\begin{Bmatrix} N_x \\ N_y \\ N_{xy} \end{Bmatrix} = \begin{bmatrix} A_{11} & A_{12} & A_{16} \\ A_{12} & A_{22} & A_{26} \\ A_{16} & A_{26} & A_{66} \end{bmatrix} \begin{Bmatrix} \varepsilon_x^{\circ} \\ \varepsilon_y^{\circ} \\ \gamma_{xy}^{\circ} \end{Bmatrix}$$

E_x(%0°@%±45°@%90°) carbon-epoxy UD laminates

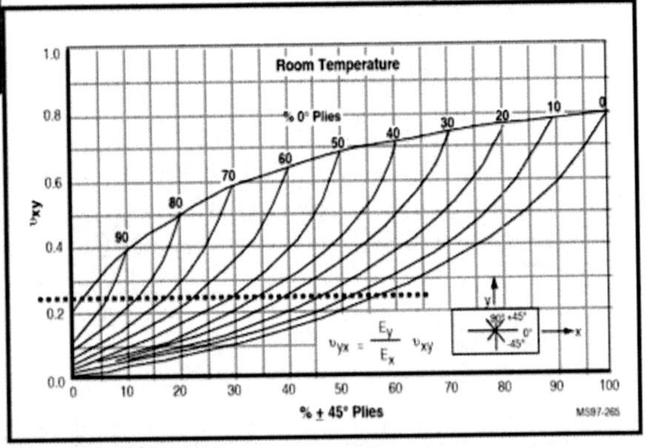

Typical specific thresholds w.r.t. max. strength or strain for damaged fibre dominated laminates loaded in compression

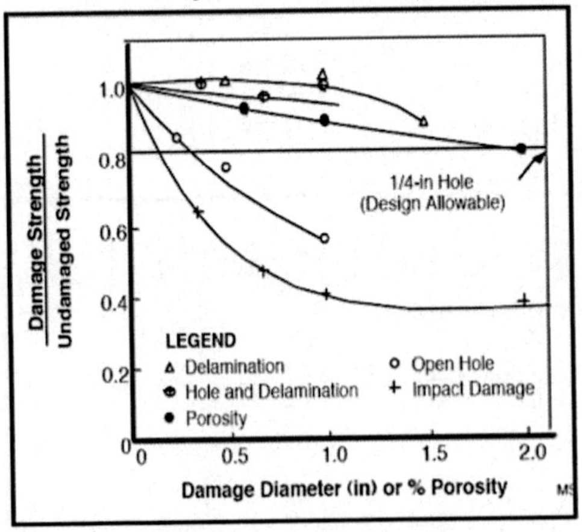

ν_{xy}(%0°@%±45°@%90°) carbon-epoxy UD laminates

Fig. 1.15 Balanced and symmetric laminates: ε, E and σ for dimensioning ν_{xy} to match mismatches un-notched, the structure load carrying capability and efficiency can be orchestrated. Like mentioned in earlier chapters quality of design and cost of manufacturing and maintenance is mainly determined by creating structure simplicity and by the elimination stress raising details or in the broadest sense by eliminating discontinuities on a macro level (notches, ex-centricities, steep stiffness variations, etc.) and very important too, discontinuities on a micro level (minimise inter-ply and intra-ply discontinuities, the more homogeneous the better). Often neglected but nasty local discontinuities are the mismatches of Poisson's ratios and thermal extension coefficients, they are a challenge for designers and engineers to overcome by tuning the adhered elements, but neglected they might turn out into a nightmare. Like mould designers practise, the simplest and cheapest approach is to stick on one "material", for example carbon-epoxy in appropriate laminates, for all adherent parts.

The last example of "rendering simplicity" is found in lugs, like the wing-fuselage mounts of the F27, a part machined out of an almost quasi-isotropic laminate. After a 135 Nm impact of a look alike detail in a undercarriage drag stay ([14], Fig. 1.16), severe de-laminations are present and for the laminates based on the philosophy to minimise inter- and intra-ply discontinuities, this comparison study shows surprising residual properties after impact.

The result after impact is a single load path "connector" that has been split into a multi load path lug retaining the original design strength and fatigue resistance of the original monolith. In the 1980s a test program was undertaken to find an alternative for the Al 2024 F27 wing–fuselage lugs, although in possess of pre-strained holes but still limited in life. The carbon-epoxy facsimile versions without bushes, showed an unlimited fatigue life and a residual strength, after fatigue, higher then the results of the static tested ones (weight reduction 40%). A phenomenon similar to metal fuselages after undergoing a 2p-cabin pressure test, but based on a different mechanism, namely plastic setting of all riveted joints to do an equal job.

Damage mechanisms and the response to damage are in composites totally different to ductile metals. The through thickness fatigue crack in metals has a niece in composite laminates with a totally different morphology, a complex combination of matrix cracks, splits and de-laminations. In the case of a simple stress raising notch located in the edge of a tensile specimen ([15], Fig. 1.17) transverse cracks and splits are generated from $\sim$1,000 micro-strain on and beyond a magnitude of about 5,000, free edge de-laminations appear. The stress concentration K_{11} varies along the edge, from ply to ply and from ply to interface. Typical for laminates, in the interface between to different layers also normal and shear stresses are generated, variable with K_{13} and K_{33}, the so-called inter-laminar free edge stresses. All stress concentrations have different distributions off-notch and are linked. Generally speaking the weakest link is in the matrix or resin, which therefore is the research domain for the improvement of ductility, fibre–matrix interface adhesion and nano-particle reinforcement.

For example reinforcement of resins by nano-particles, is based on the steep increase in surface to volume ratio of particles in the nano domain. The result is a homoeopathist dream: a very small content of particles (fibres, tubes or platelets)

Sources: Hart, Hart Smith et al.

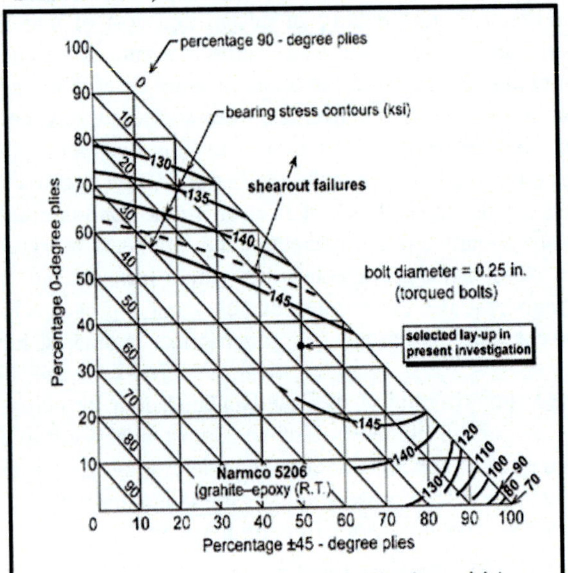

a) Bearing stress contours for bolted carbon/epoxy joints

Classical lug design after impact 135 N.m

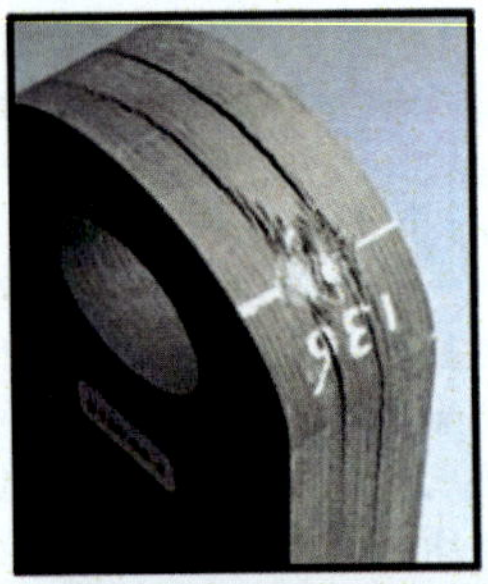

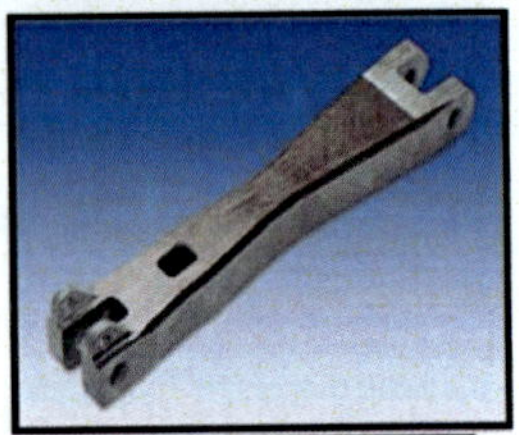

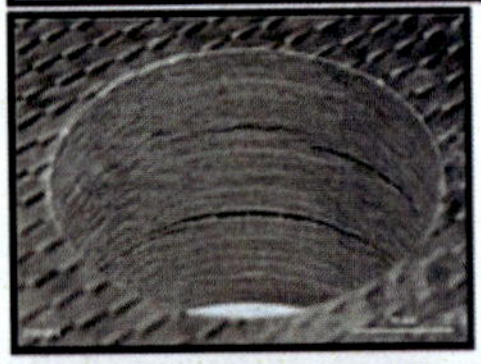

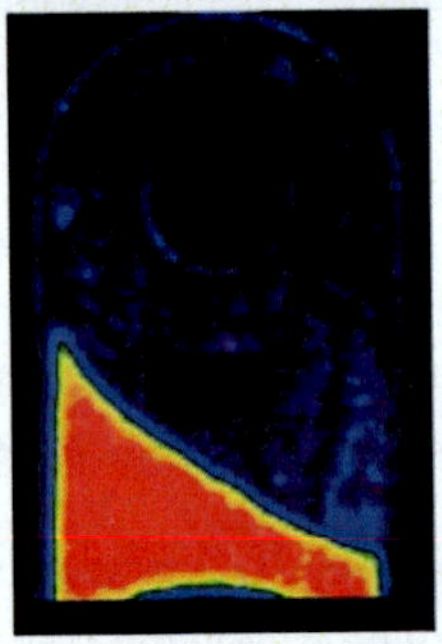

NLR program: carbon-epoxy Cycom 823/875 lugs

Cramer 823 laminate vs. Non Crimp Fabric

80/20 weave, 303 g/m^2 vs.50/50 biax, 540 g/m^2

- **Slightly less susceptible for impact than NCF**
- **Bearing stress 360N/mm^2, >20% better than NCF**
- **Fatigue level 35% σ_b, 5.10^5 cycles, no reduction**

Fig. 1.16 Lugs: balanced symmetric: reduce discontinuities: (1) quasi-isotropic and homogeneous, (2) minimise inter-ply orientation mismatch, (3) intra-ply, "lighter' fabrics are better. Residual strength almost 100%. (1) after N = 5 × 10^5 fatigue cycles (35% UL), (2) after impact lug, 135 J//, delaminated

diluted in resin do improve critical resins properties (mechanical and physical). Attempts to increase stiffness beyond the glass transition temperature and to reduce the saturation level of e.g. polyamide 6, by adding 4.6% of nano silicate, are giving promising results (Sect. 1.9, [16]).

Source:Liu, TUDelft

Notch induced splits
NIS and de-laminations NID, cross-ply laminate, tension loaded.translucent glass-polyester

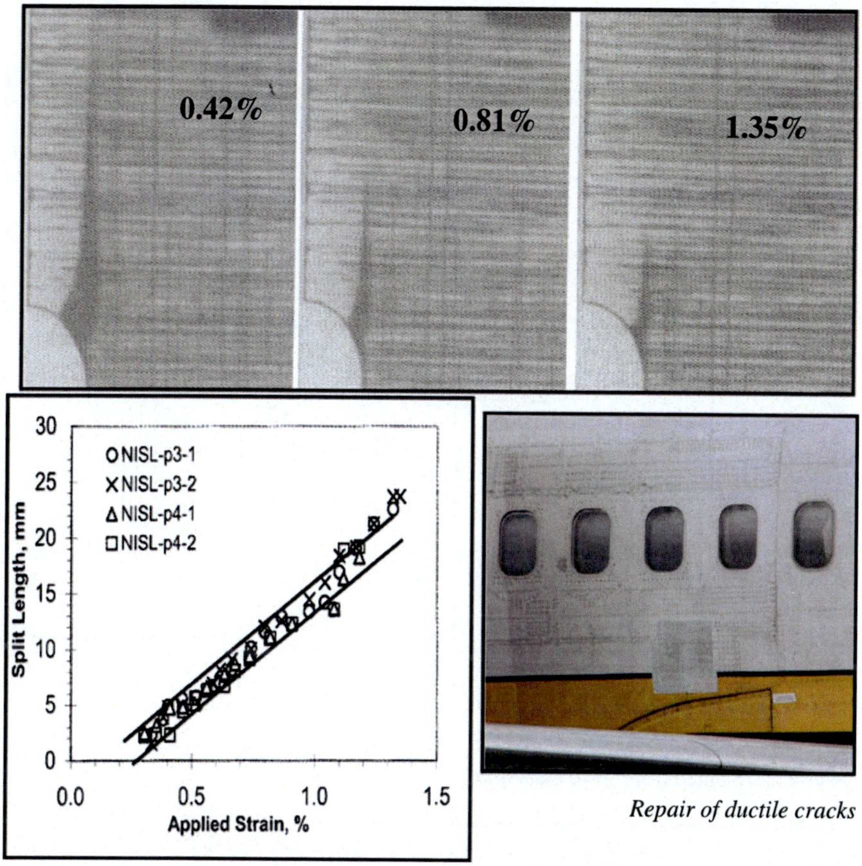

Fig. 1.17 Notchless safety less notches, fewer notch induced matrix cracks, splits and de-laminations

1.8 Simple Fibre Placement, Safe and Saving

Most important ambition for the near future is the development of downstream manufacturing techniques for the fibre structure in primary structures, dry and draped in "unlimited size" moulds and "frozen" into solid structures after vacuum assisted impregnation. Since this impregnation technology turned into a void free high quality process ([17], Fig. 1.18) for sailing yachts, bridges, wind turbine blades (all up to 60 m) and recently for aircraft parts like winglets and moving wing parts (Boeing's 737, 787) and "large" structures for "small" aircraft like the

Source: K. van Rijswijk

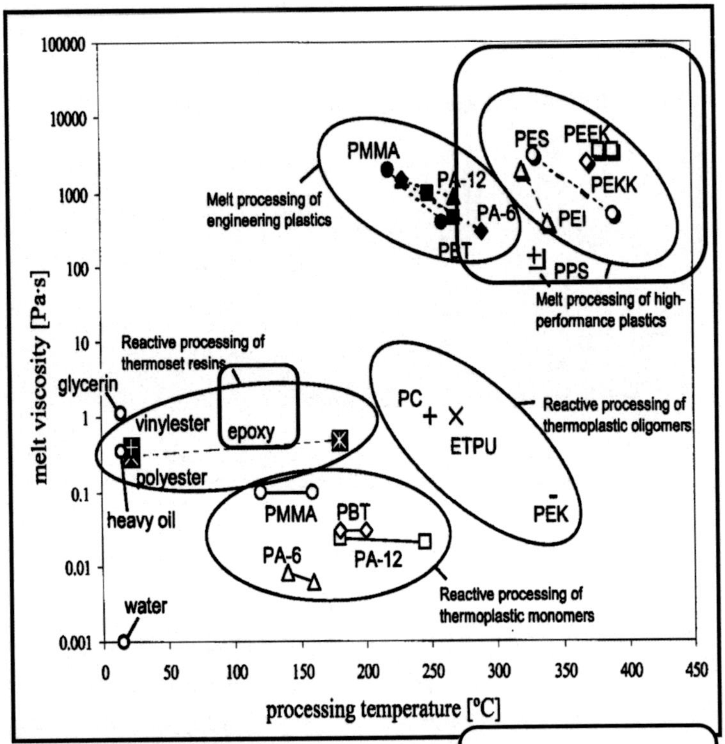

Melt viscosities and processing temperatures of most common engineering thermosetting and thermoplastic polymers

qualified and certified for aircraft

Processing temperatures, melt and reactive, for several thermoplastics

Thermoplastic matrix	Processing temperature [°C]		Temperature reduction [°C] (reactive vs. melt processing)
	Melt processing	Reactive processing	
PA-6	230-290	140-160	70-150
PA-12	230-270	180-245	0-90
PBT	250-270	180-200	50-90
PMMA	220-260	120-160	60-140
PC	265-360	250	15-110
PET	265-325	250-325	0-15
PES	330-390	300	30-90
PPS	330	300	30
PEEK	380-390	350	30-40

Fig. 1.18 Engineering polymers. 2000 processing temperatures and viscosity

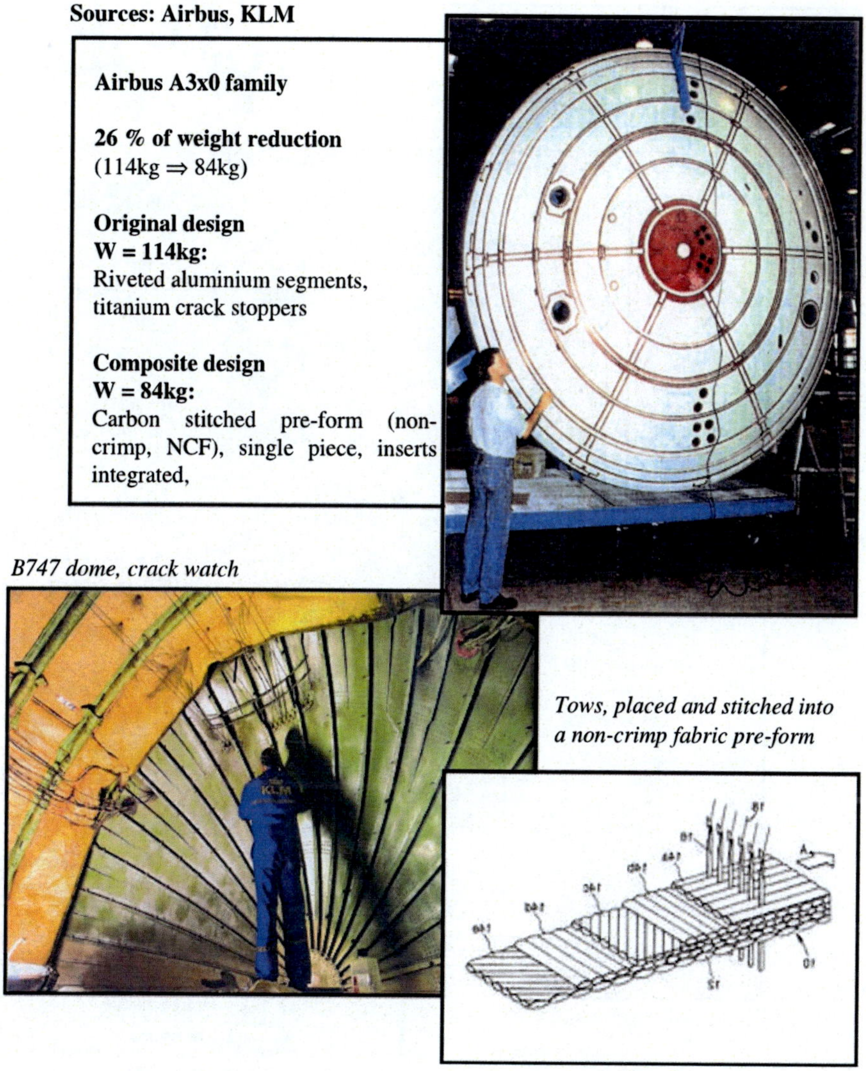

Fig. 1.19 Dedicated fabrics a composite classical, pressure domes dominated by bi-axial tension and sensitive for fatigue en corrosion

Bird of Prey (UAV) and the Diamant Business jets. Multi directional and multi-layer fabrics with tows and tapes, bound by stitches or (thermo) plastic films, are more and more applied as well. Nice and successful examples are the Airbus pressure bulkheads (Fig. 1.19), nowadays applied in the B787 too.

Pre-impregnated fibres, tows and tapes have a breakthrough thanks to the availability of capital-intensive fibre-placement robots (Fig. 1.20), changing aircraft structures manufacturing into an industrial and labour extensive activity.

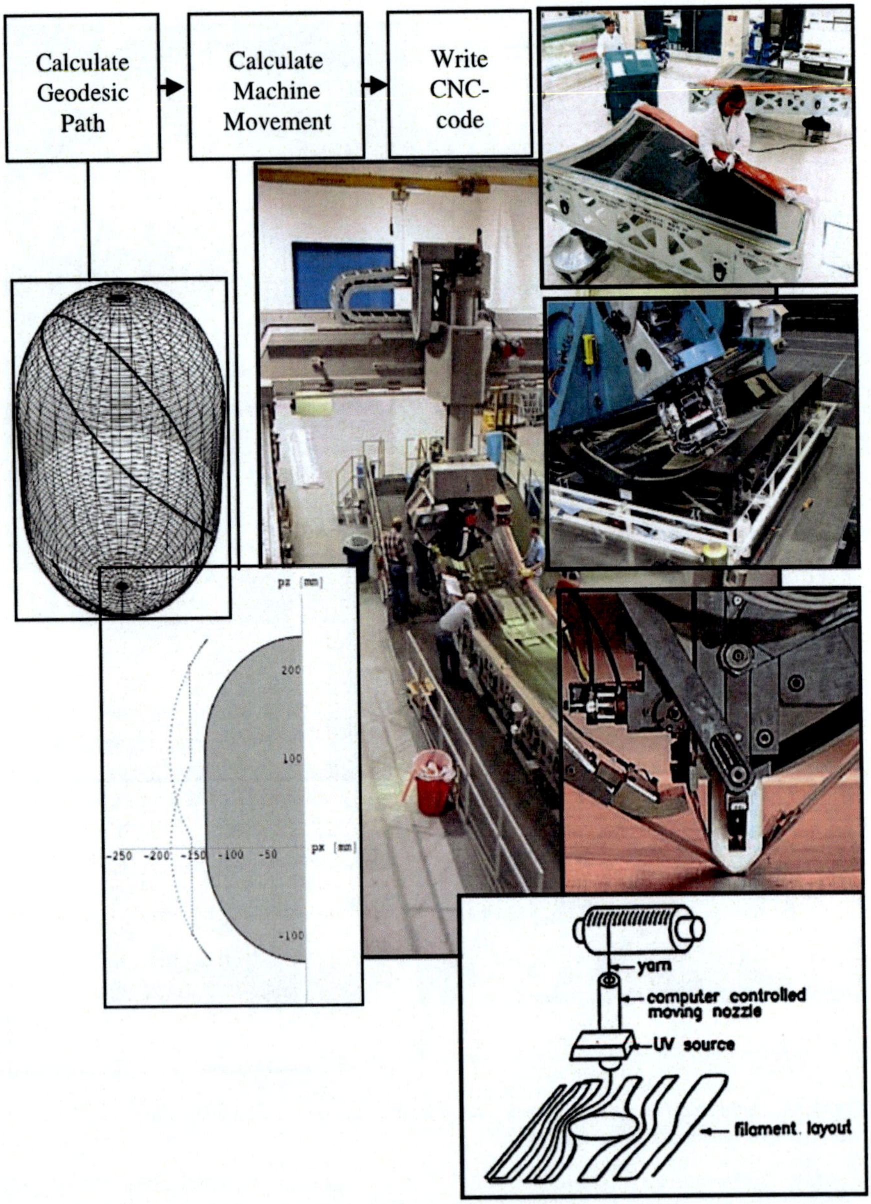

Fig. 1.20 Industrial manufacturing the faster the better reduce mass of rotating mandrels reduce mass of head place dry fibres keep them straight, simple geodetics

In the 1950s a similar break-through was noted for integral aluminium structures, e.g. blade stiffened, thanks to the introduction of numerical milling machines (Fig. 1.8).

Another machine of the 1950s, the filament winding machine, has unexpected qualities as well. When dedicated for a family of products it's a fast (multi-eye feeding) and cheap. When using "dry filaments" the winding speed can be increased with a factor of 10 and the manufacturing is changed into a clean, solvents free, process too.

By clever design and optimisation procedures wound plate, shell and cell structures can be produced (e.g. plates rotating around the diagonal). Light mandrels, multi eye feeding of fibres, a polymer binder and a minimum speed and orientation variations, makes the machine a potential laminator for "homogeneous" dry laminates [18]. An example of a change from hand laminating of aramid fabric + phenolic resin patches, via press forming of polyamide thermoplastic pre-pregs [19], to the rapid winding of dry pre-forms before a short press cycle is visualised in (Fig. 1.21). The reduction of lead time, the improvement of ballistic impact energy absorption and the material cost reduction percentages are extreme and show the advantage 3D textile forming with fast and simple equipment. Textile structure designers therefore has to skill themselves in the conformal mapping of 2D wound plate structures into 3D shapes (draping) and to create concave shapes by convex winding. Regarding details like cutouts, the philosophy must be once again to reinforce the local notch by simple and as homogenous possible thickness increments, which literally can be cut out afterward. The bio-mimic approach to follow or to create stress trajectories around cutouts (Fig. 1.20), similar to the root area of a branch growing out the trunk, is for example in fuselages not so practical for production and assembly, because the load conditions of shear and cabin pressure request for almost quasi-isotropic lay-ups and a sufficient bending stiffness along the cutout edge to reduce stress-raising curvature effects. When bending stiff edges are applied in a window (e.g. a floating window frame in a sandwich structure), the result is a reduction of the local edge stress from 9 times the nominal tangential stress for a curved solid plate edge, to 3 times in the case of a simple one centimetre thick sandwich edge, a flat plate value.

1.9 Simple Polymer Resin Systems, Safe and Saving

Generally speaking the polymer matrix and its interface to engineering fibres is the weakest link in the composite marriage. With respect to ductility, physical properties and price, the families of modern fibres are still limited in number and possibilities for advanced applications. Like blending of polymers and alloying metals, property variation and tuning of fibres can be realised by mingling different fibres in possess of the required properties and with more or less the same diameters.

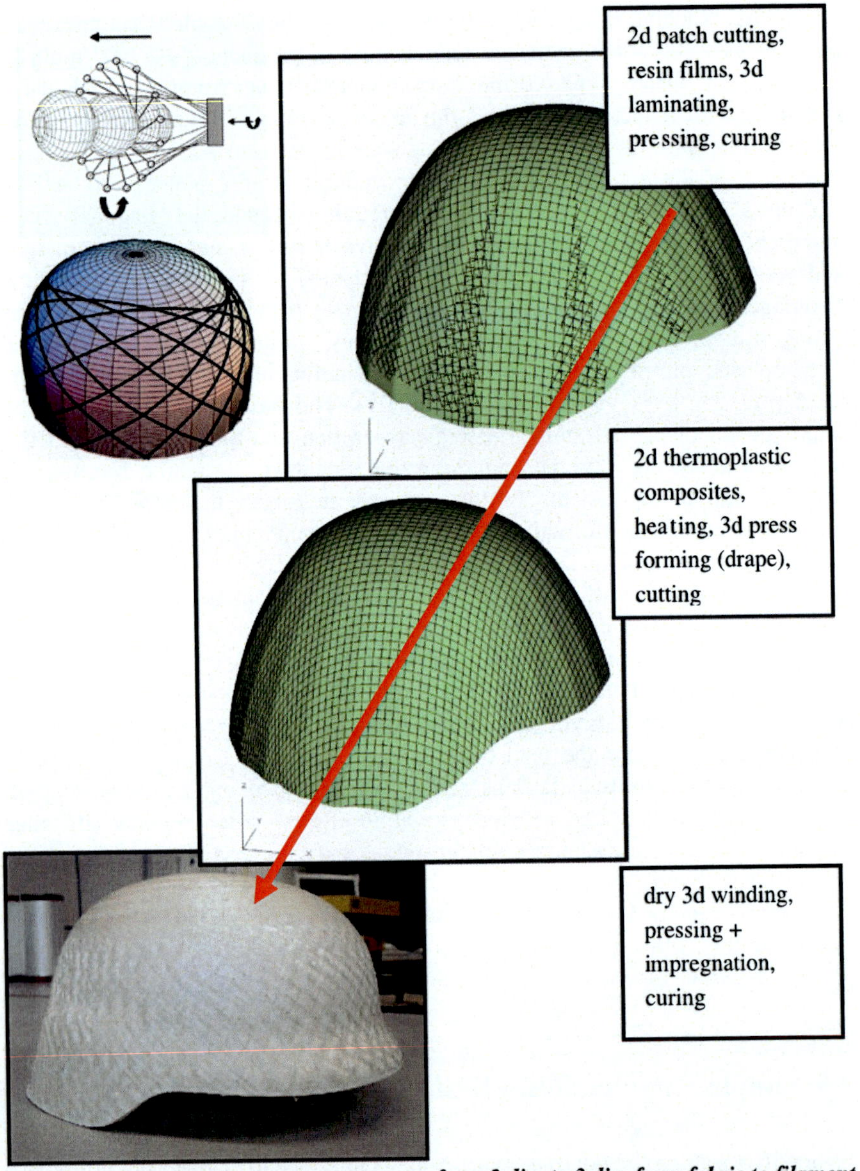

Fig. 1.21 Progress by process development: e.g. composite helmets: < 80%, lead time reduction > 30%, energy absorption < 70%, material cost reduction

In regard the number of polymer resins, the variety is enormous, however once temperature of processing and operation, chemical and physical resistance are part of the selection, in aerospace, the proven, qualified and certified polymers are limited to epoxies and phenolics (interiors) and a few thermoplastic materials.

In the last generations of aircraft, short fibre-reinforced thermoplastics have proven their attractiveness for injection moulded parts, up to 50% weight reduction and unexpectedly up to 90% of cost reduction. A few hundred small parts (<500 g) are present, different in nature and number (1–100). In Fokker F50 and F100 aircraft, about 200 different fuselage-interior brackets (PEI, 30% glass) and parts of control systems (PEEK, 30% carbon) were introduced successfully, cost and weight efficient.

In the same era of the 1990s the many continuous fibre reinforced thermoplastics entered the market of which the Ten Cate CETEX (PPS and PEI based) family did survive. Since a few years the material is success story because parallel to the material, the manufacturing and modelling development resulted in rapid and reproducible production results. Blanks, are heated and draped by bending, shearing and slipping under low pressure into 3-D shells, ribs, brackets, the building blocks for wing and interior parts and important are welded together by electrical resistance heating.

So the processing characteristics of thermoplastic composites, the transition from glassy to rubbery phase by heating, resulted in the development of rapid cost efficient press forming process of relative small parts and assembled to large structures by bonding, riveting or resistance welding. Another manufacturing advantage of thermoplastic composites is the storage at room temperature (metal workshop alike).

Despite their potential for cost efficiency it took about a quarter of a century before the thermoplastic composites became seriously implemented into aircraft structures. The reason was the high costs of the available thermoplastic composites and lack of "fool" proof and low cost manufacturing processes. In the 1970s and 1980s the research was focused on the APC-2® thermoplastic composites. This composite is based on PEEK, a thermoplastic resin with excellent properties, however, for "open" melt processes a "impossible" paramount T_g of 390°C.

The low glass transition temperature and low cost PP and PA composites are easy to process, unfortunately the properties are too low for usage in aircraft structures. A PEEK composite with properties very well suited for highly loaded primary aircraft structures, however with a high T_g and processing temperature >400°C and very high costs. In between are the composite materials based on PEI and PPS resins. The PEI grade was developed in the 1970s and 1980s and is, due to its low resistance to fuel and synthetic hydraulic oil, mainly used in aircraft interior applications. The PPS grade, in possess of required resistance, due to its semi-crystalline structure, was especially developed in the 1980s 1990s for structural aircraft applications. Its lower costs and ease of processing made it an attractive material to be used for a variety of aircraft parts; approximately 5 tonnes of the material is being used on an A380.

The thermoplastic composites would be used to their full potential if being applied to the larger primary aircraft structures like fuselages, empennages and wings. The limiting factor in this case is the existence of the 'perfect' material. The PEEK laminates are too expensive whilst the properties, especially the temperature resistance, of the PPS laminates are not fully convincing for these types of structures, so an in between polymer is requested.

Cytec is developing laminates based on PEKK resin, whilst TCAC is developing laminates based on novel derivatives of the PAEK (PEKX) and PPS (PPSX) families. In the latter case the resins are specifically developed for continuous fibre reinforced thermoplastic composites. The properties of the resins are, therefore, optimised for composite use which may result in a potential cost optimisation. This in contrast with the existing thermoplastic composites which are all based on resins already available for injection moulding applications.

Upgrading thermoplastic composites by adding nano particles is another approach. One specific nano-filler, namely nano-clay, this is for very good reasons. Research on the reinforcement of PA6 with 3–5% of clay particles result in an increase in relevant mechanical and physical properties [16]. Attempts to increase stiffness beyond the glass transition temperature and to reduce the saturation level of e.g. polyamide 6, by adding 4.6% of nano silicate, are giving promising results. The nano-silicate particles are not only reducing or delaying the water absorption but also increase the properties to the dry as moulded level. As can be seen in Table 1.6, the properties of PA6 in its dry as moulded condition are good in comparison with PEI and PPS. Consequently, if the game of clay exfoliation and impregnation of the continuous fibres is played well, a low cost easy processable three-phase composite can be created which could be suitable for semi-structural applications.

For the years to come the expensive intermediates, the preimpregnated materials, might get competition from downstream impregnation techniques like Vacuum Resin Infusion which by its applied low pressure "unlimits" the size of parts and the necessary but simple moulds [wind turbine blades, yachts, (cadre)]. Low cost resins, like vinylesters and reactive processable monomers like anionic polyamides (nano-particle reinforced) and high temperature PEK, might be infused in dry assemblies of textile structures including smart fibres and inserts to increase the integration of parts and functions (Fig. 5.2 and metal fibre).

So if all the cards are played well, the aerospace community will experience the development of cost efficient primary aircraft structures. However, there is one draw back, namely the manufacturing of thick composites (>1 cm thickness). Press forming technologies are not and automated fibre placement AFP is questionable suited for manufacturing of thermoplastic composite parts of considerable thickness (>1 cm). In a full composite aircraft especially wide body, there will be primary aircraft structures of considerable thickness, like in centre section areas. The current techniques and developments to produce thick composite parts are hand lay-up, AFP and RTM. Especially low pressure RTM, like vacuum assisted infusion, is a process with a potential for cost efficiency for large structures due to the consistent high quality [17] and the possibility to produce integrated structures thus reducing the assembly costs.

Resin infusion is, however, only suitable for low viscous thermoset polymer composites. A guideline that is commonly used for resin infusion is that the maximum viscosity of the resin for infusion is 1 Pa·s. (Fig. 1.18). As can be seen

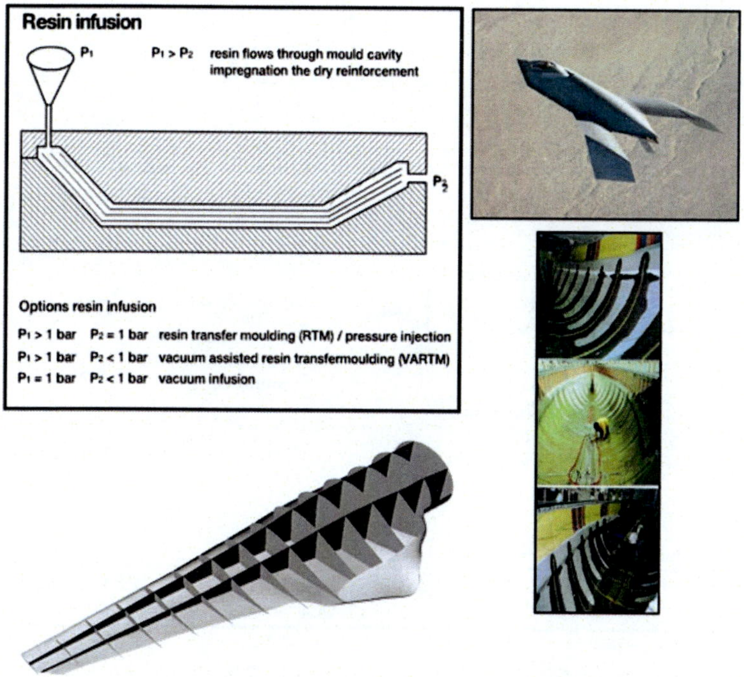

Fig. 1.22 Low pressure, low cost void free infusion free of autoclaves

the thermoset resins like epoxies do have a viscosity below 1 Pa·s as well as a relatively low processing temperature. The melt process able thermoplastic resins like PPS, PEI, PEEK on the other hand have high viscosities as well as high processing temperatures.

There is luckily also another family of thermoplastic resins namely the reactive processable or Ring Opening Polymerisation thermoplastics (Fig. 1.22). As the name already suggests, ring-opening polymerisation (ROP) is based on a polymerisation mechanism in which ring-shaped molecules (cyclics) are opened into linear monomers or oligomers and subsequently connected into high molecular weight polymers without generating by-products, see Fig. 1.23 for APA6.

As can be seen in Fig. 1.18 these reactive thermoplastics have viscosities in the order of 10–100 lower than thermoset resins with only a moderate increase in processing temperature. These resins are thus potentially suitable for resin infusion processes. Currently, research is being performed on several of these systems, namely Cyclics a cyclic PBT, anionic PA12 and anionic PA6. The research is mainly focused on automotive and wind turbine rotor blades. However, when a three-phase nano-clay APA6 composite could be developed, this thermoplastic composite resin infusion system may become applicable for future aircraft structures (Table 1.6).

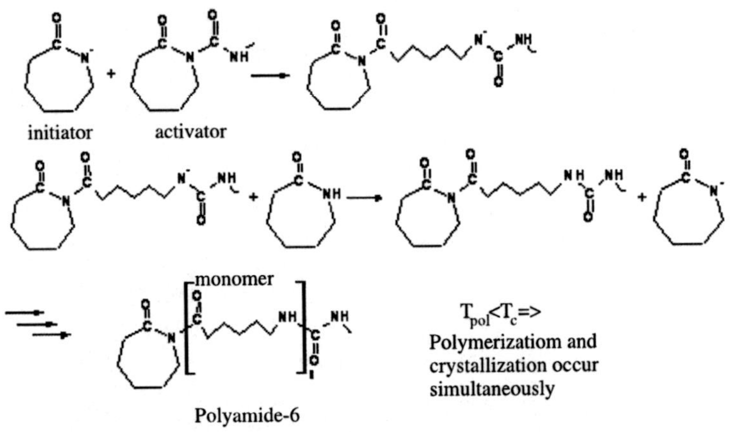

Fig. 1.23 Polymerisation process (APA-6)

Table 1.6 Polymer composites properties

Polymer	HPA6	APA-6 (170C)	PEI	PPS	PEKK	PEEK
Mechanical properties						
Modulus of elasticity (GPa)	3.0	3.7	2.96	3.4	3.4	3.7
Yield strength (MPa)						
Tensile strength (MPa)	65	85	105	85	90	100
Tensile strain (%)	10	19	6	3.0	80	100
Flexural modulus (GPa)	2.7	–	3.3	3.7	3.3	3.9
Flexural strength (MPa)	113	–	145	147	140	131
Compressive strength (MPa)	–	–		110	207	
Physical						
Density (g/cm^3)	1.12	1.17	1.27	1.35	1.30	1.32
Average level of crystallinity (%)	37	37	Amorphous	50	30–35	40
Thermal properties						
Melting temperature (°C)	220	213	None	280	338	340
Glass transition temperature (°C)	69	62	217	85	156	143
Service temperature (°C)	–	–	150	80	121	121
Processing parameters						
Processing temperature (°C)	230–290	140–180	360	340	370	380–400
Viscosity (Pa·s), processing temperature 10/s rate	200	0.01	2,000	3–5	2,500	3,500

1.10 Manufacturing, Assembly and Control

When fibre reinforcing materials extend beyond glass- and carbon fibres and include yarns of metal fibres that can be shaped in the same way through available

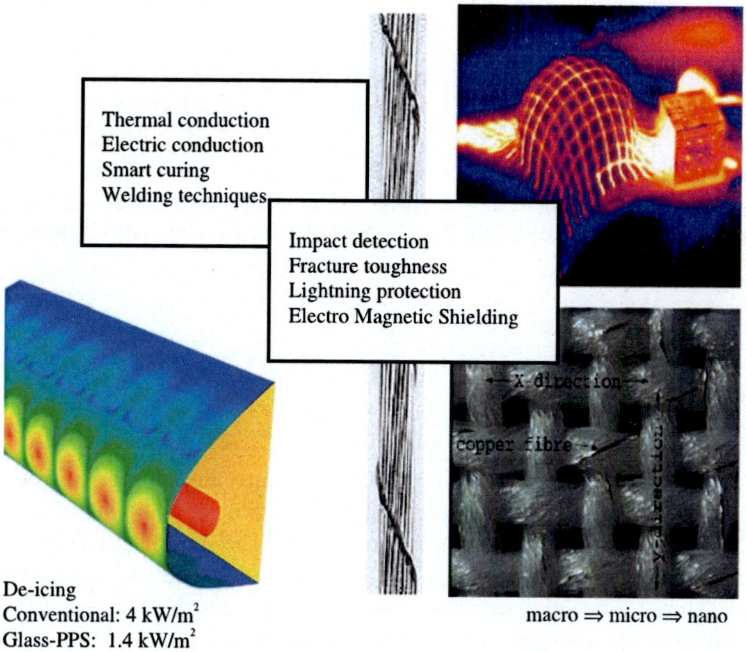

Fig. 1.24 Metal meshes multifunctional laminates

textile fibre placement techniques (weaving, tape laying, filament winding, etc.), a new range of applications should emerge. If steel and aluminium mills could produce appropriate steel and aluminium yarns, the unprecedented textile-like formability affords complex three-dimensional shell structures and unlimited in size. Any mechanical, physical and electric magnetic property can be realised by blending. Expressed in textile terms, by inter-mingling, co-mingling and laminating with fibres and yarns of metals, minerals and polymers the number of applications will become infinite. The added value of metal meshes is starting in the manufacturing: fast heating by induction to cure or to melt, not energy intensive via the mould but with minimal energy, from the inside. For assembly metal meshes enables jointing by welding of thermoplastic composites, with unexpected static and fatigue strength, in spite of an embedded discontinuous "defect" and lack of fillets. Probably the steep stress distribution of classical bonded lap joints, bathtub curve alike, is transferred into a serrated type of stress distribution, more peaks, lower levels. A recent fatigue performance characterisation of resistance-welded thermoplastic composites (GL/PEI, CF/PEI and CF/PEKK) showed indefinite fatigue lives at 25% of the static lap joint strength for the carbon fibre CF specimens. The static lap joint strength of the resistance-welded CF/PEKK and CF/PEI specimens surpassed with 52 N/mm^2 and 47 N/mm^2 the average 41 N/mm^2 of epoxy IM6/3501. Compared to the same epoxy adhesive the resistance-welded carbon specimens were better in fatigue performance too, in terms of absolute values [20].

Additional functionalities introduced by metal wires are electro magnetic shielding, heating, transport of energy and signals. Most unexpected effect in using hybrid fibre reinforced polymers is the high fidelity to detect defects with infrared thermography, even in "field conditions", after resistance heating. If material parameters are known, application of predetermined heating time and power makes it possible to detect each defect location and defect size [21] (Fig. 1.24).

1.11 Conclusions

In the first chapters we identified whether future air transport is relevant and sustainable or not and which energy supply technologies could play a durable role. In the future subsonic aircraft performance will be improved tremendously and become more sustainable, especially when international environmental regulations are tightened. For public transport over long distances there is no other transport system that can compete with aircraft, unless people are willing to invest, en masse, in travelling time, in days instead of hours. When in future hydrogen technology will emerge in road transport, will it settle in air transport as well? If it will, then the layout of aircraft will be affected tremendously. When lightweight solutions are developed for hydrogen-tight liners with equal thermo-isolating properties, dry iso-tensoid fibre placement strategies will result in safe and lightweight pressure vessel solutions. Failsafe segmented fuel storage will become a keystone technology [18].

On the other hand, the use of liquid fossil or bio fuels could be far more practical if a worldwide low cost fuel supply is guaranteed and future environmental rules are met.

Whatever happens, in transport in general the dematerialisation on a system level (structure ++) and miniaturisation of electronics and control systems will continue, not for the sake of weight reduction but to increase the performance per unit weight and volume.

As mentioned the relevance and unique role of air transport, especially for intercontinental travelling, is proven by the low specific drag ($D_{spec.}$). Even in the high subsonic velocity domains the fuel efficiency per unit weight in combination with the productivity of aircraft can compete with all other types of transport and can still be improved with tens of per cents. Although the vehicle efficiency of contemporary aircraft is not bad, $W_{empty}/W_{payload} \approx 4$ on a system level, on a structural level the efficiency can be improved up to 24% which is about 12% of the total operational empty weight (OEW). When realised it reduces the average OEW/MTOW ratio from 5.6 to 5.0 without a trade-off in passenger comfort and safety.

That the durability of aircraft structures will be improved by the application of composites is not doubtful anymore. Contemporary comparisons have proven reductions on inspection and maintenance cost of more than 30% (B777 vs. 767).

If we design for integration and structure simplicity with freedom of shape unexpected advantages will occur as well, like the application of low cost (low pressure) infusion techniques in combination with the manufacturing of dedicated textile structures with, bound by solvable stitches or adhesives. Textile preform manufacturing like weaving, fibre placement and stitching could be extended with dry filament winding, the improvement related to cost and properties for ballistic impact protection are exceptional (>50% for both parameters), Down stream manufacturing is the biggest challenge to reduce cost, the transfer of flat and dry fibre bundles into pre-forms, the impregnation with low cost resins. Development of modified vinyl esters or even more ambitious of low viscosity thermoplastic monomers or oligomers prepared for reaction into a composite structure after infusion (cure of material and structure in one shot). The use of "small" industrial pressed thermoplastic parts will become more attractive if the welding capabilities are used. Resistance-welded joints using metal meshes show very promising static strength and fatigue properties. Unexpected is the fact that the stress raising metal mesh is reducing the limiting peak stress in lap joints, the bath tub curve is transformed to a serration. Semi-crystalline thermoplastics like PPS, PEKK and PEEK approved for the melt impregnated carbon composites, could get competition from lower T_g materials like tough and low cost PA-6/12, if both the glass transition temperature and sensitivity for humidity are modified by blending or filling. Nano-clay fillers do have an effect on both properties at low weight percentages (<6%), not enough but the tendency is promising.

When composites are settled and accepted by manufacturers and operators, a rapid improvement of polymer and metal fibres in combination with new resins, will make structures tougher and more fire and damage resistant. The problems that will surely arise are challenges for designers and engineers, open-minded and enterprising, who are used to solve problems in structural design just like the aviation pioneers more than 70 years ago.

References

1. Lee JJ et al (2001) Historical and future trends in aircraft performance, cost, and emissions. J Annu Rev Energy Environ 26:167–200. doi:10.1146/annurev.energy.26.1.167
2. Condit PM (1996) CEO of The Boeing Company: airline costs on the rise while yield slips. AIAA World Aviation Conference, Los Angeles
3. Helms H et al (2004) Energy savings by light-weighting-II. IFEU-Institut für Energie- und Umweltforschung
4. Dijkstra HS (2008) Materials for future aircraft structures. MSc Ph.D. thesis, Faculty of Aerospace Engineering, Delft University of Technology, The Netherlands
5. Schatzberg E (1994) Ideology and technical choice: the decline of the wooden airplane in the United States, 1920–1945. Artic Technol Cult 35(1):34–69

6. Rothwell A (1992) Introduction to aircraft structural design, part II. Lecture notes, Delft University of Technology, The Netherlands
7. Rouchon J (1996) Fatigue and damage tolerance of aircraft structures. Centre d'Essais Aeronautique de Toulouse, TopTech Studies, Delft University of Technology, The Netherlands
8. Beukers A et al (2003) Aircraft structures in the century ahead. Royal Society of Aeronautics, London
9. Krakers LA (2008) Parametric fuselage design: integration of mechanics, acoustic & thermal insulation. Ph.D. thesis, Faculty of Aerospace Engineering, Structures and Materials Laboratory, Delft University of Technology, The Netherlands
10. Tooren MJ (1998) Sandwich fuselage design. Ph.D. thesis, Structures and Materials Laboratory, Delft University of Technology, The Netherlands
11. Bailie JA et al (1997) A summary and review of composite laminate design guidelines. Langley RC, Hampton
12. Nijhof AHJ (2004) Vezelversterkte kunststoffen, mechanica en ontwerp. Delft University Press, The Netherlands
13. De Goeij W (1999) Implementation of bending-torsion coupling in the design of a wind-turbine rotor-blade. J Appl Energy 63(3):191–207. doi:10.1016/S0306-2619(99)00016-1
14. Hart WGJ et al (2003) Damage tolerance properties of carbon epoxy lugs made from resin transfer moulded plates. NLR, Marknesse
15. Liu C (2004) On the prediction of damage and fracture strength of notched composites. Ph.D. thesis, Delft University of Technology, The Netherlands
16. Vlasveld DPN (2005) Fibre reinforced polymer nano composites. Ph.D. thesis, Delft University of Technology, The Netherlands
17. Labordus M (2001) Voids and bubbles during vacuum infusion. SMA, EM01-352
18. Koussios S (2004) Filament winding—a unified approach. Ph.D. thesis, Delft University of Technology, The Netherlands
19. Bergsma OK (1995) Three dimensional simulation of fabric draping: development and application. Ph.D. thesis, Structures and Materials Laboratory, Delft University of Technology, The Netherlands
20. Dubé M et al (2008) Fatigue performance characterisation of resistance-welded thermoplastic composites. J Compos Sci Technol 68(7–8):1759–1765. doi:10.1016/j.compscitech.2008.02.012
21. Ahmed TJ et al (2008) Heat emitting layers for enhancing NDE of composite structures. J Compost Part A 39(6):1025–1036. doi:10.1016/j.compositesa.2008.02.017

Chapter 2
Opportunities for Polymeric-Based Composite Applications for Transport Aircraft

J. C. Halpin

2.1 Emerging New Aircraft Have the Most Efficient Structures

New airframes are made of more than 60% new-advanced materials, chosen for their superior weight and strength properties. The innovative use of Carbon Fiber Reinforced Plastic, grants weight savings via optimum fiber lay-up and skin thickness tailored to the requirements of the location and corrosion control using molded composite parts, and Titanium provides fuel and maintenance efficiencies (Fig. 2.1).

Airframes operate in a variety of discrete threat environments. Composite airframes have different capabilities than metallics, and they also have increased sensitivity to a variety of impact threats. Focusing on a group of discrete threats, such as hail, outlining a Durability and Damage Tolerance technology and safety management approach for impact events in operational fleets is a useful way to identify technology needs and opportunities.

Figure 2.2 shows a Status Matrix for aeronautical Service Induced Impact Threat environments ranging from low-velocity to relatively high-velocity impact conditions. This matrix summarizes the nature of the threat, method of characterizing the response of a material or structure to the impact, methods for the analytical simulation of the structural response to the impact event, the probability for the severity of the threat to be addressed in the structural design and substantiation, or if this is an event or incident that equipment operators and maintenance staff will be aware of (expected locations where the impact event(s) would typically occur).

In the development and introduction of new materials and processes, there is a formal qualification procedure required by the responsible airworthiness authorities.

J. C. Halpin (✉)
JCH Consultants, Inc., 7143 Hunters Crk., Dayton, OH 45459, USA
e-mail: jchalpin@aol.com

L. Nicolais et al. (eds.), *Composite Materials*,
DOI: 10.1007/978-0-85729-166-0_2, © Springer-Verlag London Limited 2011

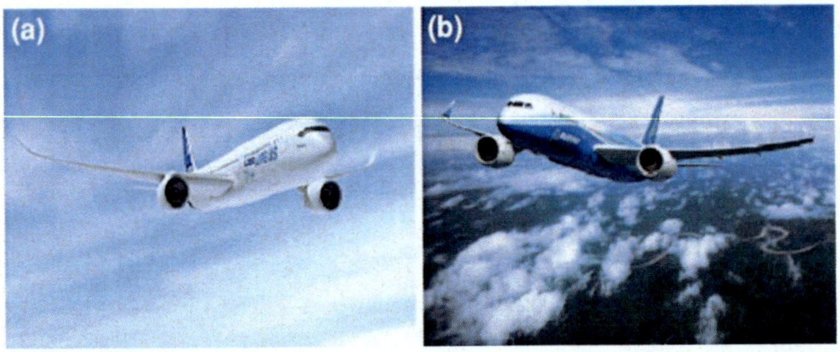

Fig. 2.1 B787 and A350XWB aircraft renderings

Threat	Test Protocol	Simulation Models	Threat Allowable	Self Evident Event	Impact Location(s); Zones 1 & 2
Bird Strike	Gel-pack	Yes	"B" FAR's (Wt. & Vel.)	Yes	YES
Hail	Simulated Hail Ice [illegible]	Yes Maturing	"B" Update MIL-HDBK [illegible]	Yes	YES
Runway Debris	Lead Ball ? Drop-tower?	?	"B" Update JSSG-2006 ?	Sometimes	Usually
Tire Rupture	Rubber Puck	?	AC25.963-1	Yes	YES
Panels Lost In-flight	?	?	?	Yes	Sometimes
Tool-drop	[illegible] Hemisphere Drop-tower	?	JSSG-2006 Structures	Sometimes	Yes
Incidents [illegible] Contact With Ground Vehicles	TBD	TBD	TBD	Sometimes ?	Yes
Others? Lighting Strike	----	----	----	----	----

Fig. 2.2 Status matrix for aeronautical service induced impact threat environment

Two approaches are used: certify by test or certify by analysis. A combination of approaches is used for the certification of an aircraft with the emphasis on characterization by test at the materials and structural element levels with a shift toward analysis at the component and full airframe level, Fig. 2.3. It is for this reason the table includes both a test protocol and a suitable simulation methodology. These are essential elements within the engineering process that facilitates the use of new polymeric-based materials technology into new vehicles. The sequence of test characterization is illustrated in Fig. 2.3. A detailed discussion of these procedures is available in the MIL CMHB-17 [1]. More on this topic is available later in this discussion.

Before proceeding into the detailed discussions, it is useful to recognize some top-level characteristics, weight and cost components, for a transport class

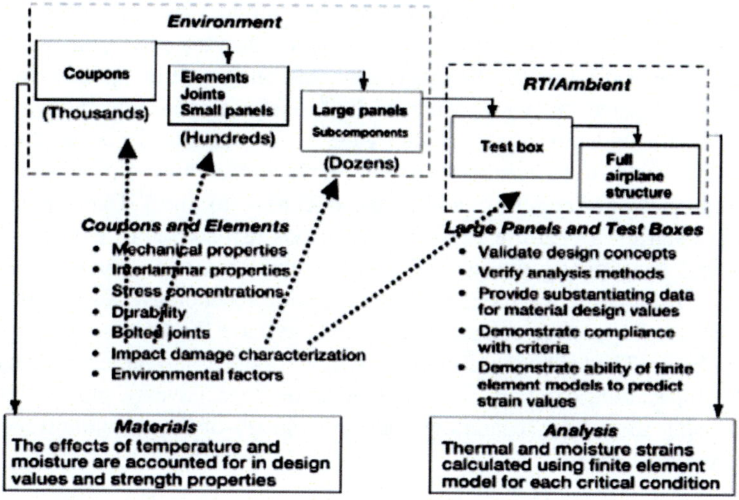

Fig. 2.3 Illustration of the building block concept for substantiation of airframe structure [1]

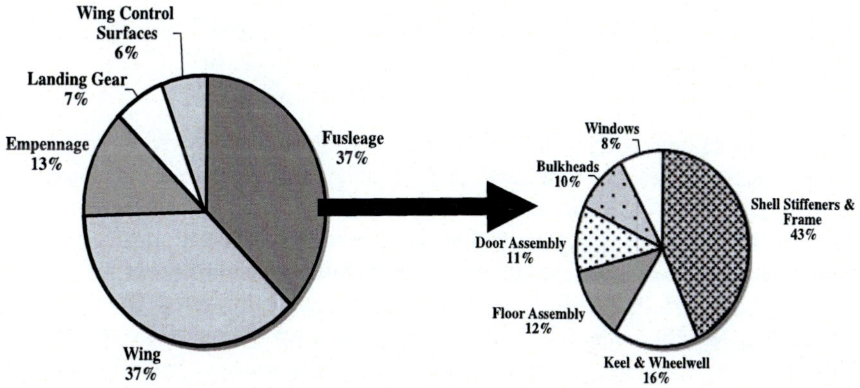

Fig. 2.4 Typical weights distribution for a commercial transport aircraft

airframes, see Fig. 2.4. Recent comments by the major airframe, "Primes" have clearly identified a challenge facing the industry for continued improvement in fuel efficiencies, [2]. The following comment is typical:

> Bair (Boeing BCA) said the 737 replacement will certainly have a carbon-fiber composite plastic structure. However, the 787 technology does not scale down well enough. For example, the top of a composite fuselage must be thick enough to withstand heavy hail (ground hail – JCH). That fixed thickness adds proportionally more weight to a small jet. Boeing is working with composites manufacturers to come up with different materials, but those are not ready yet.

The fuselage, empennage, and wing control surfaces are the cost center for the airframe with the fuselage costs about 1.5 greater than the cost of the wing per unit weight. The cost ratios for the empennage and wing control surfaces are about a factor of 1.2 versus the wing. Much of the fuselage, empennage, and wing control surfaces structures are relatively thin gage with respect to the wing. As a result, they have tended to be vulnerable to aggressive impact threat environments. These environments are requiring additional thickness to meet Damage Tolerance (Safety) and the Departure Reliability demands (economic) of the operating airlines and constraining the desired 20%+ improvement in operational fuel efficiency. Historically, the focus has been on wing technology. At present industry understands the need to enhance the technology base for the other components of the airframe. The following discussion will be divided into three sections devoted to the impact considerations including hailstone impact events, molded composite parts using short fiber technology, and a summary of the technology needs and opportunities.

2.2 Impact Considerations

2.2.1 Understanding the Hard Small Object Low Velocity Damage Experiences

The historical approach to impact damage resistance has evolved from the early experiences addressing tool drop and "runway" foreign object damage. This technology base evolved in the 1970s as technology preparations were being made for the B-2 bomber. Characterization of material resistance to transverse impact resistance utilized a quasi-static test concept, falling weight impact testing. Typically, this test method utilizes a hemispherical metallic impactor. The selection of the falling weight method with metallic impactors was judged to be reasonable at that time as the impact threats of tool drop and FOD were judged to involve "low impact velocities," involving "hard" objects, and localized impact conditions. Very early (1975–1985 time frame) in the characterization of material resistance data appeared suggesting that there was a level of impact kinetic energies for which a specific laminated composite plate would not experience delamination, resin cracking or fiber failure. At higher impacting energy levels damage occurred, increasing in severity with increasing impacting energies until penetration. By the late 1980s, it was apparent that the observation of a defined damage threshold was consistent among a variety of industrial teams and in open referred journal papers [1, 3–5]. It was also apparent that this damage threshold was strongly dependent on laminate thickness (bending stiffness) and the fracture toughness of the matrix. Figures 2.5, 2.6, 2.7, and 2.8 are typical examples.

In Figs. 2.5 and 2.6, the Damage Thresholds are either referred to as the Failure Threshold Energy, FTE, or the Damage Threshold Load, DTL. The work of Davis

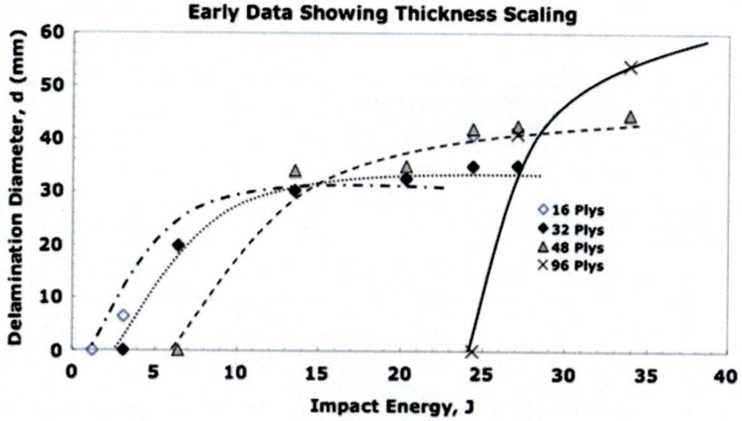

Fig. 2.5 Early (1980s) falling weight data for AS4(45/0/-45/90)$_{SM}$ laminates

Fig. 2.6 Damage resistance of [45/0/-45/90]$_{SM}$ AS4/3501-6RFI using 0.5 in. (12.7 mm) diameter indenter

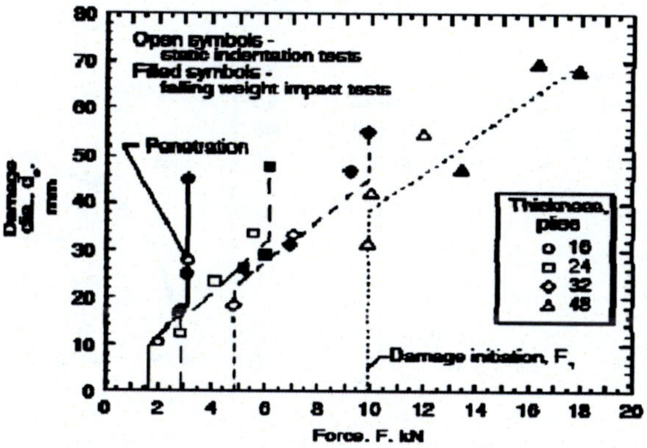

and coworkers and Olsson and coworkers [6–11] articulated the dependence of the Threshold conditions in terms of the laminate thickness and interlaminar Mode 2 fracture toughness:

$$P_C \approx t^{3/2}\,[(64\pi^2 EG_c/9(1-\nu^2))]^{1/2} \rightarrow Ct^{3/2} \rightarrow DTL \qquad (2.1)$$

where G_c is the mode 2 critical energy release rate, G_{2c}. Schoeppner [11] and many others have confirmed the dependence on thickness for quasi-isotropic laminates. This historical testing has provided data in terms of critical incident impacting energies or the critical contact force. Transformations between force and energy are complex as they involve the local dynamic stiffness of the target. The reader is referred to Jackson and Poe [12]. The energy format is useful for developing requirements and comparing materials, while the force format is better suited for structural analysis; both are need and useful concepts. Equation 2.1 is only intended to illustrate the physics of the topic. The influence of toughness is illustrated in Figs. 2.7 and 2.8.

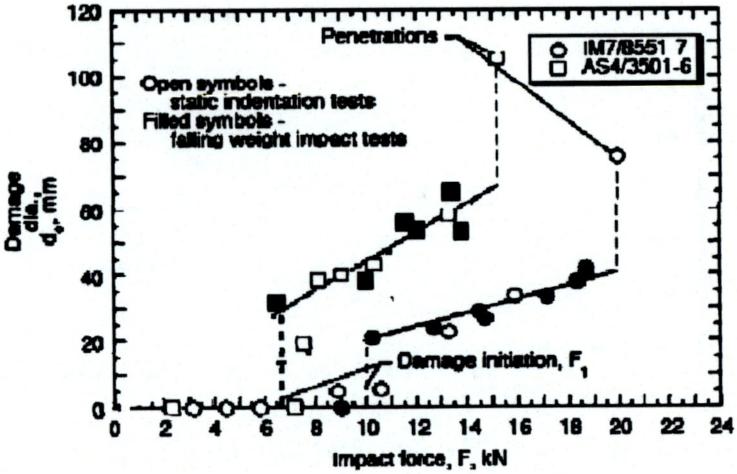

Fig. 2.7 Impact tests for untoughened and toughened carbon/epoxy

Fig. 2.8 Example of toughness influence for an untoughened graphite/epoxy and a thermoplastic graphite laminates

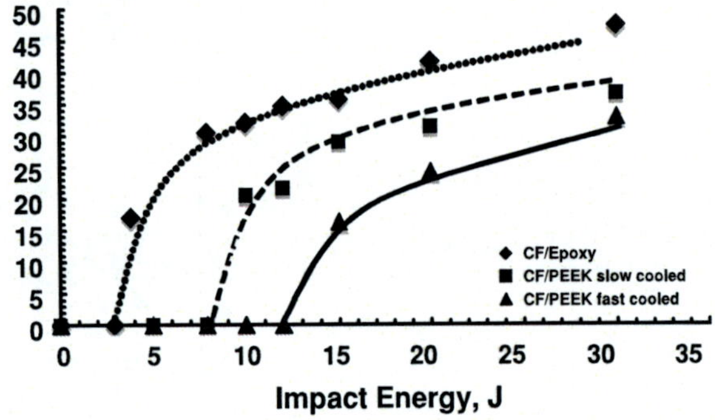

A consequence of the induced damage is a loss of compression strength capacity. The residual strength capability follows similar strength reductions to that observed in "notched" laminates. This stress penalty is typically a function of induced damage state, "fiber dominated" and has tended to be insensitive to matrix toughness, Fig. 2.9.

In summary: The past 30 years have provided a useful understanding of small hard object, low-velocity impact conditions. The current recognition of this threat to airframe structures is discussed in detail in [1]. Unfortunately, there are also some misunderstandings derived from these experiences that must be addressed.

For example, within the CMHB-17 the following comment occurs:

> Several methods for improving the performance of impacted composite panels and components have been proposed. One approach is to increase the inherent toughness of the composite by using tougher resin matrices; this is only appropriate for medium to thick gage laminates as increased toughness has little benefit for thin laminates or sandwich face sheets. Although this method improves damage resistance and reduces maintenance costs,

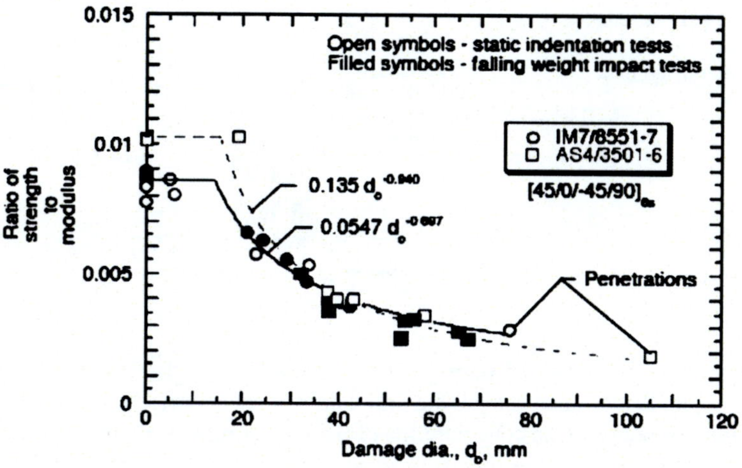

Fig. 2.9 Compression after impact test results for untoughened and toughened carbon/epoxy laminates [1, 5]

increased material costs, reductions in matrix stiffness at elevated temperatures, and potential reductions in large notch residual strengths must be considered in the final selection.

These comments are a part of the reasons for the limited application of this material option in current aircraft deigns. The airframe community believed that the toughened thermosets were sufficient to satisfy their needs as the thermoplastic composite technology offered involved sometimes difficult processing and fabrication conditions due to stiff prepregs with limited "tack" and the perceived increased material costs. In the later part of the 1990s and early in the 2000 time frame, there was pressure by the operation airlines to limit the number of composite materials used in the construction of the airframe; a legitimate logistic concern for airline maintenance. It was a natural choice to select a toughened thermoset matrix system. (Note, a variety of aluminum alloys of varying toughness, strength, and corrosion resistance are used in metallic aircraft.) The reference to thin gage materials and sandwich construction speak more directly to the inherent limitations of *honeycomb* sandwich design and a misunderstanding about the nature of the impact phenomena.

Sandwich construction exists to provide stiffness in bending and torsion, E/I and G/J capabilities, in the same manned as an "I beam," see Fig. 2.10.

In Fig. 2.10, the "thin" face sheets are also exposed to the surface impact threat environment. The trade studies have overlooked the phenomena of beam on an elastic foundation, BOEF, constraint when the face sheet is under an impact load, Fig. 2.11. Low Velocity Impact and a "quasi static" response are words used to describe a simple plate or beam that can deflect in response [13, 14] to the dynamic impulse, Fig. 2.11. That is why the thickness scaling, $t^{3/2}$, correlation is observed in the data presented above. The core, under the face sheet resists the deflection and as a consequence concentrates the incident energy within the impact contact

Fig. 2.10 Honeycomb sandwich usually wins stiffness critical trade studies

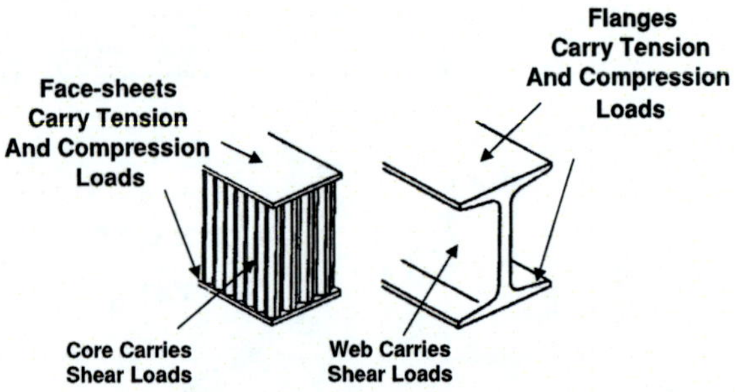

area, Fig. 2.11. Localized damage occurs as a "shear plug" under the contact with a significant increase in the interlaminar shear stresses. Penetration is a common response to the concentration of the impacting energy, or forces, Figs. 2.7 and 2.8. Note that as the impacting diameter is reduced in size, localized shear plug penetration occurs versus the larger area delamination in Figs. 2.5, 2.6, 2.7, and 2.8. It is for this reason that the thin sheets are fragile with respect to the impact threats at a reduced energy or force level that if the sheets were tested separately (Fig. 2.12).

There are alternative design geometries providing a shear transfer mechanism and the separation of the face sheets. Utilizing alternative "core" structure concepts with carbon/thermoplastics could provide some interesting options for new and replacement stiffness critical structures. The complex core geometries suggest a "moldable" material such as a *short fiber thermoplastic*. Minimum gage components are stiffness critical and suitable for this material option. In localized areas, strength considerations can be addressed through a *combination of chopped fiber with continuous fiber materials*. In any event, a new approach is required for material and design geometry options as the airframe industries strive to enhance weight efficient Damage Resistant/Tolerant designs.

The threshold conditions, DTL and/or FTE cited earlier, where reported in research paper but there use in the engineering design process did not occur. Work in the 1980s and 1990s implemented a design requirement for tool drop and foreign object damage, FOD, by bounding the impacting kinetic energy, an energy cut-off [1]. Structural damage tolerance management focused on compression after impact, CAI, and visual inspection. Discreet source impact conditions for both bird strike and tire rupture were implemented in this time frame, as summarized in the discussion of Fig. 2.2.

2.3 Hail Impact

Severe weather conditions including hailstones are regular occurrences in various parts of the world. Work is underway to characterize the frequency of hailstorms, sizes of the hailstones, and their geographical occurrence.

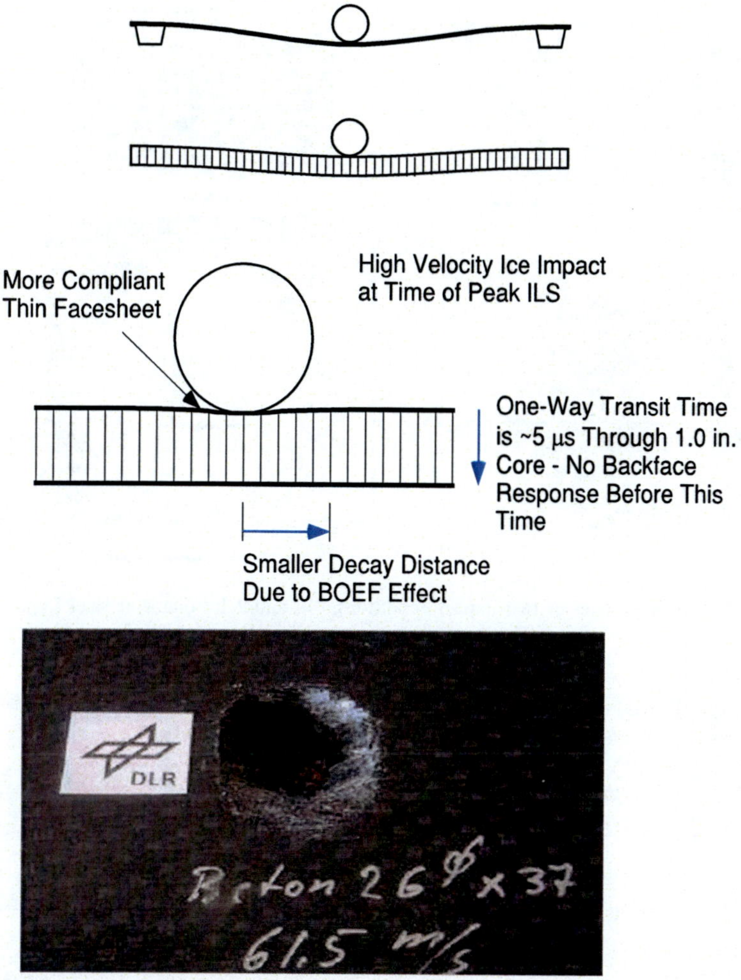

Fig. 2.11 This figure is an illustration of a global stiffing and the local response concentrating the force (*S*). Figure 4c is from Aktay et al. [15]

Extreme hailstone sizes are produced when large vertical wind shears are generated in storm systems. The hail is kept suspended, aggregating small ice particles and water, until the weight of the hailstone cannot be supported by the local wind shears, Fig. 2.13. Hail sizes, Fig. 2.14, monitored on the ground are a good indicator of the size of hail falling during the storms, minimum melting occurs as the hail descends at their terminal velocity. In-flight hail events do occur, they are damaging, but of decreasing frequency as Air Traffic Management and weather observation technology has improved. The principle challenge to the airframe is ground hail. In-flight hail, typically involves forward facing surfaces at

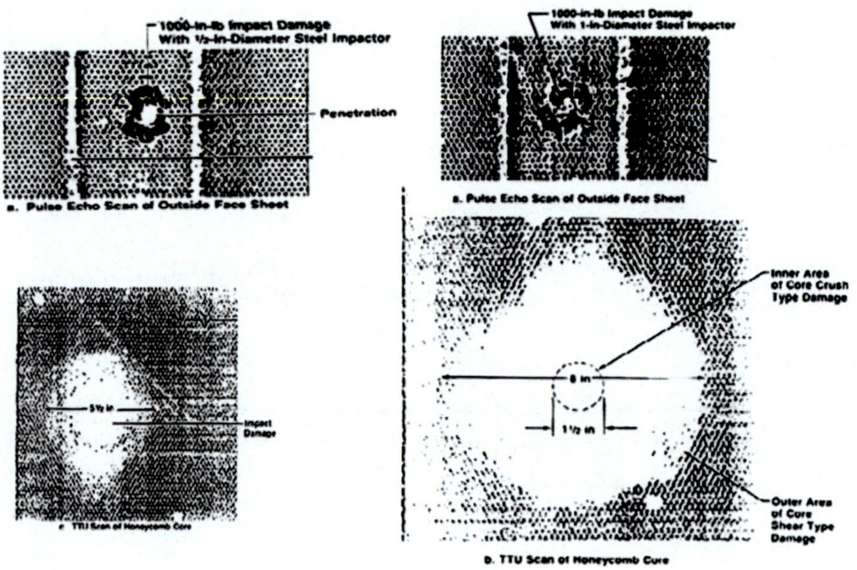

Fig. 2.12 Comparison of two impact conditions, 1/2 and 1 In. diameter steel impactors for a common sandwich construction: note diameter size effect Boeing 1986 fuselage study [16]

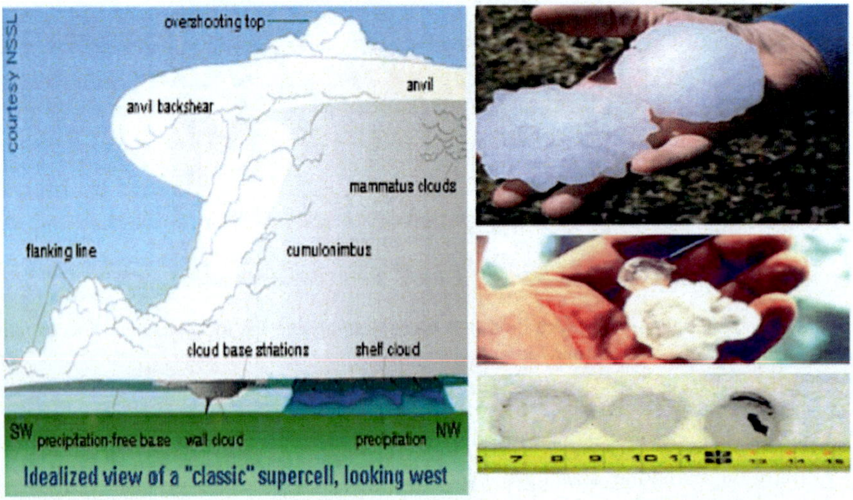

Fig. 2.13 The production of hailstones is associated with severe weather conditions

impacting velocities determined by the closing speed of the aircraft and the descending hail ice. Upward facing surfaces are challenged by ground hail, such as the fuselage, wing, control surfaces, and horizontal stabilizers.

Note the location of several US hub airports is in severe hail conditions. Similar conditions exist for different continents.

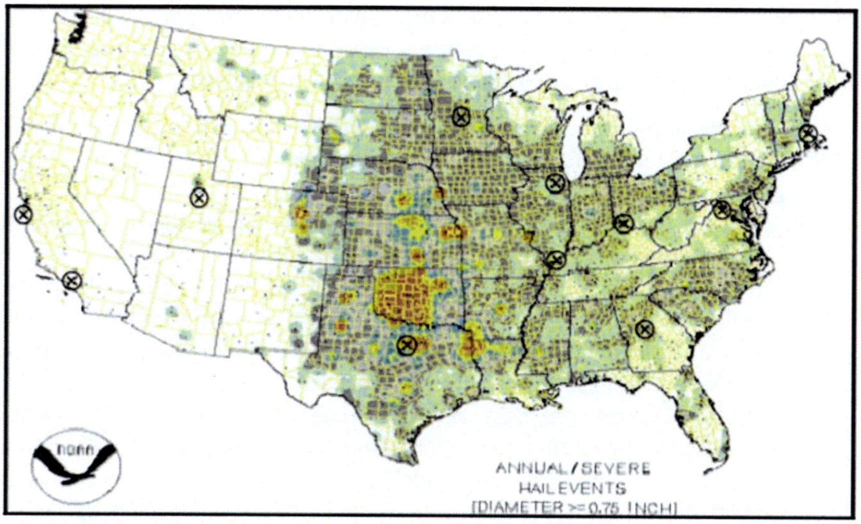

Fig. 2.14 This figure summarizes the US hail database and some hub airport locations

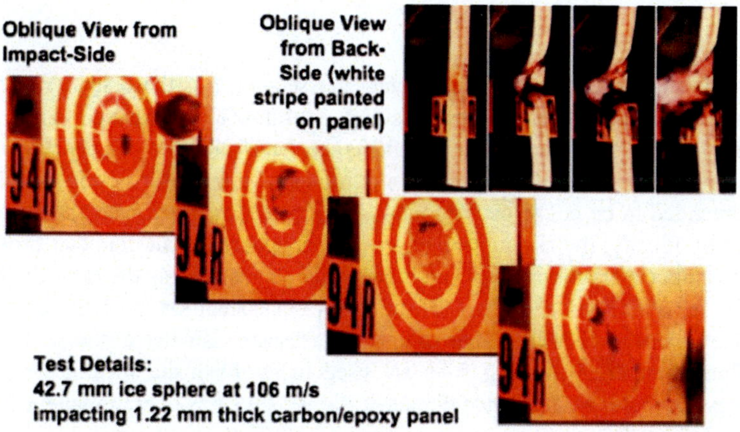

Fig. 2.15 High velocity simulated hail ice ball impacting a toughened graphite-epoxy panel [17–19]

Over the past 10 years, there has been work generated first by the jet engine community to understand the consequences of hail ingestion and more recently by some in the airframe community to support their Damage Tolerance and Departure Reliability activities. In the Fig. 2.15, there is an example of a hail impact test by Kim and coworkers [17–19]. Please note two points:

(1) Unlike the metallic ball falling weight test, the impacting object is fragmenting due to the dynamic impact pressures. This reduces the induced contact force experienced by the plate if a hard object had impacted the plate.

(2) Note that the impact event is at a high velocity, the test panel cannot deflect within the time span of the contact, a deformation pocket is created, and the panel is damaged by a localized "shear plug" mechanism.

The morphology of the damage changes with velocity, a cone shaped damage for the "Low Velocity" falling weight testing, versus a cylindrical damage shape through the thickness. This is analogous to the previous discussion of honeycomb sandwich construction, but for a different reason. (You are correct to observe that honeycomb sandwich construction is more vulnerable to severe hail.)

Figure 2.16 is a table that converts the consolidated "raw" hail database into a table suitable for Damage Tolerance evaluation, [4, 5]. The irregular shapes for hailstones are shown in [17, p. 92, Fig. 4-1]. This table includes suggested terminal velocities. Section 4.3 (p. 98) of [17] discusses the various efforts to relate drag coefficients to hailstone size, mass, and shape. The terminal velocities calculations were obtained by converting the reported hail sizes, irregular shapes, into an equivalent spherical geometry and modeled them as a smooth object to obtain "drag coefficients" for the determination of the terminal velocity, see pp. 98–107 of [17]. Equation 4-1, p 107 of [1] was used to estimate a conservative terminal velocity:

$$V_T = Kd^{1/2} = 14.0\,m^{1/6} \tag{2.2}$$

V_T is the terminal velocity in meters per second, d is the diameter in cm, and m is the mass in grams. This expression is within 6% of measured values when a value of $K = 15$ is used for spherical shapes. Maximum ice density was assumed for the hail weight. Natural hail has a porous structure, the mass cited in the table are intended to be conservative to assure a conservative estimate for the terminal velocity. Finally, the assumption of a compact spherical hail diameter provides an additional conservativeness as the induced damage scales as the ratio of D/H. See below for a discussion of the D/H ratio. For equivalent kinetic energies a smaller contact diameter is MORE damaging than a larger diameter at the same KE.

Data summaries like Fig. 2.16 are used to establish the specification Kinetic Energy for Damage Tolerance demonstrations as well as operational endurance as requested by the operating airlines. For bird strike the 90% probability, the four-pound bird was the selection. The data for terminal velocities is presented in Fig. 2.16 as a component of a potential impact energy requirement. The higher velocity used in Fig. 2.15 is due to the additional velocity component of an aircraft in flight and/or the tip velocity of a rotating fan blade. Kim and coworkers have developed a preliminary procedure for the scaling of plate thickness utilizing the FTE concept [18–20]. Test data have been reduced into "Normalized FTE" and the ratio of the diameter of the impacting ice sphere, D, to the plate thickness, H. The reduced data is presented in Fig. 2.17.

Using the data from [19] the following relationship are developed:

$$\mathrm{KE}(\mathrm{TV}, J) \rightarrow \mathrm{FTE} = \alpha * 506382 * \mathrm{D}^3 \tag{2.3}$$

Diameter, inches	Diameter, cm	Volume, cub inchs	Volume, cc	Mass, lb.	Mass, gm	Terminal Velocity, ft./sec	Terminal Velocity, m/sec	Kinetic Energy, inch-lbs.	Kinetic Energy, inch-lbs.	Cum Probability US	Cum Probability US & Intrer
0.25	0.64	0.01	0.13	0.0003	0.12	32.29	9.84	0.05	0.006		
0.50	1.27	0.07	1.07	0.0021	0.97	45.66	13.92	0.83	0.094		
0.75	1.91	0.22	3.62	0.0072	3.26	55.93	17.05	4.21	0.476	0.22	0.17
1.00	2.54	0.52	8.58	0.0170	7.72	64.58	19.68	13.31	1.505	0.48	0.39
1.20	3.05	0.90	14.83	0.0294	13.34	70.74	21.56	27.61	3.120	0.65	0.54
1.25	3.18	1.02	16.76	0.0333	15.08	72.20	22.01	32.51	3.673	0.68	0.58
1.50	3.81	1.77	28.96	0.0575	26.06	79.09	24.11	67.41	7.617	0.81	0.72
1.70	4.32	2.57	42.15	0.0837	37.94	84.20	25.66	111.21	12.566	0.88	0.80
1.75	4.45	2.81	45.98	0.0913	41.39	85.43	26.04	124.88	14.111	0.90	0.82
1.76	4.47	2.85	46.78	0.0928	42.10	85.67	26.11	127.76	14.436	0.90	0.82
2.00	5.08	4.19	68.64	0.1362	61.78	91.33	27.84	213.04	24.073	0.94	0.88
2.04	5.18	4.45	72.84	0.1446	65.56	92.24	28.11	230.60	26.057	0.95	0.89
2.25	5.72	5.96	97.73	0.1940	87.96	96.87	29.52	341.24	38.560	0.97	0.93
2.40	6.10	7.24	118.61	0.2354	106.75	100.05	30.49	441.75	49.918	0.98	0.95
2.50	6.35	8.18	134.07	0.2661	120.66	102.11	31.12	520.11	58.772	0.99	0.96
2.75	6.99	10.89	178.44	0.3541	160.60	107.09	32.64	761.49	86.048	0.99	0.97
2.76	7.01	11.01	180.40	0.3580	162.36	107.29	32.70	772.63	87.307	0.99	0.98
3.00	7.62	14.14	231.67	0.4597	208.50	111.85	34.09	1078.49	121.870	1.00	0.99
3.25	8.26	17.97	294.54	0.5845	265.09	116.42	35.48	1485.48	167.859	1.00	0.99
3.50	8.89	22.45	367.88	0.7301	331.09	120.82	36.82	1998.04	225.779	1.00	1.00
3.75	9.53	27.61	452.47	0.8979	407.22	125.06	38.12	2633.04	297.534	1.00	1.00
4.00	10.16	33.51	549.13	1.0898	494.22	129.16	39.37	3408.57	385.169	1.00	1.00
4.25	10.80	40.19	658.67	1.3071	592.80	133.13	40.58	4343.98	490.870	1.00	1.00
4.50	11.43	47.71	781.87	1.5516	703.68	136.99	41.75	5459.87	616.966	1.00	1.00

Fig. 2.16 Table of ground hail probabilities and terminal velocities

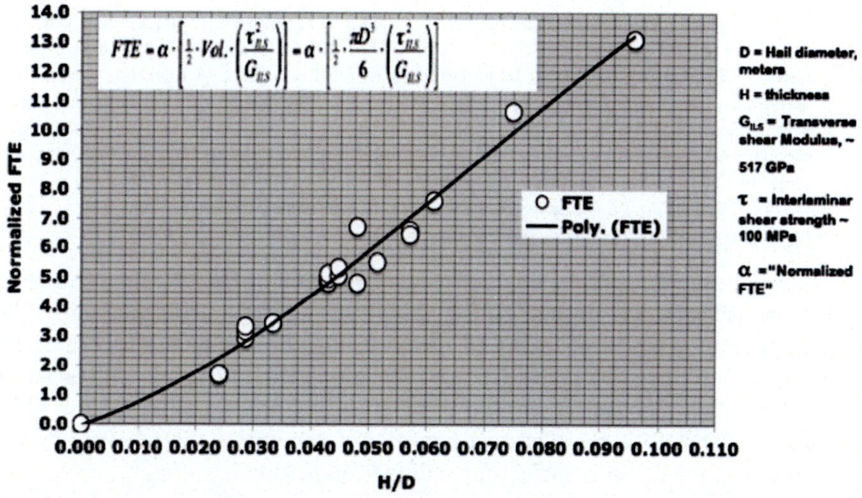

Fig. 2.17 Data reduction for hail ice impacting a graphite plate

Rearranging the equation α is defined as a function of the specified hail diameter:

$$\alpha = \mathrm{KE}(\mathrm{TV}, J)/\{506382 * \mathrm{D}^3\}$$

Using the graph in Fig. 2.17, the *H*/*D* ratio is defined by α. Some typical results are shown in Fig. 2.18:

Cumulative Probability (%)	Hail Diameter, inches	Impacting Velocity, ft/Sec	Impacting Kinetic Energy, Joules	"Normalized" Impacting Kinetic Energy, α	H/D	Damage Withstanding Thickness, inches
98	2.4	100	50	0.435	0.038	0.0912
95	2.04	92	26	0.369	0.0355	0.072
90	1.76	85.6	14.4	0.318	0.0313	0.0551
~ 50	1.0	65	2.7	0.241	0.025	0.025

Fig. 2.18 Estimates of wall thickness required to endure a hail strike at the FTE level

These are interesting numbers, but remember the comments made regarding the use of Eq. 2.1. However, these numbers are good qualitative order of magnitudes. Current dual aisle fuselage skins are of the order of 0.070–0.090 inches in thickness. As the industry scales down from a dual a isle design to a single isle design the diameter of the pressurized fuselage shell reduces about a factor of 0.725–0.76. In a pressurized shell, the wall thickness would normally be reduced by a corresponding factor, depending on other design requirements. These results confirm Bair's comments [2], additional material (weight) for the smaller diameters, and the need for improved material toughness to facilitate composite fuselage construction in the future long haul and regional aircraft designs.

The downsizing of the fuselage by about a factor 0.75 suggest a target for Mode 2 toughness should be at least $(0.75)^{-1} \sim 1.3$ to 1.5 of the current toughened resin capabilities. The fragility of current honeycomb sandwich has a damage tolerance threshold about 1/2 of a solid laminate. Capturing an additional structural margin for both Damage Tolerance and Safety Maintenance Management suggests a goal of 2X improvement with comparable in-plane capabilities and processability for the current toughened resin systems. In addition, application of selected composite materials at various locations in the airframe, depending on the design requirements, is a necessary action. No one system will be optimum for the various design needs.

The dependence of the sizing for hail as a function of H/D should also suggest that the industry has misunderstood the nature of the hail impact topic. The industry is in need of an improved database, digital simulation procedures that could take advantage of the FTE, or DTL conditions, and materials with enhanced toughness with practical processing capabilities. As noted earlier, the use of the Damage Threshold concept has not transitioned into engineering design practice. The rational for this is a subject for a further discussion.

Again the physics of the hail impact indicates a strong function of the Mode 2 Energy Release Rate, G_{2c}, and the Interlaminar fracture toughness, τ_{ILS}. The industry MUST change its interpretation of the hail impact threat in terms of the Low Velocity FOD and Tool Drop legacy. This means additional test capabilities, typically gas gun technology, and the use of frozen Simulated Hail Ice. Metallic or other hard impactors, like a cotton-reinforced ice, do not simulate the damage state that will occur in service. Inappropriate testing compromises both the dimensioning of the affected airframe location and the Damage Tolerance substantiation by test and analysis, see Fig. 2.3 and [1]. The reader can gain additional insight by comparing a laminate sizing calculation using both the falling weight and hail ice data described earlier.

2.4 Molded Short Fiber Parts and Components

As new commercial airframes convert to polymeric-based composite technology, there is an increasing interest in the replacement of cast metallic parts with molded discontinuous parts and components. Potential weight savings, inconsistent quality, and the corrosion incompatibility of cast metallics with graphite laminates are creating this application interest. There are about 6–7,000 piece parts suitable for conversion from cast metallic's to molded composite components. Metallic castings have had a history of poor process control resulting in significant design penalties. Suitable graphite molding material systems have been slow to emerge due to physical–chemical differences relative to the glass polyester system. The acceptance of cast short fiber parts mostly addresses the challenges of process control, Damage Tolerance and economics. Product and process design needs to provide an "allowables-based" approach to design and certification.

1. Recently, a strong scientific-technology base exists to understand chopped fiber prepreg concepts.
2. There is a lack of engineering data available for chopped fiber systems variability and the associated stress concentration, bolt bearing response and combined load strength envelope. These characteristics will strongly influence part and component applications.
3. An "allowables" based strategy will provide engineering acceptance by the structures component within the Prime's structures organization (provides the basis for substantiation by analysis at higher levels of assembly, Fig. 2.3).
4. Capturing the potential economic advantages suggests a focus on commercial process-quality control compatible with traditional materials allowables management.
5. Qualification and individual part certification will be complicated by inconsistent process critical technology associated with compression molding.
6. The NCAMP concept for the certification of allowables and facility certification should be implemented by the technology suppliers with the assistance of the Primes, see [1, 21].

Looking forward, the natural evolution for this activity would be the development of an "allowables-based" materials certification, combined with part and application certification by a combination of test and analysis to enable an open competition for global suppliers. As these activities progress, new guidance from the FAA and EASA will evolve to replace the rules for metallic castings. This guidance is to incorporate into the "Building Block" certification concept for Composite airframes, Fig. 2.3. The airframe primes will look to the lower Tier suppliers to mature this technology and to provide certification options. A strong collaborative development between the technology provider, the parts supplier(s) and the prime air framers must occur to transfer this technology base.

2.5 Summary and Conclusions

Hail Impact; the Impact Matrix Chart, Fig. 2.2, and the Building Block development, Fig. 1.3, clearly identifies the need for a method of test and analysis for the hail following along a similar path to that used for bird strike and tire rupture:

- Defining a threat level,
- Qualifying a test procedure (and simulation test object for natural hail—like the "gel pack" for bird strike), and
- The development and qualification for the digital simulation of the impact on engineered structures.

These steps are essential, as a "PRIME" will certify by a combination of test and analysis, Fig. 2.3. There is a need for and R&D investment here. The CMH-17 does a miss service as it discourages (down plays) the need for improved technology.

Hail impacts have been confused with the Low Velocity falling weight characterization approach. This is a misunderstanding of the dynamic nature of the physics. Hail impact is a Medium to High Velocity event with an impacting object that fragments on impact. An understanding of these phenomena and the use of the Threshold Damage concepts will yield weight efficient designs.

Both industry and the CMH-17 [1] have misrepresented (or misunderstood) the importance of matrix toughness and the need for additional investment in alternative approaches to tougher materials and sandwich design geometries. As pointed out, the sandwich honeycomb construction provides macro E/I and G/J stiffness advantages but localizes the impact induced deflections (a micro response) to the impact point making the construction much more sensitive, vulnerable, to in-service impact events. We need to reopen this topic, there is an opportunity for thermoplastic material based composite and stiffing concepts that do not use the honeycomb technology base. It is the localization of the impact energy that defeats the improvements provided by better materials. This is why thicker laminates benefited form improved material toughness when used in unsupported solid laminate applications.

Specific recommendation for the needed improvement in the toughened resin, and/or thermoplastic-based composite has been made.

Mixed material solutions in the airframe will provide an optimum solution, a single material solution is neither practical nor useful in meeting operational efficiency and the Damage Tolerance, and Safety Maintenance Management needs.

Molded chopped fiber technology needs to mature in terms of interfacing with the Damage Tolerance, Safety Maintenance Management practices for air vehicle applications. The NCAMP process does provide an affordable method to the certification of Material Allowables and the associated Design Allowables. There is work in the USA to reenergize the TSO process to facilitate the transition of nonmetallic molded parts and components into airframe application, see the FAA Web Site for the TSO concept.

References

1. Composite Materials Handbook MIL-HDBK17, (now CMH-17) (2002) The composite materials handbook. ASTM, Conshohocken
2. Gates D (2008) Seattle Times aerospace reporter. Bair pilots Boeing effort to replace best-selling 737, *The Seattle Times*, Thursday, July 17
3. Poe CC (1992) Impact damage and residual tension strength of a thick graphite/epoxy rocket motor case. J Spacecr Rocket 29:394–404
4. Halpin JC (1980) UCLA lecture notes(Unpublished)
5. Dost EF, Ilcewicz LB, Avery WB, Coxon BR (1991) Effects of stacking sequence on impact damage resistance and residual strength for quasi-isotropic laminates. In: O'Brien TK (ed) Composite materials: fatigue and fracture, vol 3, ASTM STP 1110, American, pp 476–500
6. Davis GAO, Robinson P (1992) Predicting failure by debonding/delamination. In: Debonding/delamination of composites, AGARD-CP-530, vol 5, pp. 1–28
7. Olsson R (2001) Analytical prediction of large mass impact damage in composite laminates. Compos Part A 32:1207–1215
8. Olsson R, Donadon MV, Falzon BG (2006) Delamination threshold load for dynamic impact on plates. Int J Solid Struct 43:3124–3141
9. Davies GAO, Zhang X, Zhou G, Watson S (1994) Numerical modeling of impact damage. Composites 25:342–350
10. Davies GAO, Zhang X (1995) Impact damage prediction in carbon composite structures. Int J Impact Eng 16:149–170
11. Schoeppner GA, Abrate S (2000) Delamination threshold loads for low velocity impact on composite laminates. Compos Part A Appl Sci 31:903–915
12. Jackson WC, Poe CC (1993) The use of impact force as a scale parameter for the impact response of composite laminates. J Compos Technol Res 15:282–289
13. Timoshenko S, MacCullough GH (1935) Elements of strength of materials. Van Nostrand Company, New York, pp 326–329
14. Zhang X (1998) Impact damage in composite aircraft structures experimental testing and numerical simulation. Proc Inst Mech Eng G: J Aerosp Eng 212:245–259
15. Aktay L, Johnson AF, Holzapfel M (2005) Prediction of impact damage on sandwich composite panels. Comput Mater Sci 32(3–4):252–260
16. Smith PJ, Thomson LW, Wilson RD (1986) Development of pressure containment and damage tolerance technology for composite fuselage structures in large transport aircraft. NASA contractor report 3996
17. Gokhale N (1975) Hailstoms and hailstone growth. State University of New York Press, Albany
18. Kim H, Kedward KT (2000) Modeling hail ice impacts and predicting impact damage initiation in composite structures. AIAA J 38:1278–1288
19. Kim H, Kedward KT, Welch DA (2003) Experimental investigation of high velocity ice impacts on woven carbon/epoxy composite panels. Compos Part A 34:25–41
20. Kim H, Nightingale J, Park H (2008) Impact damage resistance of composite panels impacted by cotton-filled and unfilled ice. In: ICCM16, Kyoto Japan
21. Clarkson E, Ng Y (2008) Comparison of various material acceptance criteria. J Adv Mater 40:69–83

Chapter 3
Composite Materials for Marine Applications: Key Challenges for the Future

R. A. Shenoi, J. M. Dulieu-Barton, S. Quinn, J. I. R. Blake and S. W. Boyd

3.1 Introduction

Polymeric composite materials have been used in boats, ships, submersibles, offshore structures and other marine structural applications for about 50 years. Considerable progress has been made in this period on understanding the behaviour of these materials and the tailored structures under mechanical, thermal and fire-induced load scenarios. Processing and production considerations too have received much attention leading to a capability of constructing quite complex, multi-material, large, three-dimensional assemblies capable of sustaining extreme loads. Nevertheless there is still an air of conservatism and even hesitation in specifying polymer composite-based solutions for several applications. This is owed to doubts about new ways to use existing materials or to use new and existing materials in new applications. This implies the need for further work for enhanced application and use of composite materials in marine applications.

The key challenges for the future are twofold. First, on an economic front, there is need to ensure that CAPEX (Capital expenditure) and OPEX (Operating costs) of ships, boats and other marine artefacts are optimised and the material specification leads to such a goal. Secondly, with ever growing concern for sustainability, it is important to appreciate and understand life cycle issues from an environmental impact viewpoint. Thus, one could argue that these twofold economic- and energy-based outcomes lead to the following five technical challenges:

1. Enhanced levels of fundamental understanding of the load transfer mechanisms in layered orthotropic structures using empirical, physical means to ensure enhanced confidence in theoretical modelling capabilities.

R. A. Shenoi (✉), J. M. Dulieu-Barton, S. Quinn, J. I. R. Blake and S. W. Boyd
School of Engineering Sciences, University of Southampton,
Southampton, SO17 1BJ, UK
e-mail: r.a.shenoi@soton.ac.uk

L. Nicolais et al. (eds.), *Composite Materials*,
DOI: 10.1007/978-0-85729-166-0_3, © Springer-Verlag London Limited 2011

2. Better appreciation of the modelling of safety concerns that account for potential variabilities and uncertainties in material and structural behaviour.
3. Life cycle assessment of composite structures, leading to cradle-to-grave design concepts, that are better able to account for environmental impact based on energy considerations.
4. Development of concurrent engineering approaches that account for design–production interaction leading to specification of optimal design choices from a costing viewpoint.
5. Identification of apt inspection, intervention and repair strategies for ensuring continued structural health of the artefact through its life.

3.2 Load Transfer Mechanisms

In recent years, there has been an increasing demand for large high-speed marine vehicles such as passenger/vehicle ferries. In these vessels, structural weight is of great importance; lighter weight leads to greater speeds, payloads, and/or fuel economy. Fibre reinforced polymer (FRP) materials offer potential savings in structural weight and have been successfully employed in the construction of a variety of boats and small ships. However, the current wet layup production techniques have a number of disadvantages; construction of a mould is both expensive and time-consuming, storage of the mould requires substantial space (often at a premium in modern shipyards), whilst emissions from the polymer resins during the curing process can have significant health and safety implications for the workforce. The adoption of a construction technique utilising standard parts based on pre-formed components could reduce or even eliminate some of these disadvantages.

In an effort to simplify the construction of relatively high-speed craft, there has been a move towards the use of extruded aluminium components in substantial parts of their structure. There are now a variety of standard and proprietary extruded planks, which incorporate stiffeners and edge details to allow rapid and economic lightweight construction. Similar concepts have been developed in civil and aerospace engineering applications utilising FRPs in the form of pultruded planks in the construction of lightweight structures such as bridge enclosures and footbridges. However, whilst the planks in these structures are bonded along their edges, structural butt joints are generally not required, either because the structures are sufficiently small that joints are not needed, or because the structure can be built in such a manner that joints are staggered, and longitudinal loads can be carried over a joint by neighbouring planks.

Some interest has developed in the possible use of pultrusions in ship construction. However, transfer of the civil engineering technology to ship construction is not without challenges. Typical ship lengths of interest are much greater than the maximal length of plank that can be economically transported, whilst ship construction practice often requires butt joints to be aligned to allow construction of the ship in discrete "modules". Finally, present marine design practice requires effective stressed skins in all in-plane directions in order to resist longitudinal and transverse bending of the hull girder. There is thus a requirement for strong and efficient butt joints between plank components if pultrusions are to be used in this context. Initial work on pultruded joints [1] considered butt joint design and the limits of existing materials and joining techniques. Finger joints in glass reinforced plastic (GRP) material, which model pultruded construction, have also been considered [2]. Various joint geometries were examined, and the full-field stress distribution over the joint from thermoelastic stress analysis (TSA) was compared with load displacement behaviour. TSA is a well-established full-field, non-contact stress analysis technique based on infra-red thermography. It was shown that by increasing the fingertip angle there is a decrease in load carrying capacity, a decrease in shear stress and an increase in stress concentration factor at the finger joint tip. The results from the experimental work were used to validate a numerical model that provides data for initial joint optimisation.

Continuation of this study considered the load transfer in adhesively bonded joints manufactured from pultruded composite materials. A numerical model has been developed to represent the through thickness layers in a pultruded material, and the material data for this model were obtained using the TSA technique [3]. Figure 3.1 shows the stress plots obtained from the TSA and finite element analysis (FEA) results obtained for an adhesively bonded double-lap joint.

Figure 3.2 shows the correlation between the TSA and FEA results. Two FEA results are shown based on assumptions regarding the through thickness thermoelastic constant. The results indicate that the two assumptions, which can be considered to be true upper and lower values, bound the experimental results.

Further work is continuing on the determination of through thickness thermoelastic properties for the constituent materials in the pultruded layup. This data is

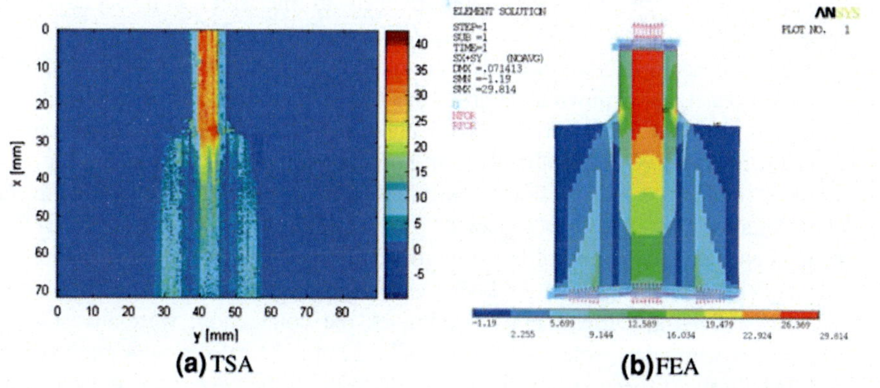

Fig. 3.1 TSA and FEA stress data (MPa) for a double-lap joint in tension. **a** TSA. **b** FEA

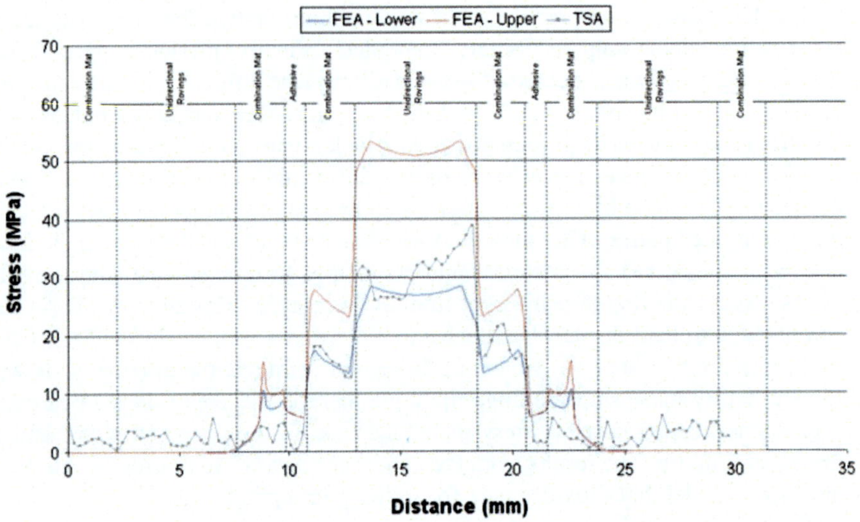

Fig. 3.2 Comparison of TSA, and upper- and lower-bound FEA stress data from a line through the joint near to the end of the straps

essential for the application of the modelling approach for adhesively bonded lap joints where the load transfer is in the through thickness direction. Initial results indicate that the assumptions made, as shown in Fig. 3.2, bound the actual results.

The use of lightweight materials for the construction of the superstructure and other associated structures such as communication masts for marine vehicles and in particular naval vessels has been under investigation since the late 1980s. Initial work naturally focused on the advantages of using GRP such as the weight savings and the lowering of the centre of gravity of the ship, as well as the risk to key operational aspects such as air blast, fire, radar signature and infra-red signature. It was not until the late 1990s and early 2000s that the vital topic of how the composite superstructure should be attached to the steel hull began to be investigated.

Joints consisting of an aluminium or steel section laminated into a composite sandwich panel, also known as hybrid joints, have been found to be most suitable. The joint that has been subject to the most attention and is thus the focus of research attention at the University of Southampton is that shown in Fig. 3.3, which is used in the construction of the helicopter hangar on the French La Fayette class frigates. This study was supported by the UK Ministry of Defence (MOD) to gain a better understanding of the strength and durability of the steel to composite connection shown in Fig. 3.3. Some aspects, such as the static compressive strength and fatigue life characterisation of the connection, were investigated through the European project EUCLID RTP3.21 and the results were published in Ref. [4]. Further aspects, such as the consideration of the performance of the joint after artificial hygrothermal ageing, the numerical modelling and prediction of

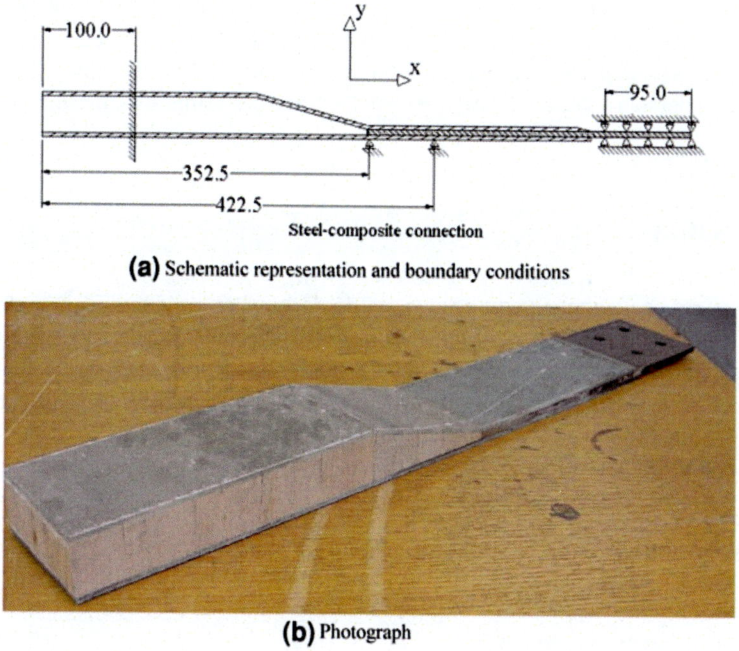

Fig. 3.3 Hybrid steel–composite connection. **a** Schematic representation and boundary conditions. **b** Photograph

failure of the connection, and the optimisation of the connection for the applied loads is provided in Ref. [5]. The results of this study identified the static and fatigue characteristics of the joint to provide information on how the connection behaves under axial loading, as well as the location of initial failure under static loading. In addition, a statistical function was used to correctly represent the fatigue characterisation curve. The long-term accelerated ageing program, to investigate the influence of moisture on the connection, found that the in-plane tensile performance of the joint was unaffected by the accelerated ageing process. The research also investigated the behaviour of the steel–composite joint, providing information vital to the understanding of the mechanisms of stress distribution within the joint and the progression of failure. The progressive damage modelling used a new method of defining the degradation of the material properties post-maximum stress.

In addition, the model for the degradation was based on a new method of incorporating fracture toughness energy as the variable to describe the mathematical function of property degradation. Genetic algorithms were used to investigate the design space of the steel–composite joint and provided a number of possible improvements to the performance of the joint through geometric changes alone. The main objective of the study was reduced joint weight. This highlights the importance of optimisation as a tool for the structural engineer in an area where little research has been conducted. A large step change in performance in terms of weight was achieved through the use of this optimisation technique. Overall, the research provided valuable information that can be used by the naval architect to better understand the application of steel–composite joints in a marine structure.

3.3 Safety

One of the challenges in composites, particularly when products such as ships and boats are made-to-order, with each being of a different design and specification, which militate against extensive testing and prototyping, is the mechanism to manage variability and uncertainty. The variabilities could be related to fabrication-driven, strength-driven, and through-life-driven factors.

On the fabrication side, one has to consider the following:

- Process type [spray-up, HLU (Hand Lay-Up), VARIM (Vacuum Assisted Resin Infusion Moulding), prepreg];
- Topology (single skin monocoque, single skin stiffened, sandwich, hybrid);
- Reinforcement type [CSM (Chopped Strand Mat), CFM (Continuous Filament Mat), weaves and stitches];
- Reinforcement material type (glass, kevlar, carbon, hybrid);
- Resin variability (polyester, vinyl ester, epoxy, phenolics)—even from component to component in one structural piece;
- Core variability [balsa, PVC (Polyvinyl Chloride), honeycomb]—densities vary from part to part.

On the strength side, the factors that would typically need quantifying would be:

- Variation of loads—leads to uncertainties;
- Difficulty in prescribing fixity at boundaries—leads to uncertainties;
- Variability in material properties—process and operator dependence; affects strength calculations;
- Variety of failure limits [e.g. y% of "ultimate strength" as per ABS (American Bureau of Shipping) rules or 30% failure strain implicit in LR (Lloyd's Register of Shipping) rules];
- Variety of failure models (independent stress/strain or interactive criteria).

On the through-life side, the typical factors are threefold:

- Fatigue calculations noting variability of loads + load sequence effects and validity of linear Miner's Rule, S–N response, failure modes;
- Durability issues (laminate versus core material versus structure);
- Fracture and life estimation including such issues as consistency of crack initiation locations/causes, crack propagation mechanisms and directions, modelling parameters and validity of Paris equation.

One approach to address these variabilities and uncertainties is through the use of partial safety factor approaches such as those suggested in some civil engineering codes [6–8]. These seek to ensure that for any given limit state, the calculated effects of destabilising loads (S) are less than the resistance of the structure (R) by a margin commensurate with the required probability of failure. To achieve this, design variables subject to statistical uncertainty are factored by partial safety factors. This can be expressed as:

$$S(x_{L,i} \quad \gamma_{fL,i})\gamma_{f3} \prec R(a_d \quad x_{M,i}/\gamma_{M,i}) \tag{3.1}$$

where $x_{L,i}$ are the load variables, a_d are the design values of the geometric data and $x_{M,i}$ are the material variables. The partial safety factors can be stated as, $\gamma_{fL,i}$ on the ith applied loads, γ_{f3} allows for uncertainty in the design and $\gamma_{M,i}$ on the ith material property.

An alternative is a full level 3 probabilistic approach [9, 10] where the reliability of a structure is defined as the probability that the structure will perform its intended function without failing. Defining a performance function, or limit state function, g(x), as the difference between structural "capacity" and "load" then:

When $g(x) > 0$ then the structure is safe, "capacity" is greater than "load".
Conversely, when $g(x) < 0$ then the structure has failed.
$g(x) = 0$ defines the boundary between survivability and failure, the limit state itself.

The reliability index or safety index is effectively a measure of how far inside the "safe" zone the structure is operating—approaching a zero value, the probability that a structure will fail approaches 100%. As an example, when "capacity" and "load" are normally distributed then Table 3.1 below describes the decreasing likelihood of failure with increasing safety index:

Some work has been done to date in the strength assessment of single skin [11, 12] and sandwich structures [13] as well as fatigue and lifting of composite structures [14–16]. However, it is clear from these and other current studies that a variety of hypotheses about materials and structural modelling as well as believable materials data sets need to be challenged and new approaches developed.

Table 3.1 Safety index versus probability of failure (normally distributed variables)

Safety index	Probability of failure
1.28	10^{-1}
2.33	10^{-2}
3.09	10^{-3}
3.71	10^{-4}
4.26	10^{-5}
4.75	10^{-6}
5.19	10^{-7}
5.62	10^{-8}
5.99	10^{-9}

Other collaborative work has the strategic goal to develop a new stochastic approach to the design of composite structures that is able to account for variations in material properties, geometric indices and processing techniques, from the component level to the full system level. The research focus at the University of Southampton is on the mechanics of composite structures and supplying details of variabilities in composite materials/structures. Other partners focus on stochastic modelling and reliability predictions for use in design. The four phases of the work are:

Phase 1	Identifying the merits of reliability-based approaches in composite structures
Phase 2	Application of the reliability approach to stiffened marine composite structures
Phase 3	Use of general purpose FEA coupled with reliability models for stiffened single skin and sandwich panels
Phase 4	General design formulations and recommendations

The first two phases of this study have been completed to date. At the conclusion of Phase 1 various models on time-variant reliability were put forward and an example showing how FE methods can be interfaced with FORM (First Order Reliability Models)/SORM (Second Order Reliability Models) provided. A sensitivity analysis of a laminated plate showed that the influence of load had the greatest influence on the probability of failure, followed by material property.

In Phase 2 the work of Phase 1, modelling of unstiffened composite plates under loading and the subsequent reliability of those plates in withstanding those loads before first ply failure, was extended to the modelling of stiffened composite plates under loading. A practical grillage methodology, using the Energy Method, was identified and extended by the use of equivalent elastic properties for composite modelling. This methodology was applied to the reliability analysis for a composite stiffened plate. Phase 2 demonstrated the importance of accumulating good qualitative data in forming target structural reliability and, therefore, efficient design. This was revealed by consideration of the effects of the probability density functions, representing the behaviour of the random variables, on the derived structural reliability. As an example, load is typically considered to be a subjective uncertainty as often the phenomenological behaviour, such as wave loads, is not wholly understood. Thus during Phase 2 a change was made in the definition of all the variables, from normal distributions to Weibull distributions.

The benefit of using reliability analyses to identify which random variables are more influential on the resulting performance of the finished composite product was also shown. In terms of manufacture or repair this may have the more obvious advantage of allowing the engineer to concentrate on these more important areas—for example, geometry, fibre angle as cloths are stacked, process technique to maximise fibre volume fraction and so forth. The application of a grillage analysis for composite stiffened plates in Phase 2 has led to the definition of subsequent structural reliability that has been applied for the two limit states of stress and deflection. The results from these tests show the versatility in the reliability approach and the ability to better define partial and full safety factors for composite design purposes.

3.4 Life Cycle Assessment

The understanding of the environmental impact of a product will encourage better industrial practice and be more adaptable in order to exceed current legislation which is becoming increasingly strict and requires the manufacturer to take more responsibility for their production and products. The marine industry has been investigating the use of thermoplastic matrix composites (TMCs) as an alternative to thermoset composites for a number of years. The marine industry cannot use costly high-performance materials which require specialised curing cycles. Therefore, there has been increasing interest in the use of cheaper and lower performance polypropylene thermoplastics and glass reinforcements as a recyclable and durable structural material.

There is recognition of such environmental impact issues through, for instance, the issuance of standard procedures (ISO14040) [17]. A typical life cycle comprises sourcing of base materials, processing and production of components that form the ship/boat, manufacturing of the ship/boat, lifetime operations of the ship/boat and disposal or recycling of the ship/boat at the end of its useful life. Life cycle assessment (LCA) approaches can be used for materials selection in which intrinsic properties that may have an impact on how they are implemented in design are considered. Whilst much is being done in many areas of engineering application, it is felt that such approaches could be usefully adapted and extended to marine structure design too, particularly noting the increasing interest in such features by the IMO (International Maritime Organisation), which is currently developing a convention to provide globally applicable ship recycling regulations for international shipping and for recycling activities [18]. The Marine Environment Protection Committee (MEPC) at its 57th session from 31 March to 4 April 2008, made substantial progress in developing the draft text of the International Convention for the Safe and Environmentally Sound Recycling of Ships, a new convention which will provide globally applicable ship recycling regulations for international shipping and for recycling activities. The new convention will provide regulations for the design, construction, operation and preparation of ships to facilitate safe and environmentally sound recycling, without compromising the safety and operational efficiency of ships; for the operation of ship recycling facilities in a safe and environmentally sound manner; and for the establishment of an appropriate enforcement mechanism for ship recycling, incorporating certification and reporting requirements.

Current work is investigating the life cycle of a marine structure from raw material to full disposal using an embodied energy approach [19]. A grillage structure is used to highlight the issues concerned. Four materials were considered, steel, aluminium, glass reinforced epoxy (GRE) and TMC. Plate thickness and stiffener dimensions were determined in order to ensure that the stress in the grillage did not exceed 60% of the yield stress of the material and that the mid-point deflection of the panel did not exceed 1% of the panel width. The dimensioning was conducted using Vedeler's analytical model for grillage structures. The initial results were presented as a weight value and showed that steel (107 kg) and aluminium (38 kg) were the heaviest options. Both GRE and TMC were lighter at 28 and 23 kg, respectively. Data were collected regarding the energy required to manufacture the raw materials for all four material choices. Manufacturing methods were explored and the associated energy consumption calculated for cutting and joining. Post life disposal methods were examined, recycling as the option for both steel and aluminium and mechanical and incineration options explored for the composite materials. The results of the energy analysis are shown in Fig. 3.4. Two results are provided for the energy required to produce the raw materials, the high value is for virgin material the low value is for material obtained using recycling. The results show a large difference between virgin and recycled metallic materials, most possibly due to the process maturity of recycling metals. This is not reflected in the composite results. However, one cannot specify only recycled steel for construction and so the question remains—How much energy does steel manufacture consume? This will vary depending on the amount of recycled scrap used in the process and the type of furnace that is used for steel manufacture. For the composite results there is little difference between virgin and recycled materials. In general, recycling in this study was the generation of energy through incineration of the used composite which can offset the energy required to manufacture new material.

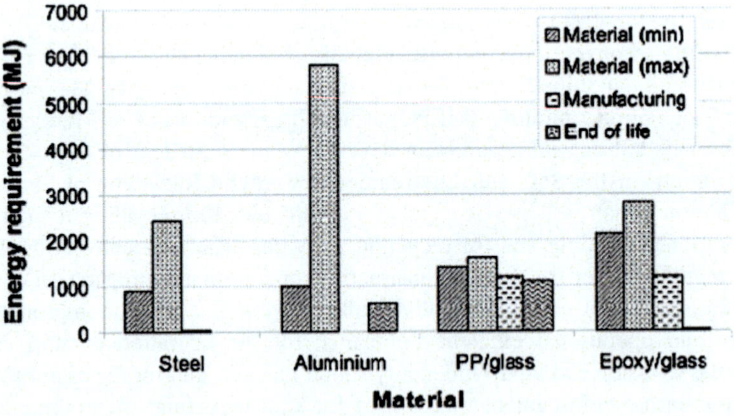

Fig. 3.4 Results of embodied energy analysis for candidate materials

3.5 Concurrent Engineering

In the ship and boat design process, appraisal of alternatives plays a key role in obtaining a successful result. An incorrect decision at the initial appraisal stage can have a significant effect on the costs of building a boat or ship. This is compounded in the marine industry by a number of commercial factors.

- The margins between a profitable and non-profitable design and build are small.
- The competition between yards in different countries is very high.
- There is a need to get out new models on a regular basis.
- It is important to be seen to market products having "high tech" credentials.
- There is a good availability of new materials with potential for better performance.
- There is growing commercial and regulatory pressure to introduce new processing techniques.

There is intense competition in the boat and ship building market. This requires companies and yards to be innovative and capable of adapting new materials, structures and production technologies in order to generate new, market-leading designs that are cost-efficient to manufacture. There is a long history of approaches applied to steel ship structure design from the 1960s [20] through to the 1980s [21].

There is a need to try and address such issues from a composites viewpoint. Possible approaches will need to be comprehensive in addressing all pertinent facets. Figure 3.5 shows such a relationship. Some of the key specific objectives could be argued as below.

- To assess materials data base requirements on the basis of existing, validated publicly available literature and to compile this into a standard and accessible format;

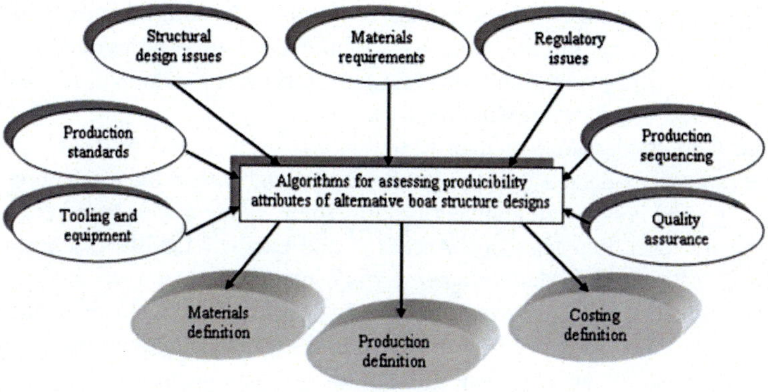

Fig. 3.5 Issues to be considered in concurrent engineering approaches

- To examine availability of design codes (e.g. classification societies, ISO (International Organisation for Standardisation), RCD (Recreational Craft Directive)) and develop linking modules from these into structural analysis software and FEA codes, materials databases, processing information etc., perhaps through a novel web-based procedure for wider application by boat and ship builders and other composites structures fabricators at different sites;
- To formulate producibility parameters relevant to new processes such as vacuum assisted resin infusion moulding and develop production models for linking to design suites;
- To identify and incorporate parameters affecting variability in materials properties that affect design and processing considerations;
- To encourage innovation and evolution by reducing risks associated with new processes/materials.

A possible way ahead is to deploy analytical/numerical codes for structural synthesis that are coupled with simulations of the production process that include tooling selection, consumables and the manual/machine interventions in fabrication and which, together are linked to optimisation tools that, in the case of composites, are best based on genetic algorithm (GA) based approaches. An example of early work in this regard deals with stiffened single skin structures [22].

Small FRP boat design and production in the leisure industry has also been considered. This is inefficient by being sequential in practice and in a highly competitive market attention has been turned to alternative successful design and production techniques employed in other sectors. Improving the design process can have a significant impact on the cost of the final product—whilst around 5% of the final product cost comes from design costs, design value can affect the final product cost by up to 80%. In the aerospace and automotive industries concurrent engineering uses parallel instead of sequential design processes, thereby allowing simultaneous changes necessitated by inputs from, for example, production engineers, quality assurance, structural engineers, outfitters and classification societies to lead to a rapid optimal design, reducing design and production times and increasing quality with little penalty in cost. The aim of current work is to assist the UK boat building industry to embrace modern integrated design and production techniques to help maintain and improve its competitive position and speed up new product introduction.

The work undertaken to date [23–25] has concentrated on four main areas, namely materials database issues, design codes and standards, production process modelling and concurrent engineering principles. Using a web-based environment with easily accessible Microsoft Access™ and Excel™ facilities, concept design, detailed design and production can be fully integrated, as shown in Fig. 3.6.

One aspect of the concurrent engineering tool being developed is the optimisation of stiffened FRP panels typically found in small boat construction. Using a materials database, an analytical grillage analysis, production cost modelling and Lloyds Register Special Service Craft Rules and ISO 12215-5 rules, candidate

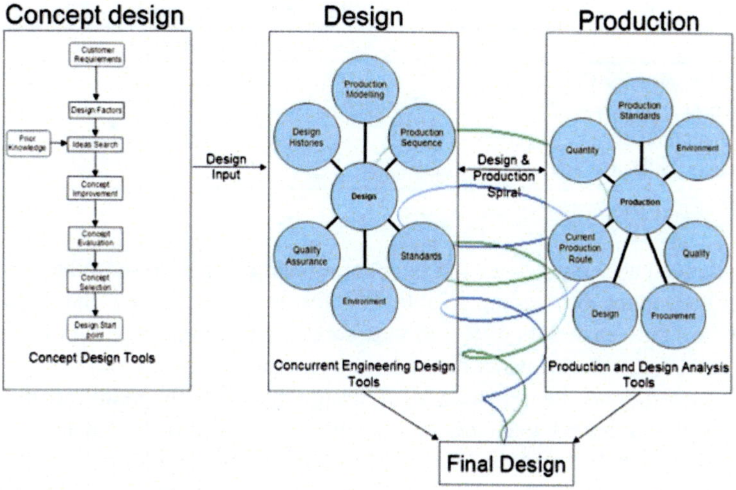

Fig. 3.6 Schematic illustration of a concurrent engineering approach, utilising parallel design processes

Table 3.2 Weight minimisation of unidirectional stiffened FRP plate subject to stiffness and strength constraints (FI is failure index)

		Case-WUl	Case-WU2	Case-WU3	Case-WU4
Constraints	δ_{max}(mm)<	∞	10.0	10.0	1.0[a]
	FI_{max}<	∞	1.0	0.1	0.1[a]
Girder spacing	(mm)	750.0	750.0	750.0	750.0
Base plate	Fibre angle	[−45]s	[0]s	[0]s	[0]s
	Fibre types	[UHM]s	[UHM]s	[UHM]s	[UHM]s
	A_w (kg/m^2)	[0.2]s	[0.2]s	[0.2]s	[0.2]s
Web	Fibre angle	[45]s	[90]s	[90]s	[90]s
	Fibre types	[UHM]s	[UHM]s	[UHM]s	[UHM]s
	A_w (kg/m^2)	[0.2]s	[0.2]s	[0.2]s	[0.2]s
Crown	Fibre angle	[45]s	[0]s	[0]s	[0]s
	Fibre types	[UHM]s	[UHM]s	[HS]s	[HS]s
	A_w (kg/m^2)	[0.2]s	[0.2]s	[0.2]s	[0.2]s
Weight (kg)		31.4187	31.4187	31.4535	31.4535
δmax (mm)		8.8657	1.6547	0.7212	0.7212[b]
FI-US1		1.19808	0.2236	0.0468	0.0468[c]
FI-US2		0.2558	0.0023	0.0345	0.0345[c]
FI-US3		1.1865	0.0166	0.0780	0.0780[c]

[a] Input constraints
[b] Calculated deflection
[c] Calculated FIs (three locations)

design solutions can be rapidly assessed for reduced cost and weight using a genetic algorithm. Table 3.2 gives an example of optimised layup schedules for unidirectional stiffened panels under four different stiffness and strength criteria.

Table 3.3 Effect of limit state constraints on stiffened FRP panel weight and cost

	Mass (kg)	Cost (£)
Lloyd's Register SSC Rules	151.42	371.92
Analytical approach		
Strength limit state	88.11	338.56
Strength, deflection and buckling limit states	104.12	315.60

Alternative panel limit states can be incorporated using relevant failure criteria for differing modes of loading: Table 3.3, for example, shows the influence of including the constraints of four failure models including buckling on the weight and cost of a stiffened panel in the boat's sideshell (6 m^2).

To incorporate the importance of design histories in optimised design, the application of neural networks to facilitate self-learning within the concurrent engineering environment is envisaged; thereby lessons can be learnt for new designs from records of previous design successes and failures, helping to make concurrent engineering philosophies and practice a step change in the UK small FRP boat production sector and an injection for international competitiveness.

3.6 Structural Health Monitoring

In the irresistible increasingly competitive world, most engineering decisions are governed by commercial considerations. These are related to capital costs (CAPEX) and operating costs (OPEX). The previous section focused on CAPEX. Structural health monitoring (SHM) and any resulting intervention for repair and maintenance of the structure directly affects OPEX. The techniques commonly utilised for SHM purposes are non-destructive inspection (NDI), e.g. acoustic emission [26], visual- [27] and vibration-based techniques [28, 29]. Visual-based techniques have proved useful over the past 50 years or so for thin single skin, unpainted structures. However, with increasing use of sandwich topology in marine construction and the higher plate thicknesses for larger load bearing structures, it is becoming incumbent to examine alternative vibration-based approaches. This requires answers to three primary questions:

a. Does damage exist in a structure?
b. What is the location and extent of such damage?
c. What is the severity of this damage?

Once these are answered then one can use continuum damage or fracture mechanics approaches to answer a fourth question:

d. How much residual life exists in this damaged structure?

One example of work on vibration-based damage identification approaches revolved around passive smart concepts with embedded transducers and strain

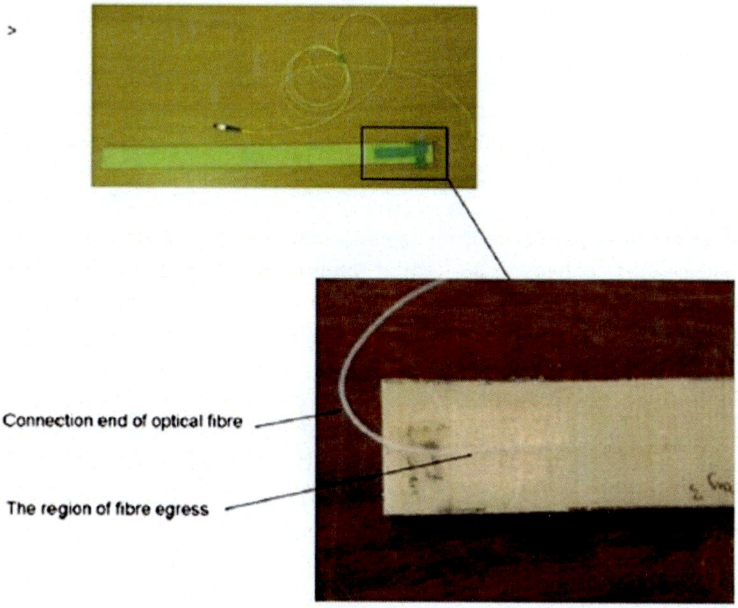

Fig. 3.7 Embedding FBG sensors in sandwich structures

gauges in sandwich structures [30]. Figure 3.7 illustrates the siting of the Fibre Bragg Grating (FBG) optical strain sensors along skin–core interfaces or in the cores of sandwich structures. The strain measurements were then used in conjunction with a damage detection algorithm which uses vibration-based data to locate and quantify damage using artificial neural network (ANN) approaches. The inputs and corresponding outputs required to train the neural networks were obtained from finite element analyses for different vibration modes for the structural components. Multilayer feed-forward and back-propagation neural networks were designed and trained by using different damage scenarios. After validation, new damage cases were investigated using both experimental and numerical analyses [31, 32], and successful application of the trained ANNs was confirmed. Such approaches have the potential for extension to more complex structural components from a practical, boat viewpoint.

Reference [29] has described a coherent strategy for intelligent fault detection that considers all of the features in detail, i.e. fault definition, operational evaluation (utilising a hierarchical damage identification scheme), sensor prescription and optimisation and a data processing methodology based on a data fusion model. More recent work presents a case study of damage detection in a curved carbon-fibre reinforced panel investigated using ultrasonic Lamb waves [33]. This study showed that multilayer perceptron (MLP) neural networks can efficiently locate damage in a stiffened composite panel, for both classification and regression networks. It was also demonstrated that outlier analysis makes an effective preprocessor of experimental Lamb wave response data for a neural network, and that prior wavelet decompositions of experimental Lamb wave data can facilitate damage detection.

In addition to these vibration-based approaches other data-rich experimental mechanics techniques have been developed at the University of Southampton for damage assessment of composite materials and structures, such as acoustic emission, thermography and TSA. These are focused on question (d), i.e. how much remnant life is there in a structure? TSA uses an infra-red detector to measure the small temperature change associated with the thermoelastic effect and is related to the changes in the sum of the principal stresses on the surface of the material. The stress data can be collected in a matter of seconds, from cyclically loaded components, and hence real time data from structures experiencing damage can be obtained.

As the thermoelastic signal is dependent on both the surface stresses and the surface temperature of the component decoupling these effects, particularly in composite materials which have an inherently low value of thermal conductivity, is crucial as there will be viscoelastic and frictional heating at any damage sites. A methodology to decouple the response is provided in Ref. [34] that involves making corrections for increases in surface temperature so that the thermoelastic signal is dependent only on the stresses. The thermoelastic response from orthotropic composite laminates differs significantly to that from homogeneous isotropic materials. The stress field associated with a typical fibre/matrix composite is essentially discontinuous and on a micro-scale cannot be considered homogeneous. The challenge has, therefore, been to apply this technique to composite structures and obtain meaningful data related to the stresses. A procedure based on the laminate strains rather than the surface ply stresses, which enables a calibration approach that accounts simultaneously for the laminate mechanical response and the surface thermoelastic response, has recently been developed [35].

In the area of damage evaluation and NDE (Non-Destructive Evaluation) using infra-red thermography progressive damage under fatigue loading has been considered [36, 37]. Figure 3.8 shows maps of the principal strains around a central circular hole in a glass epoxy plate obtained using TSA subject to progressive damage under fatigue loading [37]. The evolution of the damage is clear. To provide a quantitative damage indicator, Fig. 3.9 shows how the strain metrics

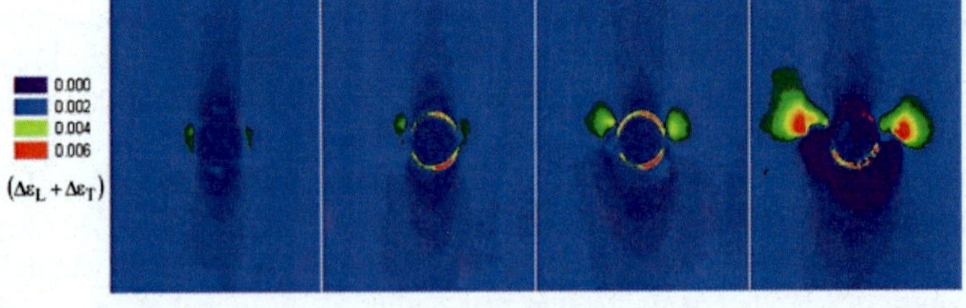

Fig. 3.8 Damage progression around a circular hole

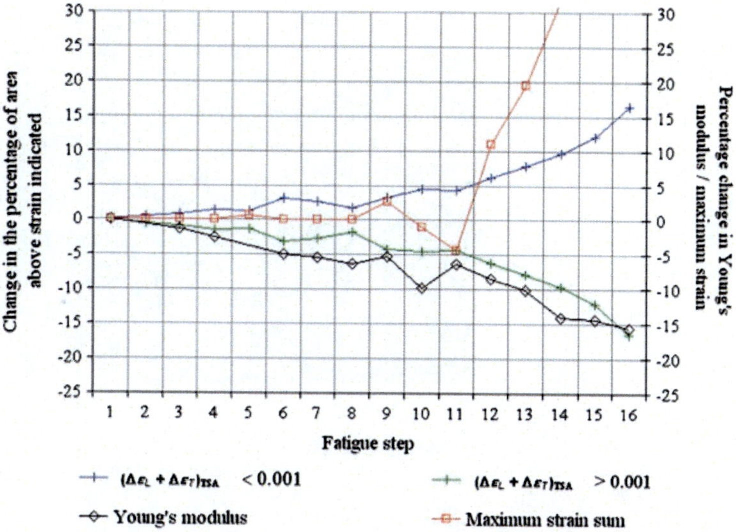

Fig. 3.9 TSA strain metrics and Young's modulus decrease during damaging fatigue

obtained from TSA increases with increasing fatigue cycles and how this can be related to stiffness decreases [37].

This demonstrates that the strain sum is a useful damage metric as after 11 fatigue "packets" this increases rapidly, indicating that it is necessary to take the component out-of-service and repair. It is noteworthy that the Young's modulus only shows a steady decrease and does not provide an indicator of when intervention is necessary.

So far, the application of TSA to composite materials has focused on non-crimp, non-woven fibres, e.g. [35]. In woven material, even under simple loading conditions such as uniaxial tension, the response will be non-uniform and dependent on the orientation of the weave. In general the heterogeneous nature of laminated composite materials produces a non-uniform thermoelastic response. Typically in laminates constructed from layers of unidirectional material, this non-uniformity is only present from lamina to lamina, i.e. through the thickness of the laminate. As the material properties are uniform within a single ply, thermoelastic measurements from the surface may assume orthotropic material properties. Therefore, woven materials commonly used in shipbuilding provide an enormous challenge to TSA. Recent work [38] at high magnification on these materials has revealed that the stresses in the woven structure can be obtained using the technique, providing the possibility of identifying damage initiators in these structures. A typical data set from a twill type weave is shown in Fig. 3.10. Here the stress concentrations because of the crimp are revealed. It should also be noted that the weave dimension was about 0.5 mm. This means that in this data interaction at the fibre-matrix scale is being revealed, which has not been seen previously, experimentally.

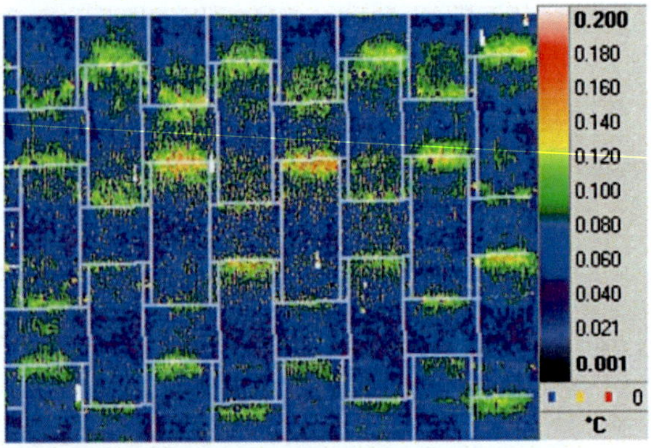

Fig. 3.10 Thermoelastic data from a woven glass epoxy material

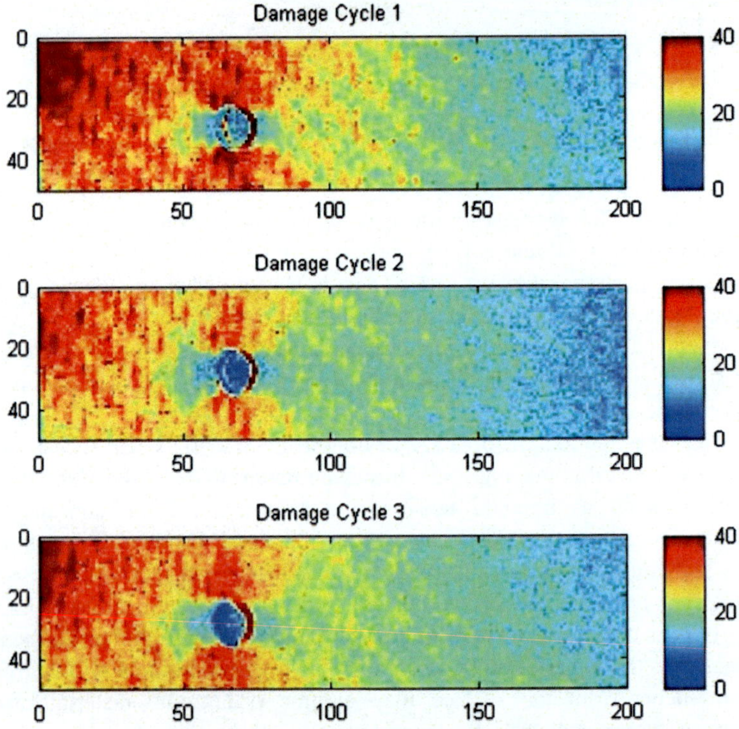

Fig. 3.11 Progression of damage around a hole in a woven GRP specimen—TSA data from an impact load on a cantilever beam

The standard setup for TSA requires a cyclic load to achieve the necessary adiabatic conditions to conduct stress/strain analysis, which has traditionally restricting its application to the laboratory. Therefore, to fully exploit these findings, the challenge is to obtain similar data by applying a transient load to the structure. This would enable the technique to be taken into the field and used to assess damage on in-service structures. Initial work, using a transient small impact/impulse loading [39], has shown that a damage detection and quantification NDE methodology based on infra-red thermography is feasible. The technique comprises the use of pulse phased thermography to locate damage and TSA under transient loading to characterise the damage. Some data from a damaged woven structure is shown in Fig. 3.11. Once again the specimen has a circular hole as a stress raiser; however, the loading is a single impact. The transient loading approach has been validated using a simple cantilever beam setup, and it has been shown that the stresses obtained correspond with theoretical values. This has provided confidence that heat transfer does not dominate the response and the small temperature change is adiabatic.

A study that considered intervention for repair has also been completed [40]. In this study a generic methodology was developed that enables vessel owners to apply a systematic procedure to make decisions regarding damaged vessels. The methodology is based on the RNLI's experience of composite vessels. From the first report of damage to the return to service a series of prompts enable the vessel owner/operator to address each stage of the repair and identify the repair procedure, yard and if applicable assessment routine. The methodology has been applied successfully to steel construction and composite construction using HMS Nottingham and an RNLI lifeboat as illustrative examples. It is intended that the procedure be made available through computer software and the potential implementation of this is also discussed in Ref. [40].

3.7 Conclusions

In conclusion it can be clearly stated that there is a future for the continued and increasing use of polymeric composite materials for structural marine applications. There is a great deal of interest from industry in new ways to use existing materials and in using new and existing materials in new applications. The performance of structures in marine craft needs regular and constant improvement, which will be driven by safety and quality issues. Economic constraints will also play an increasing role in the future, hence the requirement for development of concurrent engineering approaches. Life cycle assessment of composite structures, in order to better understand and appreciate the environmental impact of their use, is also required. Structural health monitoring and its associated inspection, intervention and repair strategies will become increasingly important to both ensure the safe operation of marine composites and to maximise and extend the life of these components.

Acknowledgments The authors are grateful to the following individuals and organisations for their financial support for this research and/or their collaboration: Aalborg University, particularly Professor Ole Thomsen AWE, particularly Mr Paul Tatum British Marine Federation, particularly Mr Nik Parker and Mr Adrian Waddams Dstl, particularly Professor Alan Groves

European project EUCLID RTP3.21 Fiberline AS Fibreforce Flemmings industrial fabrics Lloyds Register Education Trust, particularly Mr Vaughan Pomeroy and Mr Michael Franklin MOD, particularly Professor Jagath Mawella, Mr Bill Gass and Dr. Chris Cole National Composites Network Permabond QinetiQ through the MAST program RNLI, particularly Mr David Brook, Mr Steve Austen and Dr. Holly Phillips Streamline Waterjet Cutting Strongwell (USA) UK Engineering and Physical Sciences Research Council UK Technology Strategy Board University of Sheffield, particularly Professor Keith Worden Vantico

References

1. Boyd SW, Winkle IE, Day AH (2004) Bonded butt joints in pultruded GRP panels—an experimental study. Int J Adhes Adhes 24:263–275
2. Boyd SW, Dulieu-Barton JM, Rumsey L (2006) Stress analysis of finger joints in pultruded GRP material. Int J Adhes Adhes 26:498–510
3. Boyd SW, Dulieu-Barton JM, Thomsen OT, Gherardi A (2008) Development of a finite element model for analysis of pultruded structures using thermoelastic data. Composites 39:1311–1321
4. Boyd SW, Blake JIR, Shenoi RA, Kapadia A (2004) Integrity of hybrid steel-to-composite joints for marine application. J Eng Marit Environ Proc Inst Mech Eng 218:235–245
5. Boyd SW, Blake JIR, Shenoi RA, Mawella J (2007) Co-cured structural steel-composite joints for deck to superstructure connections. Trans R Inst Nav Archit Part A: Int J Marit Eng 149:83–99
6. Clarke JL (1996) Structural design of polymeric composites: EUROCOMP Design Code and Handbook. The European Structural Polymeric Composites Group, E & FN Spon, London
7. Cadei JMC, Stratford TJ, Hollaway LC, Duckett WH (2004) Strengthening metallic structures using externally bonded fibre-reinforced polymers. Constr Ind Res Inf Assoc (CIRIA) Publ C595
8. The Concrete Society (2004) Design guidance for strengthening concrete structures using fibre composite materials, 2nd edn. The Concrete Society, Camberley
9. Thoft-Christensen P, Baker MJ (1982) Structural reliability theory and its applications. Springer-Verlag, New York
10. Sundararajan CR (1995) Probabilistic structural mechanics handbook. Chapman & Hall, London
11. Jeong HK, Shenoi RA (2000) Probabilistic strength analysis of rectangular FRP plates using Monte Carlo simulation. Comput Struct 76:219–235
12. Jeong HK, Shenoi RA (2001) Structural reliability of fibre reinforced composite plates. Trans R Inst Nav Archit Part A: Int J Marit Eng 143:73–98
13. Jeong HK, Shenoi RA (2002) Probabilistic failure analysis of a FRP sandwich plate subjected to a lateral pressure load. Proc Inst Mech Eng, Part L, J Mater Des Appl 216:115–126
14. Xiong JJ, Shenoi RA (2004) A two-stage theory on fatigue damage and life prediction of composites. Compos Sci Technol 64:1331–1343
15. Xiong JJ, Shenoi RA (2004) Two new practical models for estimating reliability-based fatigue strength of composites. J Compos Mater 38:1187–1210
16. Xiong JJ, Shenoi RA (2007) A practical randomisation approach of deterministic equation to determine probabilistic fatigue and fracture behaviours based on small experimental data sets. Int J Fract 145:273–283
17. EN:ISO 14040 (1997) Environmental management—life cycle assessment—principles and framework
18. (2009) The Hong Kong International Convention for the Safe and Environmentally Sound Recycling of Ships. http://www.imo.org/environment/mainframe.asp?topic_id=818. Accessed 5 January 2010

19. Bardet RR, Shenoi RA, Boyd SW (2008) The use of life cycle tools towards sustainable thermoplastic composites in ship building. In: Proceedings of SAMPE Eur Int Conf Forum, Paris
20. Caldwell JB (1972) Design for production. Die Ingineur 84:25–42
21. Kuo C, MacCallum KJ, Shenoi RA (1984) An effective approach to design for production. Trans R Inst Nav Archit Part A: Int J Marit Eng 126:33–50
22. Sobey AJS, Blake JIR, Shenoi RA (2007) Optimisation approaches to design synthesis of marine composite structures. Ship Technol Res 54:1–7
23. Sobey AJS, Blake JIR, Shenoi RA (2008) Optimisation of composite boat hull structures. In: Proceedings of 7th Int Conf Comput Inf Technol Marit Ind (COMPIT), Liege
24. Sobey AJS, Blake JIR, Shenoi RA (2008) Comparative optimisation of first principles design methods with classification society rules for boat hull structures. Ship Technol Res 55:502–515
25. Sobey AJS, Blake JIR, Shenoi RA (2008) Optimisation of composite boat hull structures as part of a concurrent engineering environment. Proc 6th Int Conf High Perform Mar Veh (HIPER), Naples
26. Venturini Autieri MR, Dulieu-Barton JM (2006) Initial studies for AE characterisation of damage in composite materials. Adv Mater Res 13–14:273–278
27. Defence Standard 02-752 Part 2 (2005) GRP survey and repair requirements for HM ships, boats, craft and structures. Ministry of Defence
28. Doebling SW, Farrar CR, Prime MB (1998) A summary review of vibration based damage identification methods. Shock Vib Dig 30:91–105
29. Worden K, Dulieu-Barton JM (2004) An overview of intelligent fault detection in systems and structures. Int J Struct Health Monit 3:85–98
30. Dawood TA, Shenoi RA, Sahin M (2007) A procedure to embed fibre Bragg grating strain sensors into GFRP sandwich structures. Composites 38:217–226
31. Sahin M, Shenoi RA (2003) Vibration-based damage identification in beam-like composite laminates by using artificial neural networks. J Mech Eng Sci Proc Inst Mech Eng 217:661–676
32. Sahin M, Shenoi RA (2003) Quantification and localisation of damage in beam-like structures by using artificial neural networks with experimental validation. Eng Struct 25:1785–1802
33. Chetwynd D, Mustapha F, Worden K, Rongong JA, Pierce SG, Dulieu-Barton JM (2008) Damage localisation in a stiffened composite panel. Strain 44:298–307
34. Dulieu-Barton J, Emery TR, Cunningham PR, Quinn S (2006) A temperature correction methodology for quantitative thermoelastic stress analysis and damage assessment. Meas Sci Technol 17:1627–1637
35. Emery TR, Dulieu-Barton JM, Earl JS, Cunningham PR (2008) A generalised approach to the calibration of orthotropic materials for thermoelastic stress analysis. Compos Sci Technol 68:743–752
36. Emery TR, Dulieu-Barton JM (2007) Damage monitoring of composite materials using pulsed phase thermography and thermoelastic stress analysis. Key Eng Mater 347:621–626
37. Emery TR, Dulieu-Barton JM (2010) Thermoelastic stress analysis of damage mechanisms in composite materials. Compos Part A. 41:1729–1742
38. Frühmann RK, Dulieu-Barton JM, Quinn S (2008) On the thermoelastic response of woven composite materials. J Strain Anal Eng Des 43:435–450
39. Frühmann RK, Dulieu-Barton JM, Quinn S (2010) Thermoelastic stress and damage analysis using transient loading. Exp Mech. 50:1075–1086
40. Cripps RM, Dulieu-Barton JM, Jeong HK, Phillips HJ, Shenoi RA (2006) A generic methodology for post-damage decisions. J Ship Prod 22:21–32

Chapter 4
Multifunctional Polymer Based Structures for Human Tissues Reconstruction

P. A. Netti and L. Ambrosio

4.1 Introduction

Development of appropriate biomaterials needs the establishment of a philosophical paradigm. Learning from the nature, that is asking what are the physical and biological mechanisms underpinning the functions, and the performances of biological tissues which the man-made biomaterials are called upon to substitute is probably the best way to establish this paradigm. Following this bioinspired approach, major advancement in biomaterials design has already been achieved, and it holds the promise to introduce a tremendous revolution in the engineering novel smart biofunctional material platforms.

The study of biological tissue structures and mechanical performances has since long time indicated that nature builds almost exclusively multiphase, heterogeneous, and anisotropic materials, and therefore, no single homogeneous and isotropic material could be used to substitute their functions [1]. The adoption of composite technology provides a wide set of options and possibilities to engineering more appropriate and functional tissue repairing material [2]. Composite materials, indeed, are a valuable choice since the combination of a convenient selection of material characteristics (e.g., the aspect ratio, the fibers orientation, the matrix material, the fibers volume fraction) with the help of micromechanics and lamination theory allows the design of a material with the desired mechanical properties, such as elastic modulus and strength [3]. The possibility to accurately reproduce the structure and the mechanical behavior of natural connective tissues

P. A. Netti (✉)
Department of Material and Production Engineering (DIMP) and Interdisciplinary Research Centre on Biomaterials (CRIB), University of Naples Federico II, Piazzale Tecchio, 80125 Naples, Italy
e-mail: nettipa@unina.it

L. Ambrosio
Institute of Composite and Biomedical Materials (IMCB-CNR), National Council of Research, Piazzale Tecchio, 80125 Naples, Italy

L. Nicolais et al. (eds.), *Composite Materials*,
DOI: 10.1007/978-0-85729-166-0_4, © Springer-Verlag London Limited 2011

has lead to significant improvement in the design of prostheses or synthetic models for in vivo and in vitro applications [4–6]. Furthermore, the use of finite elements models (FEM) tools in combination with mathematical description of adaptive bone remodeling allows an accurate point-wise properties design of rather complex geometry and loading patterns [5–8] insuring the properties matching with the natural counterpart and the optimization of surrounding tissues conservation [9–13].

Biomaterials are used not only to replace damaged tissues but also to help and enhance tissue regeneration. Recent studies on the process of tissue regeneration in vivo, that may occur in response to a trauma, have revealed that it is a result of a complex cascade of events tightly regulated by biophysical and biochemical signals [14]. The time and space presentation of these signals is managed and controlled by the extracellular matrix (ECM) [15]. This complex interplay between cell fate and matricellular signals constitutes the foundation of the logical cellular *language* underlining the complex process of tissue morphogenesis [16]. By learning this *language*, material scientists aim at the engineering novel *cell-instructive* materials able to guide and control cell (adhesion, differentiation, migration, and biosynthesis) and tissue (growth and remodeling) functions. A key technological issue toward this achievement is to encode required biological signals within the scaffold material and control their spatial and temporal sequestration and delivery recapitulating the highly orchestrating molecular processes occurring within the ECM during morphogenesis. Modern advances in nanotechnology, bottom-up design approach, and solid free-form fabrication (SFF) in conjugation with self-assembly processes is expected to be highly instrumental to encode with the required spatial resolution biological information within the materials. There is a plethora of signals that a cell may react to, including chemical, biochemical, biophysical, and structural cues [14, 17]. The appropriate balance between microstructural features—notably, porosity and interconnectivity—and chemical–physical and biological cues may control and promote specific events at the cellular and tissue level. Over the last two decades, the concept of *cell guidance* in tissue regeneration has been extensively discussed and progressively revised as new knowledge of the complex features of cell–material interaction have been disclosed and elucidated. Part of this evolution has been the development of novel scaffold materials, compatible with the cell guidance concept and resulting from contemporary advances in the fields of materials science and molecular biology. As consequence, modern biomaterials have evolved, improving their role in guiding spatially and temporally coordinated tissue regeneration through a designed biophysical and biochemical environment able to control cell behavior. Modern biomaterials science is characterized by an increased integration with cell and molecular biology, which stimulates and promotes the identification of novel design parameters. Synthetic biomaterials endowed with matricellular cues, and able to sequester, and deliver at a given site, morphogenic factors, are emerging today to provide a multifunctional platform to control and guide the tissue regeneration process.

In the first part of this chapter, the major engineering achievements obtained by following a bioinspired approach to design and realize novel composite material for tissue repair will be presented and critically discussed. In the second part, the main achievements in multifunctional cell-instructive biomaterials design along with the future challenges will be outlined.

4.2 Materials for Tissue Repair

Reinforced polymers have gained an increasingly important role in the development of new generation biomedical materials, since they can be engineered more accurately than monolithic structures (single phase materials), thus allowing the development of more effective tissue substitutes. The main font of inspiration for designing new high performances and multifunctional materials arises from the observation and study of biological materials.

For example, the basic constituents of connective hard tissues are: the ECM (i.e., collagen, apatite, and water) and cells (namely, osteocytes in bone and odontoblast in dentine) which controls and adapts the structure performance based on a mechano-sensitivity processes [18]. The soft and ductile collagen and the stiff and brittle apatite crystals represent the constituent materials of a composite; more specific, collagen fibrils of about 100 nm in diameter are reinforced by platelet apatite crystals at a nanostructural level [19]. Since the elastic properties of collagen and hydroxyapatite are about 1.5 and 110 GPa, respectively, then it is not surprising that in mineralized tissues these constituents are conveniently organized allowing to cover a wide the range of properties [20]. Enamel, basically constituted of apatite prismatic crystals, is the stiffer hard tissue showing a young's modulus of about 100 GPa. On the other hand, spongy bone presents lower Young's modulus values [21]. However, trabecular bone is a porous material and experimental values of elastic modulus have to be interpreted as apparent values. In fact, trabecular tissue properties suggests an elastic modulus between 10 and 20 GPa [22–25] which is similar to compact bone and dentine elastic modulus.

Fiber and particulate reinforced polymeric composites represent the engineering response to tissue analogs. The continuous fiber reinforcement is particularly indicated as mechanical tailoring involves anisotropy.

The majority of the bio-structures is characterized by a complex hierarchy of structures where each different size scale, from the nanometers to the micro- and millimetric scale, presents different structural features. The remarkable properties of bulk materials, such as bone, cartilage, or tendon, are the result of these complex interaction taking place across all levels of organization, with each level controlling the next one. Designing responsive, self-healing structures, is at present one of the major objectives of materials research: particularly the identification of the materials' chemical composition and morphological features able to stimulate cells and, by a proper matrix remodeling, yield tissues with different functionality. In the continuing quest for improved performance, which may be specified by various criteria including higher bioactivity, less weight, more strength and lower cost, currently used biomaterials frequently reach the limit of their usefulness. Biocomposites represent the reply to this necessity to overcome the limitations of traditional materials (metal, polymer, ceramic): in fact by wisely combining different single-phases, it is possible to optimize the required performance and minimize the undesired drawbacks.

In future, the challenge of the material scientist will consist in the engineering of replacement materials which are able to ideally mimic the living tissue from a mechanical, but also, from the chemical, biological, and functional point of view. Given the diversity of tissue-specific orientation of fibrils (parallel and aligned in tendon, concentric weaves in bone, orthogonal lattices in cornea, and mesh-like in skin), this latter feature is yet to be fully exploited.

Access to nanotechnology has offered a completely new perspective to the material scientist to mimic the different types of extra-cellular matrices present in tissues. Techniques are now available which can produce macromolecular structures of nanometer size with finely controlled composition and architecture. Nanotechnology also improves non-resorbable biomaterials and effective manipulation of biological interactions at the nanometer level, which will dramatically improve the functionality and longevity of implanted materials. Nanomaterials and/or nanocomposites with enhanced mechanical properties could replace the materials that fatigue-fail due to crack initiation and propagation during physiologic loading conditions.

4.3 Composites for Permanent Prostheses

Traditionally, metals such as stainless steel, titanium, and Co/Cr alloys were commonly used for bone fracture fixation. Although they provide a right strength and rigidity to align and control bone motion during the healing, they are much stiffer than bone ($E_M = 100$–200 GPa and $E_B = 6$–20 GPa) carrying the majority of the load. As result of the large difference in stiffness between bone and metals, a stress protection effect usually may occur by determining the bone atrophy in the long-term period. As consequence, the stress-shielded bone does not heal completely and is susceptible to re-fracture after the removal of the metallic implant. Moreover, metallic materials, traditionally implanted into bone defects are often encapsulated by a fibrous tissue and do not adhere to bone due to lack of bioactivity, thus being isolated from the surrounding bone and remaining as a foreign body [26].

Composite biomaterials such as the hip prostheses (Fig. 4.1), fixation plates and screws, dental post, bone, and dental cements represent the efforts of advanced engineering structures for hard tissue analogs. Carbon and glass fiber reinforced thermoset polymers such as epoxies resins were the first choice for composite orthopedic prostheses [27]. Polymers matrix include poly(sulfone) (PS), poly(etheretherketone) (PEEK), and poly-etherimide (PEI) [2, 28–30]. These engineering

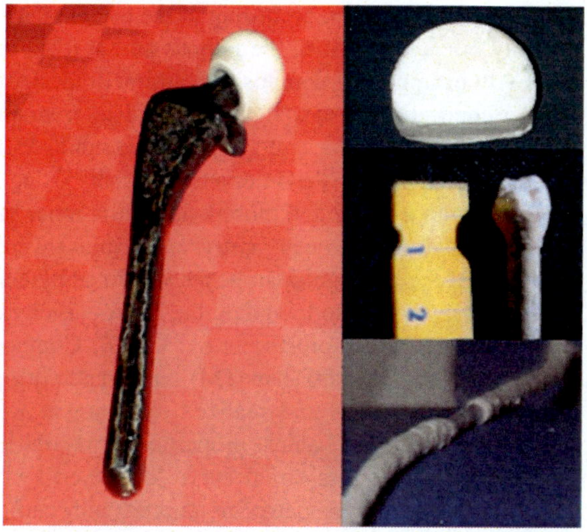

Fig. 4.1 Composite prosthesis: hip joint, intervertebral disk, dental implants, ligament

polymers are characterized by high-mechanical properties, thermal stability, very marginal water absorption, and relatively easy processing. In addition, their high level of solvents and thermal resistance allows the production of sterilisable medical devices. Moreover, the selected materials have demonstrated, at the same time, both positive and negative properties for specific applications. For instance, PEEK has excellent mechanical stability but critical processing conditions due to its temperature-sensitive semi-crystalline structure. Polysulfone has shown a reduction of mechanical properties following saturation in Ringer's solution. In vitro and in vivo, studies [31] have shown that PEI is an excellent substrate for cell spreading and growth, eliciting no cytotoxic response or hemolysis, coupled with both easy processability and resistance to sterilization capability (γ-rays and autoclave). Using PEI reinforced with drop-off plies of carbon and glass fibers, a composite hip prostheses has been developed in order to provide an adequate stress transfer between the prostheses and bone [32].

Material–structural designs for advanced prostheses requiring a stem fitting into a canal (i.e., long bone or dental root canals) may differ, although a common challenge is a stem more flexible than those made of metal in order to improve proximal stress transfer and to avoid from stress-shielding effects [33, 34]. By tailoring the stiffness of the prosthesis both along its length and through its thickness, it is possible to change the pattern of load transfer between the prosthesis and the bone. FEM combined with a mathematical description of adaptive bone remodeling suggest the high performances of composite prostheses in terms of mechanical stability and tissue conservation [9, 35].

Based on the rapid prototyping, silicon mold, and filament winding technology, the replicate of a human mandible has been obtained. The spongy bone is simulated by using Poly (methylmethacrylate) (PMMA) bone cement. The cortex of the mandible has been replicated by using glass fiber reinforcement. The orientation of the windings is chosen according to the osteons' orientation of a human mandible, mainly oriented at 45° in the ramous and at 0° in the mandible arch [20, 36, 37].

Early examples of composite biomimetic design are well documented also for dense connective tissues ligaments and intervertebral disk (Fig. 4.1). Hydrogel consisting of PHEMA and Poly(Caprolactone) PCL reinforced with PET fibers were used to mimic the intervetrebal disk. Using a filament winding, machine samples with a softer and more hydrophilic inner part (i.e., nucleus) and a harder and less hydrophilic outer part (i.e., annulus) were made. By varying the composition of the hydrogel matrix, the winding angle and the quantity of PET fibers, it has been possible to modulate the hydrophilicity and the mechanical properties of intervetrebal disk prosthesis [3, 38–40]. Composite structures based on polyurethane matrix (HydroThaneTM) reinforced with polyethylenterephtalate (PET) fibers were designed and realized by filament winding in order to model the morphology and mechanical properties of natural ligaments and to reproduce the typical J-shaped stress–strain curve, displayed by natural tendons and ligaments [36]. By using a PEI matrix reinforced with carbon fibers through the filament winding technology, a composite cage has also been developed [41].

4.4 Composites for Temporary Prostheses

The basic concept of using biodegradable composite is related to be able to control the degradation of the implant which leads to a gradual load transfer to the healing tissue, preventing the stress-shielding atrophy with the stimulation of the healing and the bone remodeling. Moreover, they avoid the employment of surgical operations for their removal reducing the pain of the patients and the total cost of the treatment with a significant advantage in terms of life quality of the patients.

The main requirements to be fulfilled by ideal prosthetic biodegradable materials, such as biocompatibility, adequate initial strength, and stiffness, retention of mechanical properties throughout sufficient time to assure its biofunctionality and non-toxicity of degradation by-products. From the mechanical point of view, degradable polymers and composites have to possess a modulus of elasticity much closer than bone one which decreases over time as the healing bone becomes stronger and stiffer [42]. It has been demonstrated that synthetic resorbable polymers like polylactide and polyglycolide fulfill several demands of ideal ostheosynthesis materials in term of biocompatibility and suitable stiffness insuring a progressive transfer of stresses to healing bone and to obviate the removal operation. However, they are too weak and flexible for safe clinical use in bone surgical applications. In order to overcome the limited mechanical response of non-reinforced materials based on of aliphatic polyesters like PLA (i.e., low bending stiffness up to 4–6 GPa in dry state at room temperature), the addition of biodegradable fibers may promote the adjustment of the bending modulus up to 50 GPa as function of the fiber content and their orientation [43]. In this context, totally degradable reinforced composites may represent the main goal in the design of new fixation materials because of the drastic decay of long-term problems induced after their digestion by living tissues.

Improved mechanical properties may be obtained by filament winding technologies. Ambrosio et al. [4] proposed a composite structure obtained by merging an Hydrotane matrix with continuous fibers of PLA and PGA helically wound by filament winding technique in order to design porous and not porous tubular constructs. The approach consists of applying the composite theory to design composite biodegradable systems made of PLA continuous fiber reinforcing PU-Hydrotane or Esters of Hyaluronic Acid, able to mimic the structural organization and performance of the living tissue [36, 38, 44].

Bidegradable polymers, including poly glicolic-lactid acid (PLGA), poly-L-lactid acid (PLLA) and polycaprolactone (PCL) have been combined with tricalcium phosphates (α-TCP, β-TCP) particles to form composite materials. They are especially attractive because they combine the controlled degradation kinetics of the polymer phase involving the formation of low molecular weight products, easily eliminable in physiologic environment, with the high-bioactive potential induced by the employment of ceramic materials which promote the formation of the mineralization sites. The proposed approach involving the combination of a polymer matrix and ceramic rigid particles allows reaching an excellent balance between strength and toughness usually improving specific characteristics compared to their separate components with a strong enhancement of the biological response of the implanted device.

On the basis of these considerations, recent studies have embossed the large extent of composites obtained by coupling degradable polymers with reactive calcium phosphates [45–48] for the repair or the regeneration of a wide set of hard mineralized tissues as function of specific properties of the final material. It has been proposed the development of a new injectable bone substitute material as bone fillers in orthopedic and dental applications by combining a ceramic material such as α-TCP or HA with an organic phase of HYAFF11® [46]. It is well known that the attractive characteristic of the calcium phosphates is their ability to form a strong direct bond with the host bone which results in a strong dynamic interface compared to bio-inert or bio-tolerant materials which form a fibrous interface. The addition of the hydrophilic phase allows to modulate the cement workability during their injection and mechanical properties during the hardening reaction of the ceramic phase giving, in a clinically acceptable time, suitable mechanical strength up to the range of cancellous bone for short-term tissue functional recovery. In perspective, biodegradable composite hydrogels could be efficaciously used to deliver appropriate drugs into the application sites with controlled kinetic release.

Roy et al. [45] have studied the performance of biodegradable composites for bone repair by the integration of beta tricalcium phosphate particles in the PLGA porous matrix evidencing a role of the ceramic phase on the degradation mechanisms of the polymer matrix. Precisely, the relatively low molecular weight of the 50:50 PLGA (only 50 kDa) promotes a fast hydrolytic degradation in vivo, with the rapid mechanical failure due to loss of structure. During the PLGA degradation via bulk erosion, the release of acidic degradation products leads to a local decrease in pH, which rapidly causes local tissue damage, i.e., bone resorption, and fibrous tissue formation. The presence of reactive calcium phosphates such as α- and β-TCP may enable to buffer the decay in pH influencing the final polymer degradation. In this direction, several studies related to in vitro degradation of a PLA composites with various additive charge of TCP particles have highlighted a pH drop at the most up to 5, corresponding to the approximate pH for activated macrophages which indicate the occurrence of a probable bone resorption [49].

4.5 Multifunctional Bioactivated Scaffolds for Tissue Regeneration

One of the most challenging goal in tissue regeneration is the design of scaffolds able to control and guide the complex cellular functions that occur during neo-tissue formation. The concept of tissue and cell guidance is rapidly evolving as more information regarding the effect of the microenvironment on cellular function and tissue morphogenesis become available. These disclosures have lead to a tremendous advancement in the design of a new generation of multifunctional biomaterials able to mimic the molecular regulatory characteristics and the three-dimensional architecture of the native ECM. The ideal scaffold should therefore possess a repertoire of cues—chemical, biochemical and biophysical—able to elicit specific cell and tissue response. Future generation of scaffolds has to provide not only the adequate mechanical and structural support but also have to actively guide and control cell attachment, migration, proliferation, and differentiation. This may be achieved if the functions of scaffold are extended to supply biological signals able to guide and direct cell function through a combination of matricellular cues exposition and bioactive molecules sequestration and delivery [50, 51]. Multifunctional scaffolds should integrate a three-dimensional and well-defined microstructure with an interconnected pore network, mechanical properties similar to those of natural tissues, being biocompatible and bio-resorbable at a controllable degradation and resorption rate as well as provide the control over the sequestration and delivery of specific bioactive molecular signals to enhance and guide the regeneration process [52, 53]

Recent research in biomaterial science has been driven by biomimicry-inspired design of materials to recreate the natural three-dimensional architecture of the ECM. Several micro- and nano-fabrication strategies have been applied in an attempt to mimic the spatial distribution of the fibrillar structure of the ECM, which provides essential guidance for cell organization, survival, and function [54–58]. These technologies include gas foaming, SFF (3D printing, 3D plotting), molecular and nanoparticulate self-assembly, electrospinning, molecular, and nano-templating [52, 54, 57–59]. Albeit the influence of scaffold micro-architecture and stereomorphology on cell function and guidance has been proved in several systems and with different cell types, the underlining mechanisms by which cells

Table 4.1 Synthetic and semi-synthetic degradable materials used as tissue engineering scaffolds

Material		Relevant features and application	References
Polymeric materials	Poly(glycolic acid) (PGA)	Hydrolytically degradable polyesters	[16]
	Poly(lactic acid) (PLA)	Musculoskeletal tissue engineering	
	Poly(lactic-*co*-glycolic acid) (PLGA)	Cartilage regeneration	
	Polylactide-*co*-glycolide (PLGA) tubular shaped foams	Fibrovascular engineering	[60]
	Poly(ε-caprolactone) (PCL)	Hydrolytically degradable polyesters Skin engineering	[61]
	Polyethylene glycol (PEG)	Synthetic hydrogel Bone formation	[62]
	Oligo(poly(ethylene glycol) fumarate) (OPF)	Cartilage engineering GFs release from gelatin microspheres	[63]
Inorganic materials	Tricalciumphosphate (TCP), hydroxyapatite (HA)	Bone substitute	[64, 65]
Semi-synthetic materials	Cross-linked thiolated HA	Neurite growth and support	[66]
	Thiolated HA poly(ethylene glycol) diacrylate co-cross-linked with poly(ethylene glycol) diacrylate	Vocal fold repair	[67]
	Non-woven meshes of esterified hyaluronan (HYAFF® derivatives)	Cartilage engineering	[68]

recognize and decode topological information are still unclear. A wide variety of biodegradable and biocompatible polymers (Table 4.1) have been processed to fabricate stereoregulated scaffolds, including synthetic polymers, such as poly(lactide) (PLA), poly(glycolide) and their copolymers poly(lactide-*co*-glycolide) (PLGA), poly(ε-caprolactone) (PCL), and natural polymers, such as collagen, protein, and fibrinogen [60–68].

4.6 Microstructural Cues

Recent literature indicates that cell can react and respond to microstructural material features such as pore size and shape and degree of interconnectivity [17, 72–74]. As reported in Table 4.2, there is a summoning experimental evidence that the microstructural features of a tissue engineering scaffolds can strongly

Table 4.2 Experimental evidence of scaffold microstructural cellular guidance

Topological property	Optimal parameter/tissue regeneration	Materials	References	Comments
Pore size	20–80 μm for hepatocytes ingrowth	Ceramic, collagen	[75, 76]	Although the complexity of the mechanism involved during in vitro and/or in vivo new-tissue regeneration process, optimal combination of pore size/material/tissue regeneration may be highlighted
	20–125 μm regeneration of adult mammalian skin	Collagen and condroitin sulfate	[76]	
	150–200 μm for fibroblast ingrowth	PCL, chitosan	[77, 78]	
	150–300 μm for rapid neo-vascularization	AlloDerm®, PLLA, PLGA, PCL/PLA	[74, 79]	
	200–500 μm regeneration of cartilage	Chitosan-based materials PLGA	[73, 78, 80]	
	100–500 μm regeneration of bone	Polyesters (PCL, PLA, PLGA) Calcium phosphate ceramics Metals (titanium, magnesium)	[72, 77, 81–87]	
Pore shape and direction	Aligned channels or fibers/nerve regeneration	Agarose Poly(2-hydroxyethyl methacrylate) (PHEMA) PLGA	[88–91]	Anisotropic scaffold micro-architectures are often necessaries to mimic the spatial organization and distribution of cells in 3D as well as to guide the new-tissue regeneration process
	Oriented pores/tooth regeneration	Calcium phosphate	[92]	
Pore interconnectivity	Degree of interconnection/tissue infiltration and fluids transport	Poly(propylene fumarate) PLGA Calcium phosphate	[82, 93–95]	Transport issues, 3D cell colonization and tissue in-growth would be inhibited if the pores are not well interconnected, even if the porosity of the scaffolds is high

Table 4.3 Technologies to emboss ordered microporosity pattern within 3D scaffolds

Technology	Processing parameters	Materials	References
Reverse templating	Templating nature, size, shape and concentration	PLA, PCL, PHEMA, zein, gelatin	[90, 97–101]
Gas foaming	Blowing agent composition, solubilization pressure and temperature, foaming temperature, pressure drop rate.	PLA, PMMA, PCL	[102, 103]
Thermally induced phase separation	Cooling temperature and rate, polymer concentration, solvent crystallization	PLA, PCL	[104–106]
Fiber spinning	Polymer concentration, applied voltage, electrodes distance, flow rate	Chitosan, PCL, PLA, zein, gelatin	[107–109]
Gas foaming/ reverse templating	Gas foaming and reverse templating parameters	PCL, PLA	[106, 110–112]
Phase separation/ reverse templating	Phase inversion and reverse templating parameters	PCL	[110, 113]
Fiber spinning/ reverse templating	Fiber spinning and reverse templating parameters	PCL	[114, 115]

influence the process of tissue regeneration and an optimal range of microstructural parameters of the porous network exist for any specific tissue (bone, liver, nerve, cartilage) as well as for scaffold vascularization [17, 74, 96]. Consequently, the setup of novel technologies for imprinting ordered porosity within polymeric matrices is emerging as a primary requirement in scaffold development. Several techniques have been exploited (Table 4.3) to imprint the ordered porous arrays including thermodynamic-based processing of polymeric solutions, such as gas foaming, phase separation, and freeze drying. With these techniques the pore dimensions and interconnectivity, can be finely controlled at the micron and sub-micron scale by modulating the process conditions. Each technique can be finely tuned to imprint a highly ordered porosity pattern with tuneable morphological orientation, and could be used in combination to realize 3D scaffolds with bimodal and highly oriented porosity and the desired high degree of pore interconnection [90, 97, 105]. The gas foaming process, for instance, has been proved to be extremely useful in the fabrication of highly porous 3D scaffolds capable also of sustain the release of fragile bioactive molecules such as growth factors (GFs) [116]. SFF encompass all the technologies which can manufacture objects in a layer-by-layer fashion from a three-dimensional computer-generated image of the object. SFF technology (3D printing, 3D plotting) results very powerful for the realization of structures with very complex internal architecture and high-reproducible architecture and compositional variation not feasible with traditional manufacturing methods. The versatility of SFF in internal architectural control is the main advantage of this technique, indeed it offers a unique way to control precisely matrix parameters, including size, shape, branching, geometry, and orientation [72, 117].

The advent of more precise and reliable nanotechnology tools allows to recreate the complex morphology and functionality of the ECM from a morphological perspective. Nano-fabricated and microfabricated tissue engineering scaffolds have the potential to direct cell fate as well as to regulate processes such as angiogenesis and cell migration. Both top-down and bottom-up technologies have been used to incorporate nanoscale control for tissue engineering scaffolds [118].

Top-down approaches, such as soft lithography, have greatly enhanced the possibility to finely control the microscale and nanoscale features such as pore geometry, size, distribution, and spatial geometry. Microfabricated approaches, for instance, have been successful used to engineer the microvasculature directly within tissue engineering scaffolds by micromolding biocompatible polymers such as poly(lactide-*co*-glycolide) (PLGA) and poly(glyceride sebacate) (PGS). Other approaches, such as the layer-by-layer deposition of cells and proteins using microfluidic channels, microsyringe deposition of PLGA polymer, and photopolymerization within microfluidic channels have been used to generate 3D structures with controlled geometries and properties.

Bottom-up approaches based on molecular self-assembly of small building blocks are becoming very popular in the engineering of nano-ordered scaffolds for tissue engineering. Strategies to achieve a 3D scaffold with nano-porosity, high pore interconnectivity plus outstanding biological recognition involve the use of amphiphilic peptide molecules, either in self-assembled, self-complementary structures, or by their self-assembly in nanofibers [119]. Self-assembled scaffolds can be easily functionalized, by incorporating peptide sequences that direct cell behavior directly onto the build-up molecule [120]. Synthetic polymeric nanofibers, obtained by electrospinning, can be used to make a highly porous non-woven structure comprising tiny fibers with morphological features closely resembling the fibrous structure of the ECM at nanometric resolution [89]. Electrospinning is increasingly being used to produce fibers from a wide range of polymers and the resulting scaffolds exhibit important advantages when compared with foams. First, the interconnectivity of voids available for tissue ingrowth is perfect, whereas in the case of foams, some cavities can be dispersed in the matrix and hence closed. Also, fenestration between adjacent cavities can be too small to allow cell permeation. Second, ultrathin fibers produced by electrospinning offer a surface/volume ratio which is unsurpassed among applied tissue scaffolds. This has important consequences for the availability and presentation of polymer-bound signaling molecules, and for degradation rates of biodegradable scaffolds. Finally, electrospinning offers new 3D scaffolds with double scale length scale features, through the combination of electrospun nanofibers and microfibers. Particular promising is the combination of electrospinning with other techniques, such as phase separation, to obtain different and interesting geometries. For instance, gels have been prepared from peptides which expressed isoleucine-lysinevaline-alanine-valine (IKVAV, an amino acid sequence found in laminin) and self-assembled to form nanofibers. Similar approaches have been used for a variety of tissues such as cartilage, bone, and cardiac applications, and show great promise in tissue engineering.

Reverse casting technique, which employs templating agents, can also produce an ordered array of pores within a polymer matrix. In particular, reverse casting using a highly organized polymeric network (e.g., micelles or self-assembling block copolymers), plus self-assembled nanoparticles or colloidal dispersions as the template, is a promising technique capable of producing highly ordered micro- and nano-patterned porosity networks, with an elevated degree of interconnectivity, high surface/volume ratio and tuneable tortuosity [90, 97].

Most of the technologies used to date suffer from the limitation that the scaffolds are preformed and cell have to be loaded within the interstitial space. Novel technologies to allow the scaffolds assembly in presence of the cellular components are at present being exploited [59].

4.7 Encoding Matricellular and Bioactive Cues into Scaffolds

Recent advances in micro- and nano-fabrication technologies offer the possibility to engineer scaffolds with a well-defined stereoregulated architecture providing a control of cellular spatial organization, mimicking the microarchitectural organization of cells in native tissues. Furthermore, combining material chemistry and processing technology, scaffold degradation rate can be tuned to match the rate of tissue growth in such a way that the regenerated tissue may progressively replace the scaffold [69–71]. Enhancing further the functionality of these already complex matrices by encoding in them the capability to expose an array of biological signals with an adequate dose and for a desired time frame, represents the major scientific and technological challenge in tissue engineering today.

Future generation of tissue scaffolds with extended functionality and bioactivity require an increased integration with cell and molecular biology, to identify novel design parameters and novel bioinspired design approaches. Synthetic bioinspired ECM should promote and control cell adhesion, migration and differentiation and should recruit peripheral host cells and facilitate their migration into the scaffold or guide morphogenetic processes taking place within its interstices through the fine tuning of the spatial and temporal gradients of bioactive signaling molecules factors [121, 122].

The ECM provides both bound or tethered matricellular signals and bioactive diffusible signals. Among the matricellular signals fibronectin, laminin, and vitronectin which control the maintenance and development of cell function within the tissue are the most studied. Integrin, a transmembrane protein, couples the ECM to the cytoskeleton inside the cell activating specific signaling pathways. Through this process, integrin molecules transmit information across the cell membrane and consequently are key regulators of cell adhesion and migration

[15]. The identification of small integrin binding oligopeptide sequences in the ECM opened up the possibility to conjugate a scaffold with biological cues creating synthetic ECM analogs in which their concentration and spatial distribution can be controlled. The matricellular signals may be encoded in tissue engineering scaffolds both by bulk and surface modification of biomaterials. This can be done, via chemical or physical methods, with bioactive molecules such as the native chain of ECM proteins as well as short peptide sequences which can specifically interact with cell receptors. Even though Gly-Arg-Gly-Asp-Ser (GRGDS)-based peptides feature the most widespread signal used to date as an adhesive motif, it is important to emphasize that non-RGD peptides, as well as peptidomimetics, are being examined as new insoluble signals with which to decorate scaffolds. The various effects of ligand density in 2D as well as in 3D, the nanoscale spatial organization, the co-regulation, the relevance of gradient and the role of material substrate can all provide insights into basic cell biology and so help to construct new guidelines in scaffold design.

The ECM also provides a tight control of the cellular microenvironment through a time and space orchestrated sequestration and delivery of mobile active biomolecules such as growth and morphogenic factors. Therefore, a clinically effective scaffold for tissue regeneration requires an encoded *chrono-program* of sequestration and release of molecular agents fulfilling the specific needs of the biointegrating tissue. This approach is part of the concept of *chrono-biotechnology* which may be accomplished through the integration of controlled release know-how with the aim of achieving the control in time and space over the presentation of the needed bioactive molecules. The latter act synergistically, with one another and with the flow of interstitial fluids, at pico- to nano-molar concentrations, thus underlining the necessity of tight control over dosing and localization of signaling molecule release [121–124].

To date, many attempts have been made to obtain systems integrating delivery devices and TE templates able to mimic ECM and directionally reorganize the ingrowing tissue. Some relevant results have been achieved by Mooney and co-workers [116], who developed PLGA scaffolds for the sequential release of multiple bioactive GFs by mixing free VEGF with empty and PDGF-loaded polymer particles and subsequently assembling them into a porous scaffold. More recently, a porous bi-layered PLGA scaffold to locally expose VEGF alone in one spatial region, and afterward deliver VEGF and PDGF in an adjacent region was also exploited [125]. In a similar attempt, PLA microparticles plasticized with PEG were sintered into scaffolds formed by protein-free and protein-loaded layers, thus allowing a release of different bioactive molecules restricted to specific regions within the scaffold [126]. These scaffolds may find utility in applications where GFs gradients or a region-dependent tissue growth are required.

Despite these encouraging results, important technological limitations exist. The major issue relies on the use of microspheres which are formed into scaffolds, thus altering their architecture and consequently release features. Furthermore, to engineer dynamic gradients of a signaling molecule, the detailed understanding of release kinetics at the single microsphere level is necessary.

An alternative approach to create microsphere-integrated scaffolds able to regulate both temporally and spatially GFs release kinetics may take advantage of micromanipulation-based techniques. The simple dispersion of microspheres within gel-like scaffolds is a well-established approach to achieve a temporal control over GFs release [127]. It has been recently demonstrated that through the fine tuning of microsphere formulation and scaffold properties, it is possible to realize platforms able to control the microenvironmental conditions in terms of time evolution of bioactive molecules delivery [128]. Possible developments of these findings may benefit from advances in micro- and nanotechnologies so as to engineer templates embedding microspheres releasing GFs at known release rates in a predetermined and optimized spatial distribution within the scaffold. Actually, devices acting as single point source may be micropositioned by 3D printing and soft lithography to obtain highly regulated structures able to trigger the extent, and possibly the architecture/structure of tissue formation [55, 129]. The combination of micropositioning systems and mathematical modeling describing the complex and multiple mechanisms governing the release kinetics from single microspheres within the scaffold can be of help to realize scaffolds with highly controlled architecture by computer-aided scaffold design [130].

A possible limitation of these integrated systems derives from their predefined nature. In fact, once pre-programed in vitro, they will not be able to interactively modify release kinetics according to the needs of the surrounding tissue. As underlined above, a more effective biomimicry could be obtained if a dual-reciprocity scheme could be encoded in the matrix. In this way, cells can trigger the on-demand development of ECM and, in turn, the engineered scaffold could stimulate cell behaviors through the controlled release of bioactive molecules. In order to achieve this goal, the use of bottom-up strategies based on molecular self-assembly appears very promising. Stupp and co-workers have developed a class of peptide amphiphile (PA) molecules that self-assemble into three-dimensional nanofiber networks under physiologic conditions in the presence of polyvalent metal ions [59]. While PA self-assembly entraps cells in the nanofibrillar matrix, the entrapped cells internalize the nanofibers and possibly utilize PA molecules in their metabolic pathways. The method is not limited to uniaxial alignment but can be used to guide self-assembling nanofibers around corners and in complex patterns. It is also versatile enough to be used in the alignment of other self-assembling supramolecular systems starting from solutions of small molecules [131].

It should also be mentioned that a multifunctional scaffold should not only provide a controlled administration of relevant biomacromolecules and their gradients, but also present such molecules in a suitable conformation state, mimicking ECM-GFs binding. Indeed, it has been shown that molecularly decorated materials enhance tissue formation through the modulation of the interaction between protein signaling and biomaterials appear to be fundamental to provide a better integration of the scaffold with the neo-forming tissue [132].

4.8 Conclusion

Nanotechnology can assist in the development of biomimetic, intelligent biomaterials, which are designed to positively react to changes in their immediate environment and stimulate specific regenerative events at the molecular level. Advances in the areas of fundamental matrix biology, nano-fabrication, synthetic molecular self-assembly, and printing technologies will enable the generation of materials that can provide enhanced 3D tissue context maps of molecular and structural information.

References

1. Netti PA, D'Amore A, Ronca D, Ambrosio L, Nicolais L (1996) Structure–mechanical properties relationship of natural tendons and ligaments. J Mater Sci Mater Med 7:525–530
2. Evans SL, Gregson PJ (1998) Composite technology in load-bearing orthopaedic implants. Biomaterials 19:1329–1342
3. Nicolais L (1975) Mechanics of composites. Polym Eng Sci 15:137–149
4. Ambrosio L, De Santis R, Iannace S, Netti PA, Nicolais L (1998) Viscoelastic behavior of composite ligament prostheses. J Biomed Mater Res 42:6–12
5. Apicella A, Liguori A, Masi E, Nicolais L (1995) Experimental techniques and design in composite materials. Sheffield Academic Press, Sheffield, pp 323–337
6. De Santis R, Ambrosio L, Di Palma L, Apicella A, Nicolais L (2004) Continuous fiber reinforced polymer as bone model: a synthetic jaw. Compos Sci Technol 64:861–871
7. Van Rietbergen B, Huiskes R, Weinans H, Sumner DR, Turner TM, Galante JO (1993) The mechanism of bone remodeling and resorption around press-fitted THA stems. J Biomech 26:369–382
8. Apicella A, Masi E, Nicolais L, Zarone F, De Rosa N, Valletta G (1998) A finite-element model study of occlusal schemes in full-arch implant restoration. J Mater Sci Mater Med 8:191–196
9. Mihalko WM, Beaudoin AJ, Cardea JA, Krause WR (1992) Finite-element modelling of femoral shaft fracture fixation techniques post total hip arthroplasty. J Biomech 25:469–476
10. Kuiper JH, Huiskes R (1997) The predictive value of stress shielding for quantification of adaptive bone resorption around hip replacement. J Biomech Eng 119:228–231
11. Huiskes R, Janssen JD, Slooff TJ (1981) A detailed comparison of experimental and theoretical stress-analyses of a human femur. In: Cowin SC (ed) Mechanical properties of bone. ASME, New York, pp 211–234
12. McNamara BP, Cristofolini L, Toni A, Taylor D (1997) Relationship between bone-prosthesis bonding and load transfer in total hip reconstruction. J Biomech 6:621–630
13. De Santis R, Prisco D, Apicella A, Ambrosio L, Rengo S, Nicolais L (2000) Carbon fiber post adhesion to resin luting cement in the restoration of endodontically treated teeth. J Mater Sci Mater Med 4:201–206
14. Kong HJ, Mooney DJ (2007) Microenvironmental regulation of biomacromolecular therapies. Nat Rev Drug Discov 6:455–463
15. Kleinman HK, Philip D, Hoffman MP (2003) The role of the extracellular matrix in morphogenesis. Curr Opin Biotech 14:526–532
16. Lutolf MP, Hubbell JA (2005) Synthetic biomaterials as instructive extracellular microenvironments for morphogenesis in tissue engineering. Nat Biotechnol 23:47–55
17. O'Briena FJ, Harley BA, Yannas IV, Gibsona LJ (2005) The effect of pore size on cell adhesion in collagen–GAG scaffolds. Biomaterials 26:433–441

18. Fung YC (1993) Biomechanics:mechanical properties of living tissues. Springer-Verlag, New York
19. Rho JY, Kuhn-Spearing L, Zioupos P (1998) Mechanical properties and the hierarchical structure of bone. Med Eng Phys 2:92–102
20. De Santis R, Mollica F, Zarone F, Ambrosio L, Nicolais L (2007) Biomechanical effects of titanium implants with full arch bridge rehabilitation on a synthetic model of the human jaw. Acta Biomater 3:121–126
21. Rho JY, Ashman RB, Turner CH (1993) Young's modulus of trabecular and cortical bone materials: ultrasonic and microtensile measurements. J Biomech 2:111–119
22. Bonfield W, Grynpas MG (1997) Anisotropy of the Young's modulus of bone. Nature 270:453–454
23. Weiner S, Wagner HD (1998) The material bone: structure–mechanical function relations. Annu Rev Mater Sci 28:271–298
24. Ziouposet P, Currey JD, Hamer AJ (1999) The role of collagen in the declining mechanical properties of aging human cortical bone. J Biomed Mater Res 45:108–116
25. Silver FH, Seehra GP, Freeman JW, DeVore D (2001) Viscoelastic properties of young and old human dermis: a proposed molecular mechanism for elastic energy storage in collagen and elastin. J Appl Polym Sci 79:134–142
26. Kokubo T, Kim HM, Kawashita M (2003) Novel bioactive materials with different mechanical properties. Biomaterials 24:2161–2175
27. Ambrosio L, Caprino G, Nicolais L, Nicodemo L, Huang SJ, Guida G, Ronca D (1987) Composite materials for bone fractures fixation. In: Marshall IH (ed) Composite structures. Elsevier Applied Science, London
28. Alexander H (1997) Composites. In: Ratner BD, Hofman AS, Schoen FJ, Lemons JE (eds) Biomaterial science. Academic Press, San Diego
29. Chang YFK, Goodman S (1998) Composite hip prosthesis design. II Simulation. J Biomed Mater Res 39:102–119
30. Akay M, Aslan N (1995) An estimation of fatigue life for a carbon fibre/poly ether ether ketone hip joint prosthesis. Proc Inst Mech Eng H 229:93–103
31. Merolli A, Perrone V, Tranquilli Leali P, Ambrosio L, De Santis R, Nicolais L, Gabbi G (1999) Response to polyetherimide based composite materials implanted in muscle and in bone. J Mater Sci Mater Med 10:265–268
32. De Santis R, Ambrosio L, Nicolais L (2000) Polymer based composite hip prostheses. J Inorg Biochem 79:97–102
33. Wilke HJ, Seiz RS, Bombelli M, Claes L, Durselen L (1994) Biomechanical and histomorphological investigations on a isoelastic prosthesis. J Mater Sci Mater Med 5:384–386
34. Chang FK, Perez JL (1990) Stiffness and strength tailoring of a hip prosthesis made of advanced composite materials. J Biomed Mater Res 24:873–899
35. Kuiper JH, Huiskes R (1997) Mathematical optimization elastic properties: application to cementless hip stem design. J Biomech Eng T ASME 119:166–174
36. De Santis R, Sarracino F, Mollica F, Netti PA, Ambrosio L, Nicolais L (2004) Continuous fiber reinforced polymers as connective tissue replacement. Compos Sci Technol 64:861–878
37. De Santis R, Mollica F, Ambrosio L, Nicolais L (2005) An experimental and theoretical composite model of the human mandible. J Mater Sci Mater Med 16:1191–1197
38. Ambrosio L, Netti PA, Iannace S, Huang SJ, Nicolais L (1996) Composite hydrogels for intervertebral disc prostheses. J Mater Sci Mater Med 7:251–254
39. Ambrosio L, De Santis R, Nicolais L (1998) Composite hydrogels for implants. Proc Inst Mech Eng H 212:93–99
40. Gloria A, Causa F, De Santis R, Netti PA, Ambrosio L (2007) Dynamic-mechanical properties of a novel composite intervertebral disc. J Mater Sci Mater Med 18:2159–2165
41. Manto L, De Santis R, Carrillo G, Ambrosio G, Ambrosio L, Nicolais L (2005) Novel composite intervertebral disc cage for spine fusion. J Bone Joint Surg Br 87-B:68-a

42. Flahiff CM, Blackwell AS, Hollis JM, Feldman DS (1996) Analysis of a biodegradable composite for bone healing. J Biomed Mater Res 32:419–424
43. Dauner M, Planck H, Caramano L, Missirlis Y, Panagiotopoulos E (1998) Resorbable continuous-fibre reinforce polymers for osteosynthesis. J Mater Sci Mater Med 9:173–179
44. Causa F, Sarracino F, De Santis R, Netti PA, Ambrosio L, Nicolais L (2006) Basic structural parameters for the design of composite structures as ligament augmentation devices. J Appl Biomater Biomech 4:21–30
45. Roy TD, Simon JL, Ricci JL, Rekow ED, Thompson VP, Russell Parsons J (2003) Performance of degradable composite bone repair products made via three-dimensional fabrication techniques. J Biomed Mater Res 66A:283–291
46. Giordano C, Sanginario V, Ambrosio L, Di Silvio L, Santin M (2006) Chemical–physical characterization and in vitro preliminary biological assessment of hyaluronic acid benzyl ester-hydroxyapatite composite. J Biomater Appl 20:237–253
47. Schmitt M, Weiss P, Bourges X, Amador Del Valle G, Daculsi G (2002) Crystallization at the polymer/calcium–phosphate interface in a sterilized injectable bone substitute IBS. Biomaterials 23:2789–2794
48. Navarro M, del Valle S, Martinez S, Zeppetelli S, Ambrosio L, Planell JA, Ginebra MP (2004) New macroporous calcium phosphate glass ceramic for guided bone regeneration. Biomaterials 25:4233–4241
49. Lin FH, Chen TM, Lin CP, Lee CJ (1999) The merit of sintered PDLLA/TCP composites in management of bone fracture internal fixation. Artif Organs 23:186–194
50. Mikos AG, Herring SW, Ochareon P, Elisseeff J, Lu HH, Kandel R, Schoen FJ, Toner M, Mooney D, Atala A, Van Dyke ME, Kaplan D, Vunjak-Novakovic G (2006) Engineering complex tissues. Tissue Eng 12:3307–3339
51. Matsumoto T, Mooney DJ (2006) Cell instructive polymers. Adv Biochem Eng Biotechnol 102:113–137
52. Hutmacher DW (2001) Scaffold design and fabrication technologies for engineering tissues-state of the art and future perspectives. J Biomater Sci Polym Ed 12:107–124
53. Tabata Y (2005) Significance of release technology in tissue engineering. Drug Discov Today 10:1639–1646
54. Sachlos E, Czernuszka JT (2003) Making tissue engineering scaffolds work. Review: the application of solid freeform fabrication technology to the production of tissue engineering scaffolds. Eur Cell Mater 5:29–40
55. Sun W, Darling A, Starly B, Nam J (2004) Computer-aided tissue engineering: overview, scope and challenges. Biotechnol Appl Biochem 39:29–47
56. Boland T, Xu T, Damon B, Cui X (2006) Application of inkjet printing to tissue engineering. Biotechnol J 1:910–917
57. Teo WE, He W, Ramakrishna S (2006) Electrospun scaffold tailored for tissue-specific extracellular matrix. Biotechnol J 1:918–929
58. Guarino V, Causa F, Ambrosio L (2007) Bioactive scaffolds for bone and ligament tissue. Expert Rev Med Devices 4:405–418
59. Beniash E, Hartgerink JD, Storrie H, Stendahl JC, Stupp SI (2005) Self-assembling peptide amphiphile nanofiber matrices for cell entrapment. Acta Biomater 1:387–397
60. Day RM, Boccaccini AR, Maquet V, Shurey S, Forbes A, Gabe SM, Jerome R (2004) In vivo characterisation of a novel bioresorbable poly(lactide-*co*-glycolide) tubular foam scaffold for tissue engineering applications. J Mater Sci Mater Med 15:729–734
61. Ng KW, Hutmacher DW, Schantz JT, Ng CS, Too HP, Lim TC, Phan TT, Teoh SH (2001) Evaluation of ultra-thin poly(epsilon-caprolactone) films for tissue-engineered skin. Tissue Eng 7:441–455
62. Lutolf MP, Lauer-Fields JL, Schmoekel HG, Metters AT, Weber FE, Fields GB, Hubbell JA (2003) Synthetic matrix metalloproteinase-sensitive hydrogels for the conduction of tissue regeneration: engineering cell-invasion characteristics. Proc Natl Acad Sci USA 100:5413–5418

63. Holland TA, Tabata Y, Mikos AG (2005) Dual growth factor delivery from degradable oligo (poly(ethylene glycol) fumarate) hydrogel scaffolds for cartilage tissue engineering. J Control Release 101:111–125
64. Paul W, Sharma CP (2004) Ceramic drug delivery: a perspective. J Biomater Appl 17:253–264
65. LeGeros RZ (2002) Properties of osteoconductive biomaterials: calcium phosphates. Clin Orthop Relat Res 395:81–98
66. Horn EM, Beaumont M, Shu XZ, Harvey A, Prestwich GD, Horn KM, Gibson AR, Preul MC, Panitch A (2007) Influence of cross-linked hyaluronic acid hydrogels on neurite outgrowth and recovery from spinal cord injury. J Neurosurg Spine 6:133–140
67. Duflo S, Thibeault SL, Li W, Shu XZ, Prestwich GD (2006) Vocal fold tissue repair in vivo using a synthetic extracellular matrix. Tissue Eng 12:2171–2180
68. Brun P, Abatangelo G, Radice M, Zacchi V, Guidolin D, Daga GD, Cortivo R (1999) Chondrocyte aggregation and reorganization into three-dimensional scaffolds. J Biomed Mater Res 46:337–346
69. Langer R, Tirrell DA (2004) Designing materials for biology and medicine. Nature 428:487–492
70. Malafaya PB, Silva GA, Reis RL (2007) Natural-origin polymers as carriers and scaffolds for biomolecules and cell delivery in tissue engineering applications. Adv Drug Deliv Rev 59:207–233
71. Sokolsky-Papkov M, Agashi K, Olaye A, Shakesheff K, Domb AJ (2007) Polymer carriers for drug delivery in tissue engineering. Adv Drug Deliv Rev 59:187–206
72. Karageorgiou V, Kaplan D (2005) Porosity of 3D biomaterial scaffolds and osteogenesis. Biomaterials 26:5474–5491
73. Yamane S, Iwasaki N, Kasahara Y, Harada K, Majima T, Monde K, Nishimura S, Minami A (2007) Effect of pore size on in vitro cartilage formation using chitosan-based hyaluronic acid hybrid polymer fibers. J Biomed Mater Res 81:586–593
74. Rouwkema J, Rivron NC, van Blitterswijk CA (2005) Vascularization in tissue engineering. Trends Biotechnol 26:434–441
75. Ranucci CS, Kumar A, Batra SP, Moghe PV (2000) Control of hepatocyte function on collagen foams: sizing matrix pores toward selective induction of 2-D and 3-D cellular morphogenesis. Biomaterials 21:783–793
76. Yang S, Leong K, Du Z, Chua C (2001) The design of scaffolds for use in tissue engineering. Part I. Traditional factors. Tissue Eng 7:679–689
77. Oh SH, Park IK, Kim JM, Lee JH (2007) In vitro and in vivo characteristics of PCL scaffolds with pore size gradient fabricated by a centrifugation method. Biomaterials 28:1664–1671
78. Lim SM, Oh SH, Park IK, Lee JH (2007) Investigation of pore size effect on cell compatibility using pore size gradient chitosan scaffold. Key Eng Mater 342:285–288
79. Beckstead BL, Pana S, Bhrany AD, Bratt-Leal AM, Ratner BD, Giachelli CM (2005) Esophageal epithelial cell interaction with synthetic and natural scaffolds for tissue engineering. Biomaterials 26:6217–6228
80. Fan H, Hu Y, Zhang C, Li X, Lv R, Qin L, Zhu R (2006) Cartilage regeneration using mesenchymal stem cells and a PLGA-gelatin/chondroitin/hyaluronate hybrid scaffold. Biomaterials 27:4573–4580
81. Petrie Aronin CE, Sadik KW, Lay AL, Rion DB, Tholpady SS, Ogle RC, Botchwey EA (2009) Comparative effects of scaffold pore size, pore volume, and total void volume on cranial bone healing patterns using microsphere-based scaffolds. J Biomed Mater Res A 89:632–641
82. Otsuki B, Takemoto M, Fujibayashi S, Neo M, Kokubo T, Nakamura T (2006) Pore throat size and connectivity determine bone and tissue ingrowth into porous implants: three-dimensional micro-CT based structural analyses of porous bioactive titanium implants. Biomaterials 27:5892–5900

83. Fujibayashi S, Neo M, Kim HM, Kokubo T, Nakamura T (2004) Osteoinduction of porous bioactive titanium metal. Biomaterials 25:443–450
84. Staiger MP, Pietak AM, Huadmai J, Dias G (2006) Magnesium and its alloys as orthopedic biomaterials: a review. Biomaterials 27:1728–1734
85. Yoshikawa H, Myoui A (2005) Bone tissue engineering with porous hydroxyapatite ceramics. J Artif Organs 8:131–136
86. Savarino L, Baldini N, Greco M, Capitani O, Pinna S, Valentini S, Lombardo B, Esposito MT, Pastore L, Ambrosio L, Battista S, Causa F, Zeppetelli S, Guarino V, Netti PA (2007) The performance of poly-e-caprolactone scaffolds in a rabbit femur model with and without autologous stromal cells and BMP4. Biomaterials 28:3101–3109
87. Montjovent MO, Mark S, Mathieu L, Scaletta C, Scherberich A, Delabarde C, Zambelli PY, Bourban PE, Applegate LA, Pioletti DP (2007) Human fetal bone cells associated with ceramic reinforced PLA scaffolds for tissue engineering. Bone 42:554–564
88. Stokols S, Tuszynski MH (2004) The fabrication and characterization of linearly oriented nerve guidance scaffolds for spinal cord injury. Biomaterials 25:5839–5846
89. Yang F, Murugan R, Wang S, Ramakrishna S (2005) Electrospinning of nano/micro scale poly(L-lactic acid) aligned fibers and their potential in neural tissue engineering. Biomaterials 26:2603–2610
90. Yu TT, Shoichet MS (2005) Guided cell adhesion and outgrowth in peptide-modified channels for neural tissue engineering. Biomaterials 26:1507–1514
91. Moore MJ, Friedman JA, Lewellyn EB, Mantila SM, Krych AJ, Ameenuddin S, Knight AM, Lu L, Currier BL, Spinner RJ, Marsh RW, Windebank AJ, Yaszemski MJ (2006) Multiple-channel scaffolds to promote spinal cord axon regeneration. Biomaterials 27:419–429
92. Du C, Moradian-Oldak J (2006) Tooth regeneration: challenges and opportunities for biomedical material research. Biomed Mater 1:R10–R17
93. Karande TS, Ong JL, Agrawal CM (2004) Diffusion in musculoskeletal tissue engineering scaffolds: design issues related to porosity, permeability, architecture, and nutrient mixing. Ann Biomed Eng 32:1728–1743
94. Moore MJ, Jabbari E, Ritman EL, Lu L, Currier BL, Windebank AJ, Yaszemski MJ (2004) Quantitative analysis of interconnectivity of porous biodegradable scaffolds with micro-computed tomography. J Biomed Mater Res 71:258–267
95. Leong KF, Cheah CM, Chua CK (2003) Solid freeform fabrication of three-dimensional scaffolds for engineering replacement tissues and organs. Biomaterials 24:2363–2378
96. Marshall AJ, Irvin CA, Barker T, Sage EH, Hauch KD, Ratner BD (2004) Biomaterials with tightly controlled pore size that promote vascular in-growth. ACS Polym Prepr 45:100–101
97. Mikos AG, Sarakinos G, Leite SM, Vacanti JP, Langer R (1993) Laminated three-dimensional biodegradable foams for use in tissue engineering. Biomaterials 14:323–330
98. Hou Q, Grijpma DW, Feijen J (2002) Preparation of porous poly(ε-caprolactone) structures. Macromol Rapid Commun 23:247–252
99. Gong S, Wang H, Sun Q, Xue S, Wang J (2006) Mechanical properties and in vitro biocompatibility of porous zein scaffolds. Biomaterials 27:3793–3799
100. Lee SB, Kim YH, Chong MS, Hong SH, Lee YM (2005) Study of gelatin-containing artificial skin V: fabrication of gelatin scaffolds using a salt-leaching method. Biomaterials 26:1961–1968
101. Yuan Z, Favis BD (2006) Macroporous poly(L-lactide) of controlled pore size derived from the annealing of co-continuous polystyrene/poly(L-lactide) blends. Biomaterials 25:2161–2170
102. Barry JJ, Silva MM, Popov VK, Shakesheff KM, Howdle SM (2006) Supercritical carbon dioxide: putting the fizz into biomaterials. Philos Trans R Soc A 364:249–261
103. Luetzow K, Klein F, Weigel T, Apostel R, Weiss A, Lendlein A (2007) Formation of poly(e-caprolactone) scaffolds loaded with small molecules by integrated processes. J Biomech 40:S80–S88

104. Nam YS, Park TG (1999) Porous biodegradable polymeric scaffolds prepared by thermally induced phase separation. J Biomed Mater Res 47:8–17
105. Liu X, Ma PX (2004) Polymeric scaffolds for bone tissue engineering. Ann Biomed Eng 32:477–486
106. Guarino V, Causa F, Salerno A, Ambrosio L, Netti PA (2008) Design and manufacture of micro-porous polymeric materials with hierarchal complex structure for biomedical application. Mater Sci Tech Ser 24:1111–1117
107. Min BM, Lee SW, Lim JN, You Y, Lee TS, Kang PH, Park WH (2004) Chitin and chitosan nanofibers: electrospinning of chitin and deacetylation of chitin nanofibers. Polymer 45:7137–7142
108. Jiang H, Zhao P, Zhu K (2007) Fabrication and characterization of zein-based nanofibrous scaffolds by an electrospinning method. Macromol Biosci 7:517–525
109. Subbiah T, Bhat GS, Tock RW, Parameswaran S, Ramkumar SS (2005) Electrospinning of nanofibers. J Appl Polym Sci 96:557–569
110. Salerno A, Oliviero M, Di Maio E, Iannace S, Netti PA (2007) Design and preparation of m-bimodal porous scaffold for tissue engineering. J Appl Polym Sci 106:3335–3342
111. Salerno A, Iannace S, Netti PA (2008) Open-pore biodegradable foams prepared via gas foaming and microparticulate templating. Macromol Biosci 8:655–664
112. Harris DL, Kim B, Mooney DJ (1998) Open pore biodegradable matrices formed with gas foaming. J Biomed Mater Res 42:396–402
113. Guarino V, Causa F, Netti PA, Ciapetti G, Pagani S, Martini D, Baldini N, Ambrosio L (2008) The role of hydroxyapatite as solid signal on performance of PCL porous scaffolds for bone tissue regeneration. J Biomed Mater Res A 86:548–557
114. Nam J, Huang Y, Agarwal S, Lannutti J (2007) Improved cellular infiltration in electrospun fiber via engineered porosity. Tissue Eng 13:2249–2257
115. Baker BM, Gee AO, Metter RB, Nathan AS, Marklein RA, Burdick JA, Mauck RL (2008) The potential to improve cell infiltration in composite fiber-aligned electrospun scaffolds by the selective removal of sacrificial fibers. Biomaterials 29:2348–2358
116. Richardson TP, Peters MC, Ennett AB, Mooney DJ (2001) Polymeric system for dual growth factor delivery. Nat Biotechnol 19:1029–1034
117. Moroni L, Hendriks JA, Schotel R, de Wijn JR, van Blitterswijk CA (2007) Design of biphasic polymeric 3-dimensional fiber deposited scaffolds for cartilage tissue engineering applications. Tissue Eng 13:361–371
118. Whitesides GM (2006) The origins and the future of microfluidics. Nature 442:368–373
119. Whitesides GM, Boncheva M (2002) Supramolecular chemistry and self-assembly special feature: beyond molecules: self-assembly of mesoscopic and macroscopic components. Proc Natl Acad Sci USA 99:4769–4774
120. Zhang S (2003) Fabrication of novel biomaterials through molecular self-assembly. Nat Biotechnol 21:1171–1178
121. Silva EA, Mooney DJ (2004) Synthetic extracellular matrices for tissue engineering and regeneration. Curr Top Dev Biol 64:181–205
122. Leach JK (2006) Multifunctional cell-instructive materials for tissue regeneration. Regen Med 1:447–455
123. Boontheekul T, Mooney DJ (2003) Protein-based signaling systems in tissue engineering. Curr Opin Biotechnol 14:559–565
124. Saltzman WM, Olbricht WL (2002) Building drug delivery into tissue engineering. Nat Rev Drug Discov 1:177–186
125. Chen RR, Silva EA, Yuen WW, Mooney DJ (2007) Spatio-temporal VEGF and PDGF delivery patterns blood vessel formation and maturation. Pharm Res 24:258–264
126. Suciati T, Howard D, Barry J, Everitt NM, Shakesheff KM, Rose FR (2006) Zonal release of proteins within tissue engineering scaffolds. J Mater Sci Mater Med 17:1049–1056
127. Ungaro F, Biondi M, Indolfi L, De Rosa G, La Rotonda MI, Quaglia F, Netti PA (2005) Bioactivated polymer scaffolds for tissue engineering. In: Ashammakai N, Rice RL, Sun W (eds) Topics in tissue engineering. http://www.oulu.fi/spareparts/ebook_topics_in_t_e_vol2/index.html

128. Ungaro F, Biondi M, D'Angelo I, Indolfi L, Quaglia F, Netti PA, La Rotonda MI (2006) Microsphere-integrated collagen scaffolds for tissue engineering: effect of microsphere formulation and scaffold properties on protein release kinetics. J Control Release 113:128–136
129. Whitesides GM, Ostuni E, Takayama S, Jiang X, Ingber DE (2001) Soft lithography in biology and biochemistry. Annu Rev Biomed Eng 3:335–373
130. Hutmacher DW, Sittinger M, Risbud MV (2004) Scaffold-based tissue engineering: rationale for computer-aided design and solid free-form fabrication systems. Trends Biotechnol 22:354–362
131. Hung AM, Stupp SI (2007) Simultaneous self-assembly, orientation, and patterning of peptide-amphiphile nanofibers by soft lithography. Nano Lett 7:1165–1171
132. Wang DA, Varghese S, Sharma B, Strehin I, Fermanian S, Gorham J, Fairbrother DH, Cascio B, Elisseeff JH (2007) Multifunctional chondroitin sulphate for cartilage tissue-biomaterial integration. Nat Mater 6:385–392

Chapter 5
Textile-Reinforced Mortars (TRM)

A New Generation of Composite Materials as Alternative to Fibre-reinforced Polymers (FRP) for Strengthening and Seismic Retrofitting of Structures

Thanasis Triantafillou

5.1 Introduction and Background

The increasing popularity of fibre-reinforced polymers (FRP) as a means of strengthening and seismic retrofitting of existing structures derives from numerous attractive features of these materials such as: high specific strength (i.e., strength to weight ratio), corrosion resistance, ease and speed of application and minimal change of cross-section dimensions. Despite these well-established advantages over other methods, the FRP strengthening technique entails a few drawbacks, which are mainly attributed to the organic resins used to bind and impregnate the fibres. The following list comprises some of these drawbacks: (a) poor behaviour at temperatures above the glass transition temperature; (b) relatively high cost of epoxy resins; (c) non-applicability on damp surfaces or at low temperatures; (d) lack of vapour permeability; (e) incompatibility of resins and substrate materials; (f) difficulty to conduct post-earthquake damage assessment beneath (undamaged) FRP jackets.

The replacement of organic binders with inorganic ones, e.g. cement-based polymer-modified mortars, would seem as the logical course of action, targeting at the alleviation of all resin-related problems. Nevertheless, the substitution of FRP with fibre-reinforced mortars (FRM) would be inhibited by the relatively poor bond conditions in the resulting cementitious composite as, due to the granularity of the mortar, penetration and impregnation of fibre sheets is very difficult to achieve. Enhanced fibre-matrix interactions could be achieved when continuous fibre sheets are replaced by textiles, resulting in a new generation of materials, which may be called textile-reinforced mortars (TRM), and may be

T. Triantafillou (✉)
Department of Civil Engineering, University of Patras, 26500 Patras, Greece
e-mail: ttriant@upatras.gr

L. Nicolais et al. (eds.), *Composite Materials*,
DOI: 10.1007/978-0-85729-166-0_5,

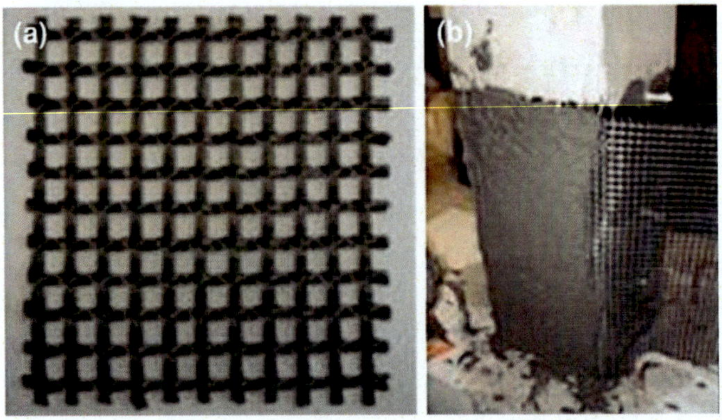

Fig. 5.1 **a** Two-directional carbon fibre-based textile. **b** Application at the base of reinforced concrete column

thought of as an alternative to FRP in the field of strengthening and seismic retrofitting.

Textiles comprise fabric meshes made of long woven, knitted or even unwoven fibre rovings in at least two (typically orthogonal) directions (Fig. 5.1). The quantity and the spacing of rovings in each direction can be independently controlled, thus affecting the mechanical characteristics of the textile and the degree of penetration of the mortar matrix through the mesh openings. The latter is a measure of the composite action achieved for the mortar-grid structure through mechanical interlock. For the polymer-modified cementitious matrix of externally applied TRM overlays used for strengthening purposes, the following requirements should be met: no shrinkage; high workability (application should be possible using a trowel); high viscosity (application should not be problematic on vertical or overhead surfaces); low rate of workability loss (application of each mortar layer should be possible while the previous one is still in a fresh state); and sufficient shear (hence, tensile) strength, in order to avoid premature debonding. In case E-glass fibre textiles are used, the cement-based matrix should be of low alkalinity.

In this chapter, the author reviews experimental studies which have provided fundamental knowledge on the use of TRM jackets: to provide confinement in plain and reinforced concrete (RC); to increase the resistance of RC members in shear and flexure; to increase the deformation capacity of old-type RC columns subjected to simulated seismic loading; and to increase the strength and deformation capacity of masonry walls subjected to out-of-plane or in-plane loading. In all cases, the effectiveness of TRM systems is quantified through comparison with equivalent FRP ones. Based on the results it is concluded that TRM jacketing is an extremely promising new technique, which will enjoy the attention of the research community and will be employed in numerous applications in the next decades.

5.2 Confinement of Axially Loaded Concrete

First we study experimentally the effectiveness of TRM versus FRP jackets as a means of confining unreinforced or reinforced concrete members subjected to concentric compression. The test plan included the following groups of specimens: (i) unreinforced cylindrical specimens with diameter 150 mm and height 300 mm (Series A and B); (ii) short column-type prisms of both reinforced and unreinforced concrete, with rectangular cross-section 200 × 200 mm and height 375 mm (Series D). Each specimen series was cast using the same ready-mix concrete batch (but slightly different from series to series, in terms of water to cement ratio). The steel used for both longitudinal and transverse reinforcement in Series D specimens (see configurations in Fig. 5.2) had an average yield stress equal to 560 MPa. The four corners of all rectangular prisms were rounded at a radius equal to 25 mm.

All specimens received textile sheets as externally bonded reinforcement, except for the Series D specimens, in which the epoxy resin-impregnated jackets comprised of unidirectional fabrics. All confining systems were applied 'as usual', that is with a single textile (or fabric) sheet wrapped around each specimen until the desired number of layers was achieved. The bonding agent was either epoxy resin or polymer-modified cement mortar, applied to the concrete surface, in between all layers and on top of the last layer. Application of the mortars was made in approximately 2 mm thick layers with a smooth metal trowel.

Specimens are given the notation Y_XN, where: Y denotes the series designation (A, B and D); X denotes the type of jacket [C for the unjacketed/control specimens, MI for Series A or B specimens with polymer-modified mortar type I jackets and MII for Series A or B specimens with polymer-modified mortar type II jackets (mortar I being of lower strength than mortar II), M for RC specimens with mortar-based jackets (mortar quality in this case being different from mortars MI and MII] and R for resin-based jackets (FRP); N denotes the number of layers.

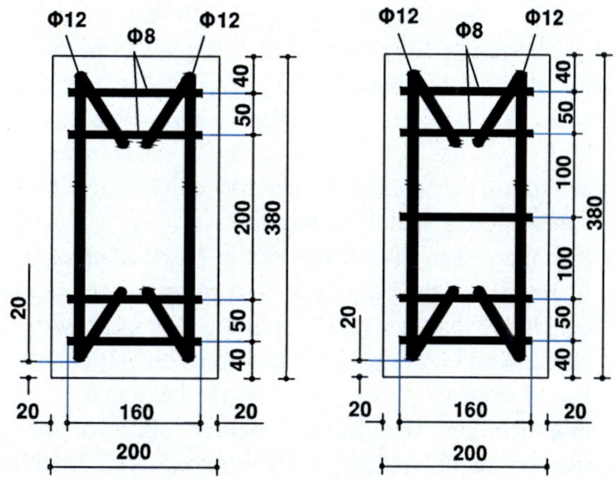

Fig. 5.2 Reinforcement configurations for specimens in Series D (dimensions in mm)

Finally, for Series D specimens only, XN is followed by the subscript Z denoting the spacing of transverse reinforcement (S200 and S100 for 200 and 100 mm spacing, respectively, U for unreinforced specimens). For plain concrete specimens, the one of Series A were used in order to investigate the effect of polymer-modified mortar quality, whereas the one of Series B were used to investigate the use of mortar versus resin. Series D specimens were used to investigate jacket–reinforcement interactions, namely the delay of rebar buckling.

Two different commercial unwoven textiles with equal quantity of high-strength carbon fibre rovings in two orthogonal directions were used. The mass of fibres in the textile used for all specimens of Series A and B (Tex1) was 168 g/m^2 and the nominal thickness of each layer (corresponding to the equivalent smeared distribution of fibres) was 0.047 mm. The corresponding values in the textile used in Series D receiving polymer-modified cementitious binder were double (in this case, i.e. in Tex2, the rovings were impregnated with a low strength polymer). The fabric used for specimens of Series D receiving epoxy resin had a unit mass of 300 g/m^2 and a nominal thickness of 0.17 mm. The guaranteed tensile strength of the fibre sheets in each direction was 3350 MPa for Tex1, 3545 MPa for Tex2 (when the nominal thickness is used) and 3790 MPa for the fabric; the elastic modulus for all carbon fibre materials ranged between 225 and 230 GPa. Mortars I and II were commercial dry polymer-modified inorganic binders containing fine cement and different fractions of polymers. The 28 day compressive and flexural strength was 8.56 and 3.28 MPa, respectively, for Mortar I; and 30.61 and 4.24 MPa, respectively, for Mortar II. The mortar used in Series D specimens had a 28 day compressive and flexural strength equal to 22.13 and 6.80 MPa, respectively.

The response of all specimens in uniaxial compression was obtained through monotonically applied loading in displacement control. Loads were measured from a load cell and displacements were obtained using external displacement transducers. From the applied load and average displacement measurements the stress–strain curves were obtained for each test (Fig. 5.3). All stress–strain plots for TRM- and FRP-confined RC specimens are characterized by an ascending branch, which nearly coincides with that for unconfined concrete, followed by a second nearly linear one, which drops at a point where the jacket ruptured due to longitudinal bar buckling at specimens' corners. The peak load of FRP-confined specimens exhibited an explosive type of failure which was not preceded by any kind of visible jacket damage, due to the release of a large amount of strain energy stored in the specimen. On the contrary, prior to strength loss, TRM jackets experienced gradual fracture and a post-peak behaviour that was distinctively more compliant than that of their resin-based counterparts.

Based on the response of confined specimens made of plain concrete, it is concluded that: (a) TRM confining jackets provide substantial gain in compressive strength and deformation capacity. This gain is higher as the number of confining layers increases and depends on the tensile strength of the polymer-modified mortar, which determines whether failure of the jacket will occur due to fibre fracture or debonding. (b) Compared with their resin-impregnated counterparts

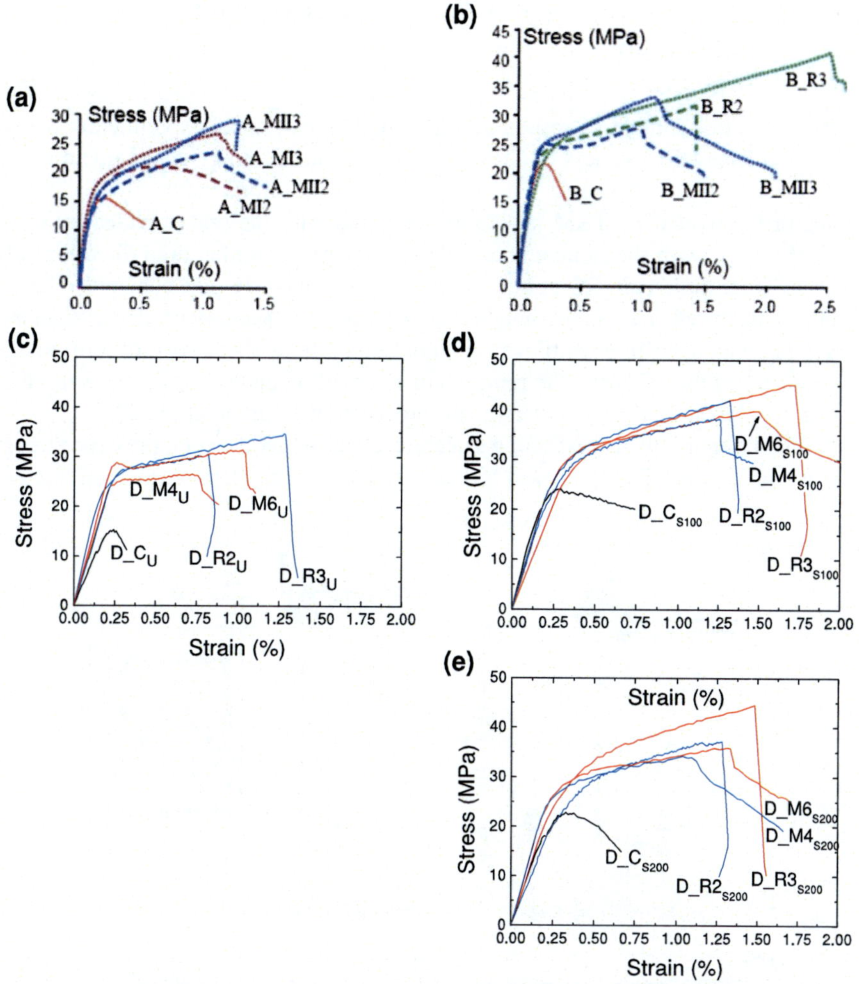

Fig. 5.3 Typical stress–strain curves for (a)–(b) series A and B specimens (plain concrete cylinders) and (c)–(e) series D specimens (plain and reinforced concrete columns with rectangular cross-sections)

(FRP), TRM jackets may result in reduced effectiveness, depending on the type of mortar. (c) Failure of mortar-impregnated textile jackets is less abrupt compared to that of their resin-impregnated counterparts, due to the slowly progressing fracture of individual fibre bundles. A more detailed analysis of the results as well as some modelling aspects of TRM-confined concrete may be found in Triantafillou et al. [1]. Generally, similar conclusions apply for the case of RC specimens; TRM jackets seem to be slightly less effective in terms of both strength increase and deformation capacity by approximately 10%.

5.3 Seismic Retrofitting of RC Columns through Confinement

In this section indicative results are presented as part of an experimental investigation of the effectiveness of TRM jacketing in plastic hinge confinement of old-type RC columns designed with poorly detailed reinforcement. The increase in ductility provided by TRM jackets is compared with the one provided by equivalent (that is with the same amount of fibres in the circumferential direction) FRP ones. Three full-scale RC columns were cast using ready-mix concrete. The columns measured 1.80 m in height and had a cross-section of 250 × 250 mm. Testing was done in a cantilever configuration with a shear span of 1.60 m. The geometry of the columns, the reinforcement detailing and the general set-up of the test are shown in Fig. 5.4. Details are provided in Bournas et al. [2].

The columns were cast using concrete of mean 28 day compressive strength equal to 25 MPa. The steel used for both longitudinal and transverse reinforcement

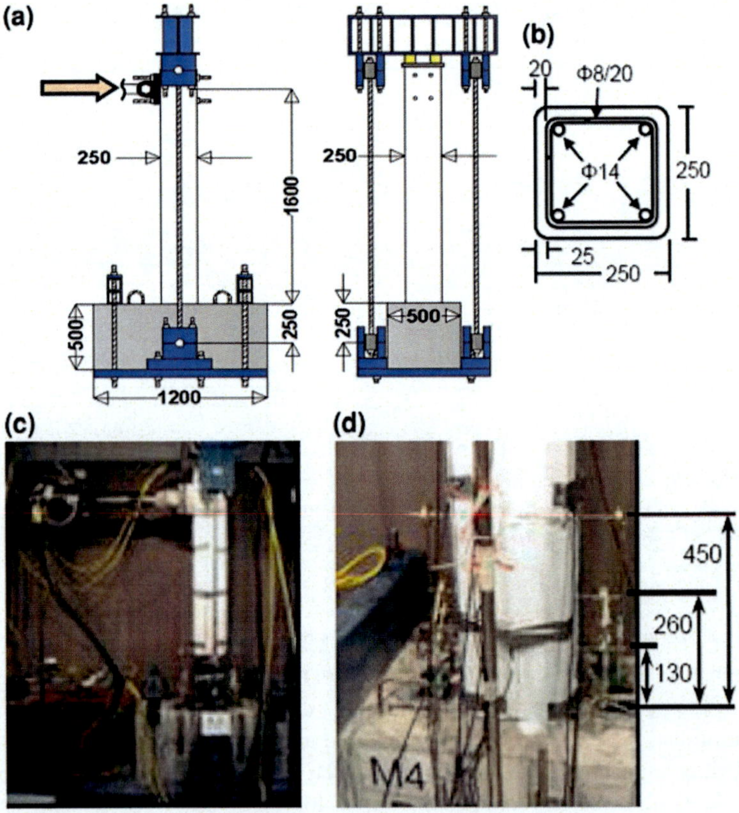

Fig. 5.4 **a** Geometry of the columns. **b** Details of cross-section. **c** General set-up of the test. **d** Position of displacement transducers (all dimensions in mm)

(both smooth) had an average yield stress equal to 372 MPa. Special attention was given to the appropriate anchoring of longitudinal reinforcement into the specimens' footings in order to minimize slippage. One column was unstrengthened (control specimen), another one received a four-layer TRM jacket in the plastic hinge region (jacket height being equal to 430 mm, accounting for the calculated height of the plastic hinge) and a third column was jacketed with two-layers of resin-impregnated carbon fibre fabric (FRP). The materials used for jacketing were identical to the ones used for strengthening specimens of Series C in the previously described experimental investigation. The columns were subjected to lateral cyclic loading (successive cycles progressively increasing by 5 mm of displacement amplitudes in each direction at a rate ranging from 0.2 to 1.1 mm/s, the higher rate corresponding to a higher displacement amplitude, all in displacement-control mode), under a constant axial load of 460 kN corresponding to 30% of the member's compressive strength. The lateral load was applied using a horizontally positioned actuator and the axial load was exerted by a set of four hydraulic cylinders. Displacements at the plastic hinge region were monitored using six rectilinear displacement transducers (three on each side, perpendicular to the piston axis, as shown in Fig. 5.4d). The load versus piston displacement curves for all specimens are given in Fig. 5.5.

The performance and failure mode of all tested columns was controlled by flexure. The unretrofitted column (Fig. 5.5a) attained a drift ratio (tip displacement divided by height) at failure of about 3.6%. The concrete cover and part of the core over the lower 200 mm of the column disintegrated and bar buckling initiated after the concrete cover spalled off at a drift ratio of about 3% (Fig. 5.6a).

The behaviour of the two retrofitted columns was very similar (Fig. 5.5b and 5.5c for columns M4 and R2, respectively), but quite different from and far better than their unretrofitted counterpart. Member deformation capacity increased by a factor of more than two, corresponding to a drift ratio at failure of about 7.5%; peak resistance was practically the same as in the unretrofitted column; and the post peak response was quite stable, displaying gradual strength degradation. Whereas the FRP jacket in column R2 exhibited limited rupture over the lower 50 mm (Fig. 5.6b) at 7.2% drift ratio (in the pull direction), the TRM jacket remained intact until the test was terminated at 7.8% drift ratio. When the jackets

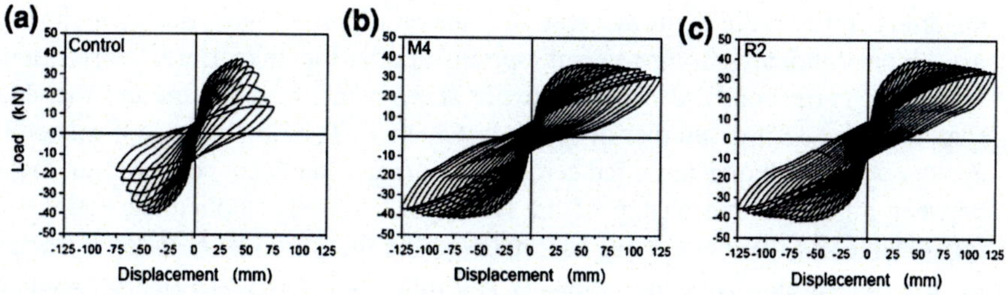

Fig. 5.5 Load-displacement curves for **a** the control specimen, **b** the TRM-confined specimen, and **c** the FRP-confined specimen

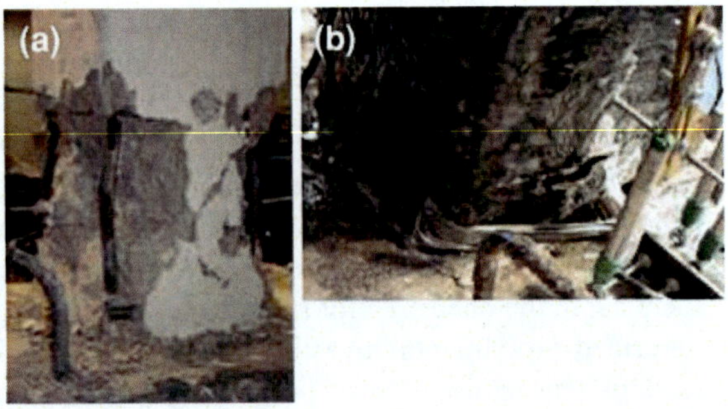

Fig. 5.6 **a** Disintegration of concrete and bar buckling. **b** Limited rupture of FRP jacket deformation capacity by approximately 10%

were removed in both retrofitted columns after the end of the tests, a completely disintegrated concrete core was exposed, one that had been kept in place by the heavy confinement provided by the jackets (both FRP and TRM).

5.4 Shear Strengthening of RC

The aim of this part of the experimental programme was to examine the effectiveness of TRM jackets as strengthening reinforcement of shear-critical RC members. The investigation was carried out on six beams deficient in shear (i.e., with a large spacing of stirrups in the shear span) in four point bending. The beams measured 2.60 m in length and had a cross-section of 150 × 300 mm. The geometry of the beams, the reinforcement detailing and the general set-up of the test are shown in Fig. 5.7.

The beams were cast using a ready-mix concrete of mean 28 day compressive strength equal to 30.5 MPa. The steel used for transverse and longitudinal reinforcement had an average yield stress equal to 275 and 575 MPa, respectively. Textile, polymer-modified mortar (type II) and resin matrices were the same materials as those in the experimental study involving confined specimens made of plain concrete. The influence of three parameters was considered in the experimental investigation, namely the use of inorganic mortar versus resin-based matrix material for the textile reinforcement, the number of layers (one versus two) and the use of conventional wrapping versus 'spirally applied' textiles. Here, 'conventional wrapping' corresponds to a single textile sheet being wrapped around the shear span until the desired number of layers is achieved. The bonding agent was either epoxy resin or polymer-modified cement mortar, applied to the concrete surface, in between all layers and on top of the last layer. 'Spirally applied' jacketing was implemented in one beam only and involved the formation of each layer through the use of a single strip, approximately 150 mm wide. The first strip was wrapped around the member in a spiral configuration, starting from one end of the shear span and stopping at the other; the next strip was wrapped in the same configuration but

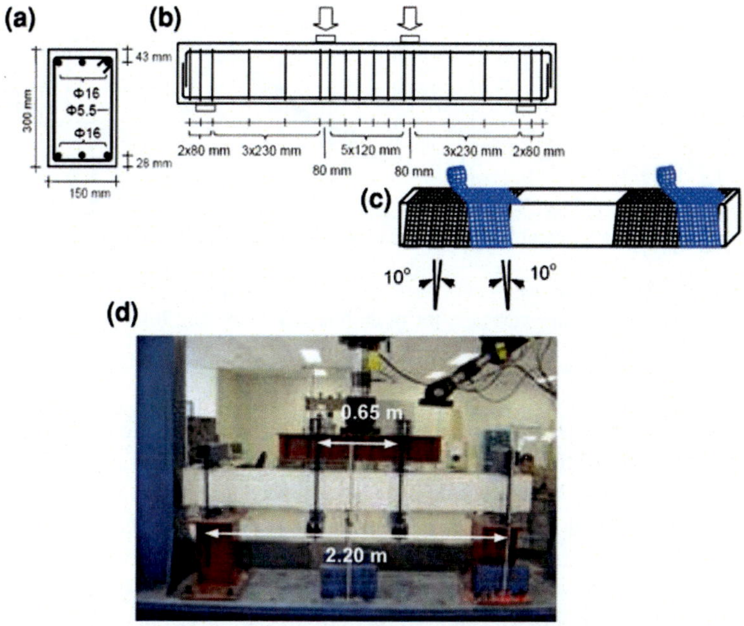

Fig. 5.7 **a–b** Geometry of the beams. **c** Spiral application of strips at the shear spans. **d** General set-up of the test [3]

in a direction opposite to that of the first strip. Both strips formed a 10° angle with respect to the transverse to the member axis (Fig. 5.7c).

Four of the beams were tested monotonically and two of them were subjected to cyclic loading. One of the four monotonically tested beams served as a control specimen (C); a second one was wrapped with two layers of mortar-based jacket in the shear span (M2); a third beam was identical to the second but with a resin-based matrix material for the textile reinforcement (R2); and a fourth beam was strengthened with jackets formed by spirally applied strips (M2-s). The next two specimens (subjected to cyclic loading a few months later than the previous four) were identical to the second and third, but with one layer (instead of two) of textile in a mortar-based (M1) and a resin-based (R1) matrix, respectively. Specimens C, M2, R2 and M2-s were tested monotonically, whereas the remaining two were subjected to quasi-static cyclic loading, all in displacement control. The load was applied using a vertically positioned actuator and the displacements were measured at mid-span using two external linear variable differential transducers mounted on both sides of the specimens. The load versus mid-span displacement curves for all specimens are given in Fig. 5.8.

The control beam (C) failed in shear, as expected, through the formation of diagonal cracks in the shear spans; the ultimate load was 116.5 kN. No sudden drop in the load was recorded after diagonal cracking, as considerable contribution

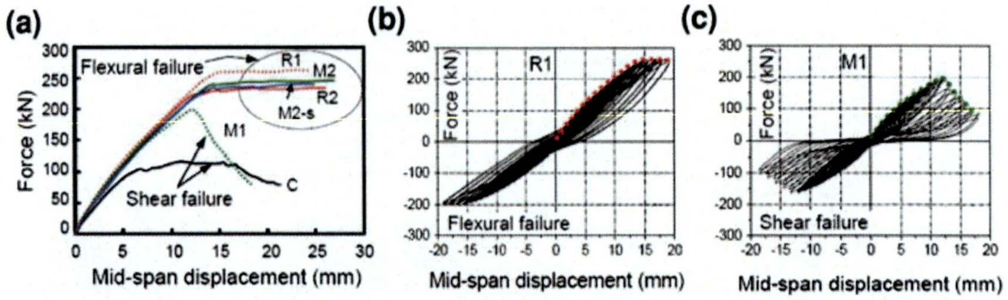

Fig. 5.8 Force–mid-span displacement curves: **a** for all beams tested (for beams subjected to cyclic loading the envelope curves in the push direction are given); **b** for beam R1; **c** for beam M1 [3]

to shear resistance was provided by both the stirrups crossing the crack and the strong dowel action (activated by the three Ø16 mm longitudinal rebars).

The behaviour of beams R2, M2, M2-s and R1 indicated that shear failure was suppressed and that failure was controlled by flexure: cracks in the constant moment region became wide and yielding of the tension reinforcement resulted in a nearly horizontal branch of the force versus displacement curve. The maximum loads in specimens R2, M2 and M2-s were 233.4, 243.8 and 237.7 kN, respectively, that is nearly the same. This confirms the fact that the shear strengthening scheme selected in this study did not affect the flexural resistance. But the increase in shear resistance was dramatic (more than 100%), regardless of the strengthening scheme: two layers of textile reinforcement (either in the form of continuous sheets or in the form of spirally applied strips) with the polymer-modified cementitious binder performed equally well to the epoxy-bonded (FRP) jacket (with two layers of textile reinforcement). Specimen R1 experienced a flexural yielding failure mode with unequal capacities in the push and pull directions (261.9 and 201.4 kN, respectively, in Fig. 5.8b), possibly due to the unintentionally larger concrete cover at the top of each beam compared to the bottom. Specimen M1 failed in shear (at a peak load of 200.1 kN); this was evident by diagonal cracking in the shear span as well as by the rather sudden strength and stiffness degradation. In this case, the application of a single-layer TRM jacket resulted in a substantial increase in the specimen's shear capacity with respect to the control specimen, in the order of 70%. It should be noted that for specimen M1: (i) fracture of the fibres in the cement-based jacket was gradual, starting from a few fibre bundles and propagating slowly in the neighbouring fibres; and (ii) contrary to conventional FRP jackets, beam cracking was clearly visible on the TRM jacket, a feature that facilitates damage assessment.

Overall, it may be concluded that the TRM jackets employed in this study were quite effective in increasing the shear resistance of RC members. Two layers of textile reinforcement (with a nominal thickness per layer equal to only 0.047 mm in each of the principal fibre directions) were sufficient to prevent sudden shear failure, whereas one layer proved less effective compared to its resin-bonded counterpart, but still sufficient to provide a substantially increased shear resistance.

5.5 Flexural Strengthening of RC

In this part of the investigation the effectiveness of TRM as externally applied flexural strengthening reinforcement of RC beam-type members was examined. The results reported here refer to testing of three under-reinforced beams in four-point bending, at a span length of 2.0 m and a shear span of 0.75 m. The beams had a cross-section of 150 × 250 mm and were reinforced with 2Ø12 longitudinal rebars on each side (top and bottom), at a cover equal to 25 mm. The shear reinforcement comprised Ø8 stirrups at a small spacing equal to 100 mm, to ensure that failure would be controlled by flexural yielding. Self-compacting concrete was used for casting of the beams (mix design and production were performed in the laboratory within the framework of a parallel experimental investigation); mean 28 day compressive strength was equal to 34.5 MPa. The steel reinforcement had an average yield stress equal to 530 MPa. Textile, polymer-modified mortar (type II) and epoxy resin matrices were the same materials as those in the experimental study involving confined specimens made of plain concrete.

One of the three beams was tested without strengthening, as a control specimen (C_fl); a second one was strengthened with four layers of textile bonded with cement-based mortar (M4_fl); the third beam was identical to the second but with an epoxy resin-based matrix material for the textile reinforcement (R4_fl). The externally bonded reinforcement had a width and a length equal to 120 mm and 1.90 m, respectively, so that its distance from each support was equal to 50 mm. All beams were tested monotonically with the load was applied using a vertically positioned actuator and a heavy spread beam; the displacements were measured at mid-span using two external linear variable differential transducers mounted on both sides of the beams. The load versus mid-span displacement curves for all beams are given in Fig. 5.9a.

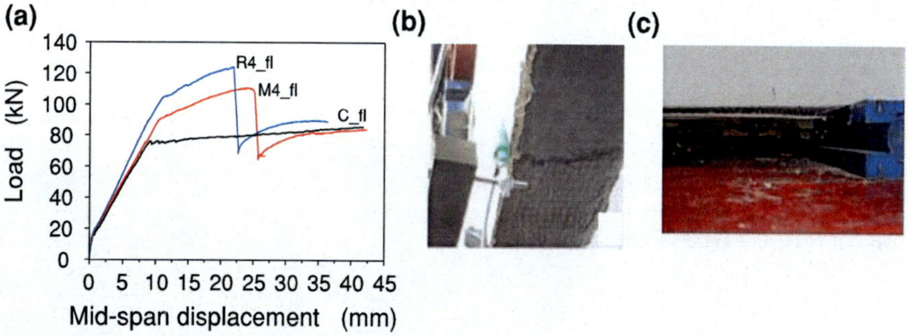

Fig. 5.9 **a** Load–displacement response of beams strengthened in flexure. **b** Tensile fracture of the epoxy-bonded reinforcement (FRP) at mid-span. **c** Debonding of the TRM reinforcement at the end (anchorage) through inter-laminar shearing

The control specimen (C_fl) displayed the standard nearly-bilinear response characteristics of under-reinforced beams. Strengthening with the epoxy-impregnated textile (beam R4_fl) resulted in increased strength (by approximately 50%) and increased stiffness, as expected; failure in this case was rather sudden, due to the tensile fracture (Fig. 5.9b) of the externally bonded reinforcement at mid-span (at a load of 125 kN). The TRM-strengthened beam (M4-fl) displayed similar characteristics to its epoxy-bonded counterpart, with four distinct differences: its response was a little more ductile; yielding initiated at a lower load; the ultimate load was lower (111 kN); and the failure mechanism was governed by debonding at the end (anchorage) of the external reinforcement due to inter-laminar shearing (Fig. 5.9c). It is believed that the slightly lower stiffness and higher ductility characteristics of beam M4_fl compared to R4_fl are attributed to the lower stiffness of the bond between the external reinforcement and the concrete, which may have resulted in reduced composite action. Overall, the TRM-based strengthening system used in this study was approximately 30% less effective in terms of strength but 30% more effective in terms of (displacement) ductility.

5.6 Seismic Retrofitting of Unreinforced Masonry Subjected to Out-of-plane or In-plane loading

TRM has also been investigated as a new method for seismic retrofitting of unreinforced masonry (URM) walls through jacketing (Fig. 5.10a). A comprehensive experimental programme was carried out on URM wall specimens subjected to cyclic loading which induced in-plane flexure combined with axial force, out-of-plane flexure and in-plane shear with axial force. The walls were strengthened using two-sided jacketing made of TRM materials (Fig. 5.10b). The main parameter under investigation was the number of textile layers (one or two), but also comparisons were made on the response of TRM-strengthened walls and identical specimens strengthened with FRP jackets. The results were obtained in

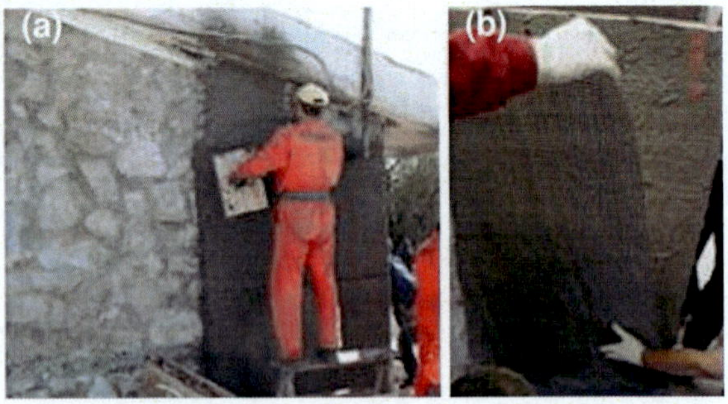

Fig. 5.10 **a** Practical application of TRM on masonry wall. **b** Strengthening of masonry specimens using TRM jackets

terms of load–displacement diagrams as well as stiffness and cumulative energy plots as a function of the loading cycles.

The investigation was carried out on three types of medium-scale, single-wythe, fired clay brick wallettes composed of running bond courses (Fig. 5.11): (a) Specimen type A (shear walls) measured 1300 mm in height and 800 mm in width; (b) Specimen type B (beam-columns) measured 1300 mm in height and 400 mm in width; and (c) Specimen type C (beams) measured 400 mm in height and 1300 mm in width. All specimens were constructed in the laboratory by an experienced mason using perforated bricks (185 × 85 × 60 mm), with the perforations running in parallel to the units' length. Details about the experimental programme and the results are given in Papanicolaou et al. [4, 5].

The first part of the investigation comprised testing of Specimen types B and C subjected to out-of-plane loading. Those specimens were used so as to assure failure parallel and perpendicular to bed joints, for the former and the latter, respectively. The test set-up (identical for type B and C specimens), along with typical failure modes, are shown in Fig. 5.12.

The second part of the investigation comprised testing of Specimen types A, B and C subjected to *in-plane loading*. Type A specimens were tested as vertical cantilevers with a concentrated force at the top, at a distance of 1.10 m from the fixed base; type B and C specimens were tested as horizontal beams in three-point

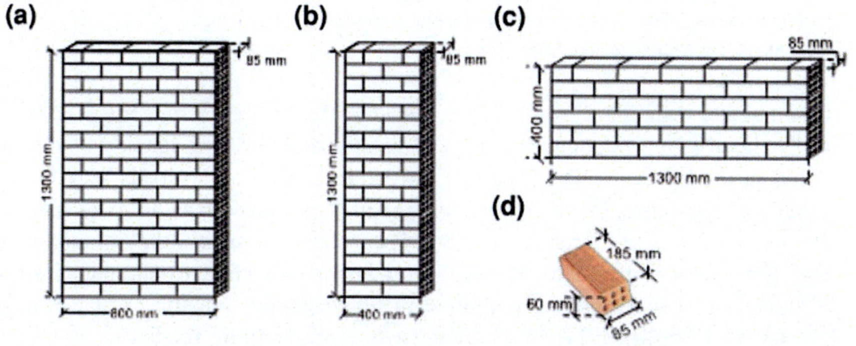

Fig. 5.11 Specimen **a** type A, **b** type B and **c** type C. **d** Six-hole clay bricks

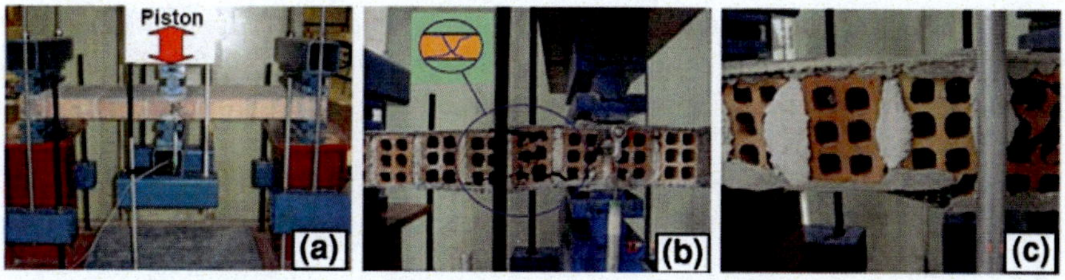

Fig. 5.12 **a** Experimental setup. **b** Diagonal cracking of masonry walls. **c** Debonding of the jacket at large displacements

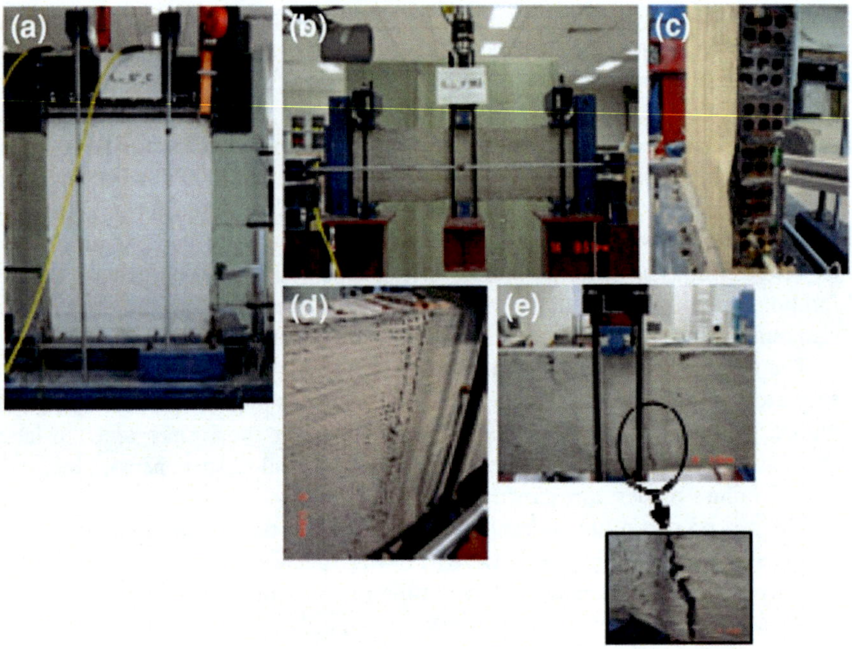

Fig. 5.13 Experimental setup of: **a** Type A walls and **b** Type B and C walls; **c** buckling of TRM jacket at the base of a shear wall; **d** flexural cracking in TRM jacket of type B wall; and **e** extensive debonding of the TRM jacket from the type C wall surface

bending, at a span of 1.17 and 1.12 m, respectively. The test arrangement of type B walls aimed at reproducing the in-plane flexure/shear seismic loading of pilasters found in the lower levels of masonry structures, where axial loads may be considerable. Therefore, during cyclic loading of these specimens an axial load was applied on their outer brick rows and kept constant throughout the duration of the test. For type C specimens, the test arrangement intended to simulate in-plane flexure/shear loading typically applied in lintels during seismic excitations. The test set-up is shown in Fig. 5.13, along with typical failure modes.

Main conclusions from this part of the study are as follows: Both TRM and FRP overlays increase the strength and deformation capacity of URM walls by several times. For the case of out-of-plane loading, TRM outperform their FRP counterparts on the basis of maximum load and displacement at failure, whereas if the failure mechanism involves tensile fracture of the textile reinforcement the effectiveness of TRM versus FRP is slightly reduced. For the case of in-plane loading, TRM (compared with FRP) results in reduced effectiveness for strength, the magnitude of which depends on the type of loading and on the number of textile layers used. In terms of strength, TRM jackets are at least 65–70% as effective as FRP jackets with identical fibre configurations. In terms of deformation capacity, of crucial importance in seismic retrofitting of URM walls, TRM jacketing is much more effective than FRP. The increased effectiveness is about 15–30% in shear walls, 135% in beam-column type walls and 350% in beam type walls. Moreover, regardless of the matrix material (polymer-modified mortar versus epoxy resin), the strength generally increases with the number of layers and the axial load, at the expense of deformation capacity.

5.7 Conclusions

A novel strengthening technique (TRM) is described in this study for strengthening and seismic retrofitting of RC members through confinement; the technique is also used in shear and flexural strengthening. Key feature of this technique is the combination of textiles with polymer-modified cementitious binders, hence it may be considered as an alternative to FRP strengthening. From the results obtained in this study it was shown that TRM jacketing of RC is nearly as effective as FRP jacketing. The authors believe that TRM jacketing is an extremely promising solution for increasing the confinement as well as the shear capacity of RC members, of crucial importance in seismic retrofitting. Extrapolation of the technique to URM walls resulted in substantial increase in strength and deformation capacity, indicating that this new generation of materials offers a promising solution in the restoration of masonry structures, including monument-type ones.

References

1. Triantafillou TC, Papanicolaou CG, Zissimopoulos P, Laourdekis T (2006) Concrete confinement with textile-reinforced mortar jackets. ACI Struct J 103(1):28–37
2. Bournas D, Lontou P, Papanicolaou CG, Triantafillou TC (2007) Textile-reinforced mortar (TRM) versus FRP confinement in reinforced concrete columns. ACI Struct J 104(6):740–748
3. Triantafillou TC, Papanicolaou CG (2006) Shear strengthening of reinforced concrete members with textile reinforced mortar (TRM) jackets. RILEM Mater Struct 39(1):85–93
4. Papanicolaou CG, Triantafillou TC, Papathanasiou M, Karlos K (2007) Textile reinforced mortar (TRM) versus FRP as strengthening material of URM walls: Out-of-plane cyclic loading. RILEM Mater Struct 41(1):143–157
5. Papanicolaou CG, Triantafillou TC, Papathanasiou M, Karlos K (2007) Textile reinforced mortar (TRM) versus FRP as strengthening material of URM walls: In-plane cyclic loading. RILEM Mater Struct 40:1081–1097

Chapter 6
Current and Future Applications of Polymer Composites in the Field of Tribology

Klaus Friedrich, Li Chang and Frank Haupert

6.1 Introduction

Polymer composites with continuous-fiber reinforcement of high volume fraction and perfect alignment are known to have very high values of specific strength and stiffness. These properties can be tailored to the load system acting on a structural part made from these materials. Besides these advantages, the wide variety of different fiber and matrix materials permits the design of composites with unique properties for different kinds of application. This is especially true if different types of fibers are used to develop the microstructure of a particular composite material (hybrid composites). The majority of material developments in this respect have been carried out to improve the mechanical properties of the composites, e.g., their resistance to fatigue conditions [1–4]. The disadvantage is that parts made of these materials usually require rather long production times due to the slow autoclave curing process or other manufacturing techniques used for this type of composites. On the other hand, discontinuous, i.e., short-fiber- or particulate-reinforced systems, especially with a thermoplastic matrix, are not able to compete with their continuous fiber counterparts in terms of strength and stiffness,

K. Friedrich (✉) · F. Haupert
IVW GmbH, Technical University Kaiserslautern, 67663 Kaiserslautern, Germany
e-mail: friedrich@ivw.uni-kl.de

L. Chang
School of Aerospace, Mechanical and Mechatronic Engineering, University of Sydney, Sydney 2006, Australia
e-mail: li.chang@sydney.edu.au

F. Haupert
e-mail: haupert@ivw.uni-kl.de

K. Friedrich
CEREM, College of Engineering, King Saud University, Riyadh, Saudi Arabia

L. Nicolais et al. (eds.), *Composite Materials*,
DOI: 10.1007/978-0-85729-166-0_6, © Springer-Verlag London Limited 2011

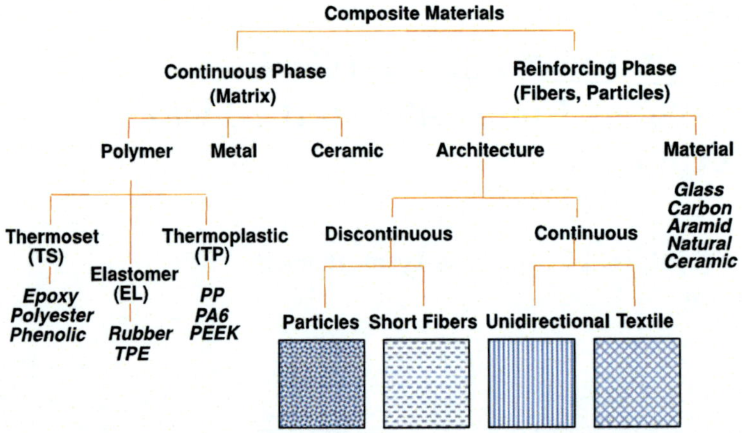

Fig. 6.1 Systematic illustration of the structural components of composite materials

but have the advantage that they can be processed into complex geometries by, e.g., injection molding, thus enabling rapid production of several thousand parts per day. In both cases the diameter of the individual reinforcing elements is in the μm-size range (e.g. glass fibers have a diameter of about 10 μm). Their length can vary between 200 μm (typical for injection moldable short glass fiber-reinforced thermoplastics), several millimeters to centimeters (long fiber filled systems), and up to meters in the case of continuous fiber composites. The principle composition of typical composite materials is demonstrated in Fig. 6.1.

More recently, new developments have shown that much smaller reinforcing dimensions can lead to special effects, which cannot be reached so easily with traditional fillers. In this class of the so-called nanocomposites, at least one dimension of the reinforcing elements is in the range of about 10–100 nm [5]. Under these conditions, the structure of the material is composed of a much larger interface between the polymer matrix and the nano-particles (Fig. 6.2), being able to create a quite different mechanical performance of the material in comparison to a traditional composite with the same filler volume fraction [6–8]. In the following part of this chapter, the term "nanocomposites" is also used when the fillers are in the sub-micron range, e.g., 300 nm.

Most of the scientific papers in the past have mainly concentrated on the mechanical property profile of various composites, i.e., their strength, stiffness and toughness characteristics [9, 10], or their long-term behavior, such as fatigue crack propagation or creep resistance [11, 12]. Little has yet been published, however, on how the various types of reinforcements influence secondary properties, as for example the composites' friction and wear behavior, although it has been shown that fiber-reinforced thermoplastics and thermosets are often used as seals, gears and dry slide bearing materials. Thermosetting resin-based composites, and especially those with continuous carbon fibers, can give better service (e.g., lower wear rates, higher strength) than those with thermoplastic matrices and short-fiber reinforcements when sliding against metals under severe conditions [13, 14].

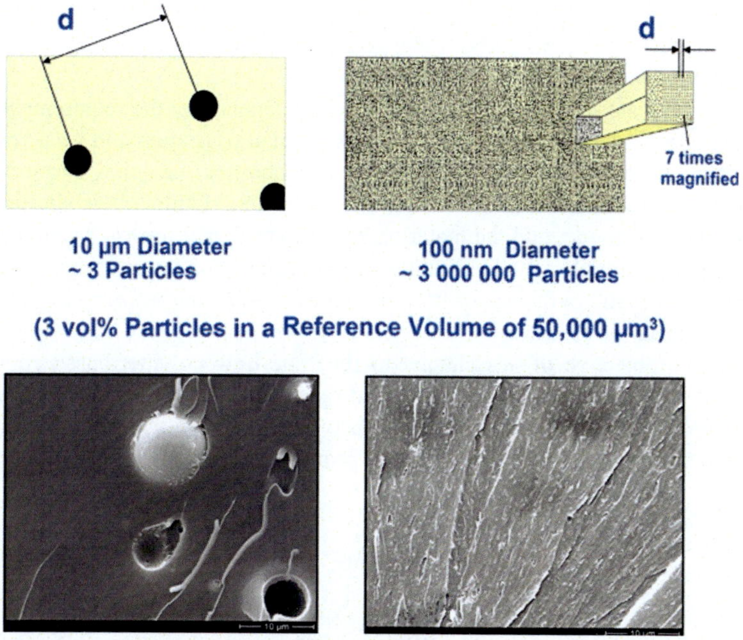

Fig. 6.2 Schematic illustration of a dramatic increase in particle number with a reduction of the particle diameter (*upper row*), and corresponding fracture surface of an epoxy resin filled with 10 μm glass spheres (*lower left*) or 13 nm sized alumina nano-particles (*lower right*) [7]

This is because the high fiber contents attainable with thermosetting composites and the preferential load bearing by the fibers ensure that their tribological properties are mainly determined by those of the reinforcements [14]. However, the majority of friction and wear loaded components are made of discontinuous reinforced polymer systems, since they allow more complex geometries and a better tailoring of their tribological characteristics for a particular application.

Figures 6.3, 6.4, and 6.5 give various examples, in which polymer composites are used as highly loaded tribo-elements. A continuous textile fabric reinforced rubber conveyor belt (Fig. 6.3) is usually loaded on its surface by sharp abrasive particles so that the requirement is that this polymer composite must have a high abrasive wear resistance. At the same time, its frictional coefficient should be high, so that the material to be conveyed does not slip downward. Figure 6.4 presents typical engineering slide pads, bearings, etc. which usually possess a short-fiber reinforcement in a thermosetting or thermoplastic matrix. They are often sliding against metallic counterparts, and must usually possess low friction and low wear. Since these parts represent most of the engineering applications, the following sections of this chapter mainly focus on such cases.

A possible medical application is demonstrated in Fig. 6.5. Here the stem of an artificial hip joint was fabricated by the use of a carbon fabric reinforced polyetheretherketone (PEEK) composite. A comparison of its fretting wear behavior relative to a titanium alloy stem was described in [15]. It was also tried out in the past, to replace the classical ultra high molecular weight polyethylene cap (UHMW-PE) by a short carbon fiber (SCF) reinforced UHMW-PE material, but this attempt was not successful enough so far.

How the materials must exactly be designed depends on the requirement profile of the particular application. That means coefficient of friction and wear resistance are no real material properties, but system properties, i.e., they depend on the system in which these materials have to function. Quite often sliding is the dominant wear mode, and the materials must be designed for low friction and low wear against smooth metallic counterparts (e.g., as gears or bearings), but sometimes also a high coefficient of friction, coupled with low wear, is required (e.g., for brake pads or clutches).

It is the objective of this chapter to illustrate how polymer-based composites can be designed for friction and wear loading situations, and to show that for future applications the combined interaction between classical tribo-fillers and newly developed nano-reinforcements provide promising solutions.

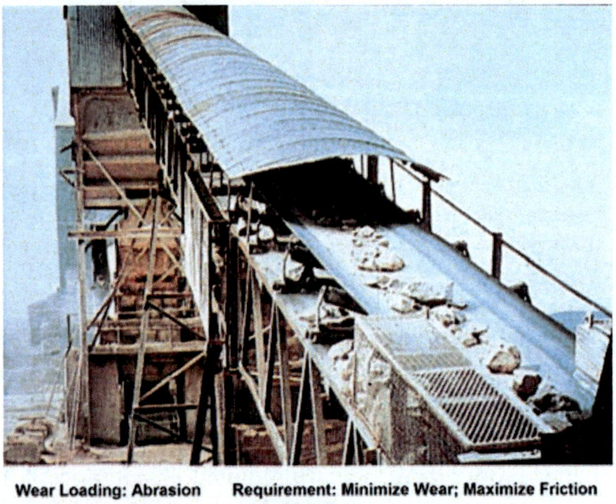

Fig. 6.3 Textile-reinforced rubber conveyor belts in civil engineering

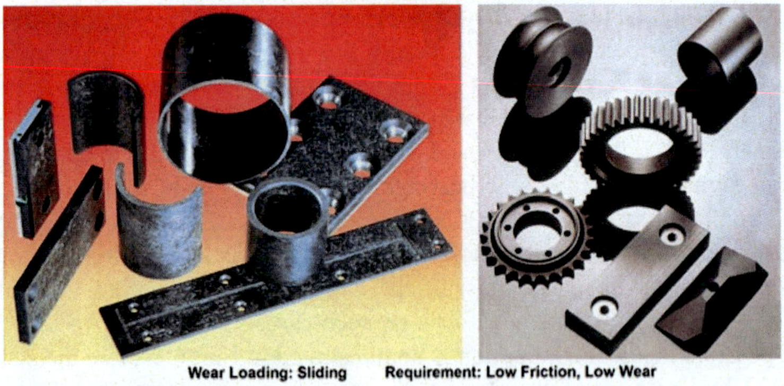

Fig. 6.4 Engineering slide pads, gears, bearings and rollers made of discontinuous fiber-reinforced thermosets or thermoplastics (*Source*: various industrial manufacturers)

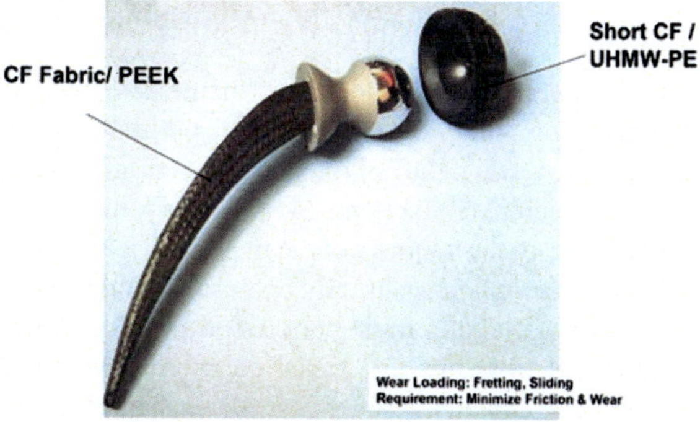

Fig. 6.5 Example of an artificial hip joint using various polymer composites (*Source*: MAN Neue Technologien, Munich, Germany)

6.2 Design Principles and Testing of Wear Resistant Polymer Composites

From several studies in the past it is well known that the friction and wear behavior of polymeric materials can be improved by a lower adhesion and a higher stiffness and strength [16–18]. This can be achieved quite successfully by using special fillers. To reduce the adhesion, e.g., internal lubricants, such as PTFE or graphite are frequently incorporated. They also allow the formation of a friction reducing transfer film on the surface of the counterpart material [19]. Continuous or short aramid, carbon or glass fibers are used to increase the stiffness and strength of the polymer system. Since friction between two mating surfaces in sliding contact generates heat, which in turn enhances the temperature in the contact area (associated with a reduction in the mechanical properties of the polymer), from the matrix point of view, a high temperature resistant polymer should be used. In addition, the tribological properties of polymers and polymer composites can be changed by the use of other thermally conductive fillers, including nano-sized particles or carbon nano-tubes. This has been demonstrated by many authors, of which only a few can be listed here (e.g., [20–23]). However, often the optimum effects for reducing both, the coefficient of friction and the wear rate, can only be achieved if the nano-fillers are used in combination with some of the traditional tribo-fillers mentioned above (Fig. 6.6) [24].

This finally leads to a complex microstructure of the composite materials, as for example illustrated in Fig. 6.7 [25].

Unlubricated sliding wear tests of these materials are usually carried out on different pin-on-disk machines, as illustrated in Fig. 6.8. The measured data allow to determine the coefficient of friction μ and the specific wear rate w_s by the following equations:

$$\mu = F_R / F_N \tag{6.1}$$

where F_R is the friction force and F_N is the normal load

$$w_s = \Delta m/(dF_N L) = \Delta V/(F_N L), \text{usually in the dimensions}\{\text{mm}^3/(\text{Nm})\} \quad (6.2)$$

where Δm is the mass loss, d is the density of the composite material, ΔV is the volume loss, and L is the sliding distance.

Before testing, the polymer composites are cut into pins (e.g., $4 \times 4 \times 12$ mm^3). In the apparent contact area (4×4 mm^2), the sliding direction should be chosen to be parallel to the majority of the in plane oriented fibers, since under these conditions CF-based composites usually possess the lowest wear rates [26]. In order to reduce the time of the running-in period, specimens are sometimes pre-worn with grinding paper (Grid 800) against the disk counterpart and then carefully cleaned with ethanol. With this method, the roughness of the specimens before testing is always the same, and at the same time the apparent area of contact with the steel disk is improved due to a better parallelism between the two mating surfaces.

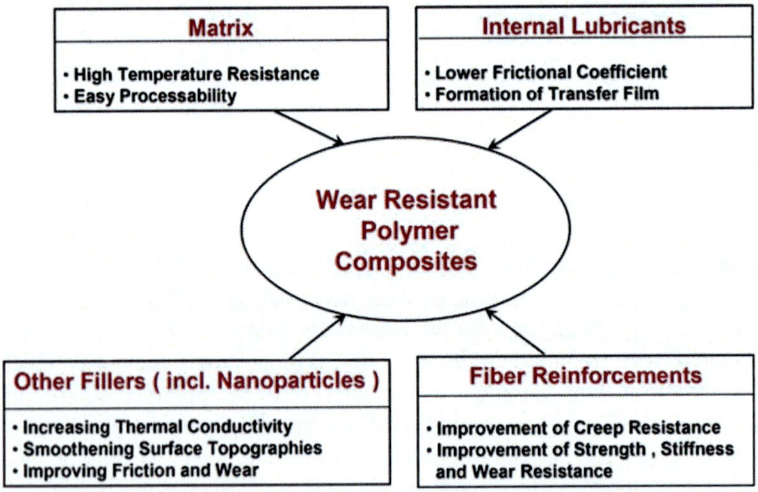

Fig. 6.6 How to design polymer composite for high sliding wear resistance

Fig. 6.7 Typical microstructure of a high temperature resistant polyetheretherketone (PEEK), filled with PTFE particles and reinforced with short carbon fibers [25]

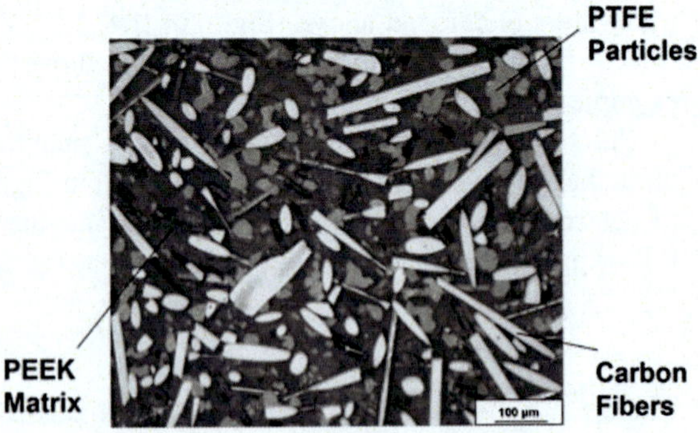

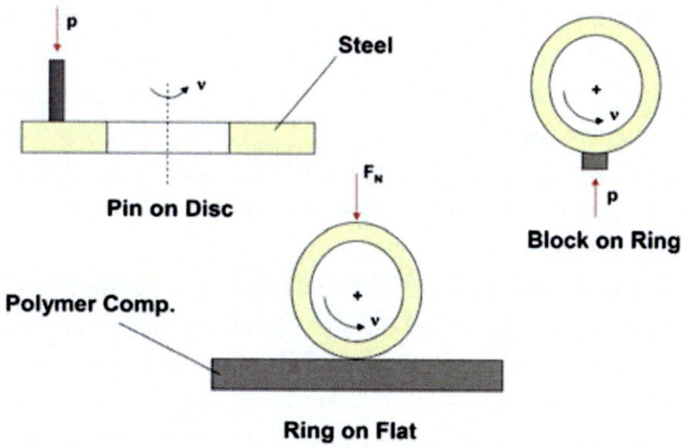

Fig. 6.8 Schematics of three different laboratory wear test configurations

For many tribological experiments, hardened (HRC 62) and polished carbon steel disks (100 Cr6; AISI 52 100) with an initial surface roughness of $R_a = 50$ nm serves as a counterpart. It is the most frequently used steel for bearing applications, exhibiting numerous advantages: high purity and strength, suitability for hardening without carburizing, and flexibility in the heat treatment.

The specific wear rate, mentioned above (also called "wear factor" of the material, k^*), can be considered as a kind of "material property," which allows to compare different materials with each other (when tested under equivalent system conditions). As long as this factor is not dramatically influenced by changes in the apparent contact pressure p or the sliding velocity v, a plot of the so-called depth wear rate w_t (reduction in specimen height per testing time) against the pv-product should show a nearly linear relationship, according to

$$w_t = w_s(pv) \tag{6.3}$$

Schematically this is illustrated in Fig. 6.9. Above a critical pv-value, however, the wear factor k^* starts to deviate from being constant, which means it is not anymore independent from the pv-product. Finally the curve goes to infinity, indicating that the very upper limit of the material's load bearing capacity is exceeded.

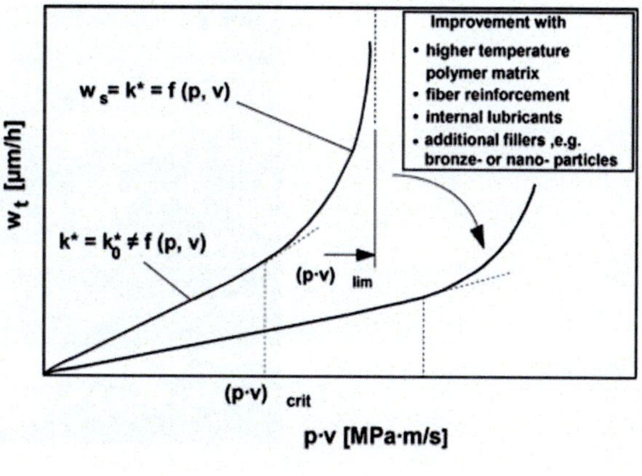

Fig. 6.9 Schematic illustration of the course of the depth wear rate versus pv-product, and possible steps how to improve the wear behavior

For the materials science people it is always the objective to develop materials with a reduced initial slope of this curve and to push the critical and limiting *pv*-levels to higher values, using different combinations of fillers and reinforcements in a given polymer matrix [27].

The depth wear rate is a convenient term for the design engineer in order to estimate the height loss of a polymeric material at various pressure and velocity conditions (assuming that the wear rate of the steel counterpart is negligible). This, in turn, can help to calculate the development of a certain clearance in journal bearings with time, and thus to predict necessary maintenance intervals in order to prevent more catastrophic failures of complete machine units.

6.3 General Aspects of Friction and Wear of Nano-particle Modified Polymer Composites

6.3.1 Incorporation of Nano-particles into Polymeric Matrices

The major processing routes which are used for incorporating nano- and micro-particles depend on the different types of the polymer matrices. In all cases, high shear energies are necessary to break up the agglomerates which are usually formed by the nano-particles (Fig. 6.10). The aim is to separate the individual particles, wet them with the polymer fluid and stabilize their separated positions during the solidification process of the matrix. The whole process can be supported by the use of additional chemical additives, such as surfactants (e.g., stearic acid or

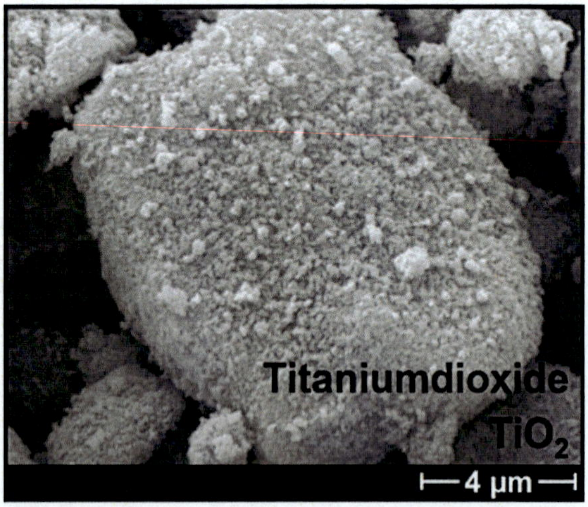

Fig. 6.10 Size of a powder agglomerate consisting of numerous TiO_2-nano-particle

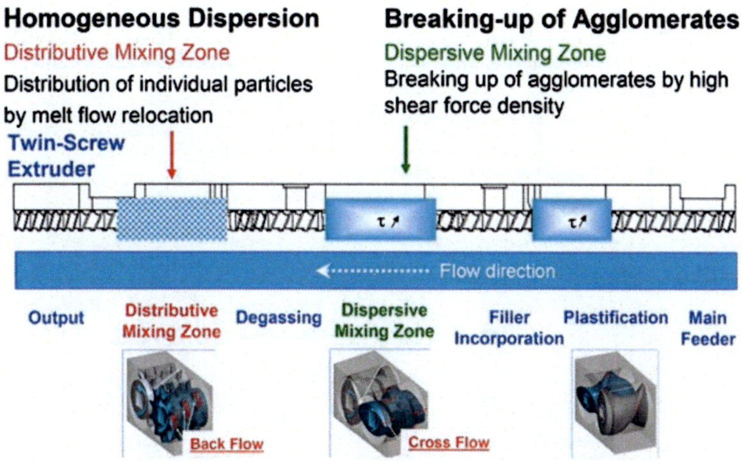

Fig. 6.11 Various zones and screw elements for breaking up nano-particle agglomerates in a twin-screw extruder and for distributing them uniformly in a thermoplastic matrix [28]

polyfunctional alcohols). When using thermoplastics as the matrix for injection moldable tribology components, a twin-screw extruder, equipped with appropriate feeders for the various fillers, is usually the best processing solution (Fig. 6.11) [28]. In the case of a high temperature resistant PEEK, filled with zincsulfide (ZnS)-nano-particles of 300 nm in diameter, this resulted in a uniform distribution of the fillers, as shown in Fig. 6.12. A dissolver disk in combination with a pearl mill can be applied in order to create the necessary shear and collision effects for destroying the nano-particle agglomerates in thermosetting resins (Fig. 6.13). In combination with other tribo-fillers, this results in a microstructure which is exemplarily illustrated in Fig. 6.14.

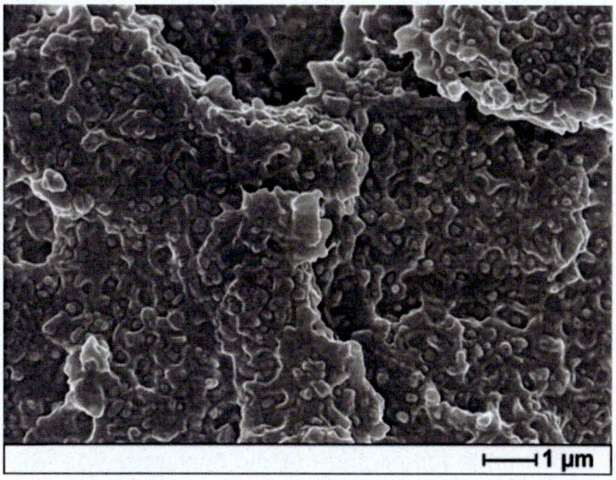

Fig. 6.12 Homogeneous and agglomerate-free distribution of 15 vol.% ZnS nano-particles (300 nm diameter) in PEEK [28]

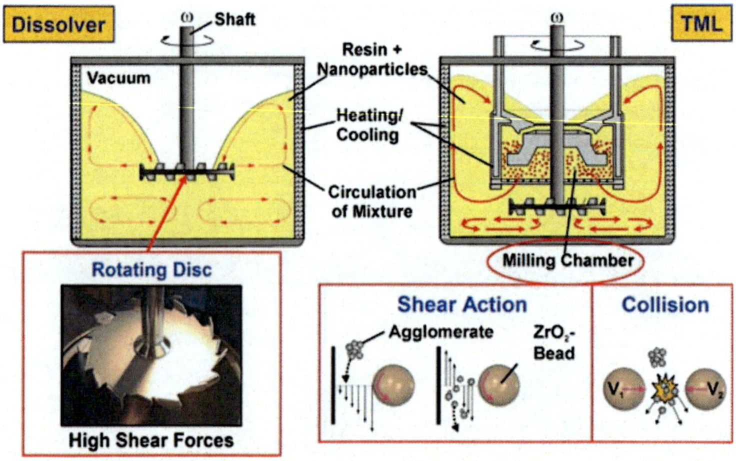

Fig. 6.13 Mechanical dispersion methods of nano-particles in a thermosetting matrix (*TM* Torrus Mill, in which zirconium oxide (ZrO_2) pearls help to break up the agglomerates) [7]

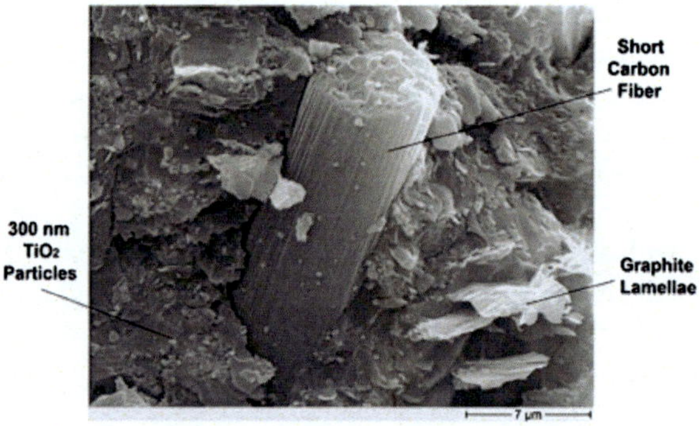

Fig. 6.14 Combination of micro- and nano-fillers on the fracture surface of an epoxy matrix tribo-compound

6.3.2 Synergistic Effects of Nano-particles and Traditional Fillers on the Sliding Wear of Different Polymer-Based Composites

When particle size is reduced to the sub-micron or nano-scale, the wear performance of composites may be significantly different from that of micro-particle filled systems [29]. One reason is that the abrasiveness of hard nano-particles decreases remarkably as a result of the reduction in angularity in comparison with micro-particles. This can have another advantage, namely that these nano-fillers, once they get freely movable in the contact region between the mating surfaces, can act as distance holders and as nano-polishing agents which smoothen the topographies and reduce the coefficient of friction. This, in turn, can also lead to a reduction in temperature of the contact region [30].

Further, it can be expected that the higher thermal conductivity of ceramic nano-particles, as compared to the polymer matrix, also increases the thermal conductivity of the composite, which can contribute to a reduction in heat development in the sliding contact area.

In general, smaller particles seem to contribute better to the improvement of tribological properties under sliding wear conditions than larger particles. One example of this relationship was detected by Xue and Wang [31]. They found that various kinds of SiC-particles, i.e., nano-, micron-, and whisker-type particles, could reduce friction and wear when incorporating them into a PEEK matrix at a constant filler content, e.g., 10 wt% ($\sim$4 vol.%). However, the use of nano-particles resulted in the most effective reduction, which was attributed to their beneficial effect on the formation of a thin, uniform, and continuous transfer film. Wang et al. [32] investigated the influence of the size of ZrO_2 nano-particles, varying from 10 to 100 nm. Effective reduction of the wear of filled PEEK by nano-particles was observed only when the particles were less than 15 nm in size. Xing and Li [33] recently compared the wear properties of spherical particle filled epoxy, in which the particle size varied from 120 to 510 nm. They also confirmed a similar trend, namely that the smaller the particles used as fillers, the better was the wear resistance of the composites. The relationship between the size of nano-particles and asperity size was also studied by Bahadur et al. [20, 34]. Regarding the wear performance of PPS filled with various kinds and amounts of nano-particles, it was found that 2 vol.% of Al_2O_3 resulted in an optimum reduction in the wear rate of the composites when the surface roughness of the steel counterpart was in the range between $R_a = 60$ and 100 nm. However, with a surface roughness of 27 nm, i.e., smaller than the particle size (33 nm on average), any amount of nano-particles increased the wear rate.

Although in most of the studies cited above the morphology of the nano-particle dispersions was not provided in detail, it should be clear that high nano-filler content leads to a reduction in wear properties, which may be due to a tendency of particle agglomeration. In general, it is necessary that nano-particles are uniformly dispersed rather than agglomerated, in order to yield a good property profile. Agglomeration is considered to be a common problem of polymer nano-composites, especially at higher nano-filler contents.

To the present, various inorganic nano-particles, e.g., Al_2O_3, TiO_2, ZnO, CuO, SiC, ZrO_2, Si_3N_4, SiO_2, and $CaCO_3$, have been incorporated into PPS [20, 34], PEEK [31, 32, 35], epoxy [33, 36–40] and PTFE [41, 42] matrices, to improve their wear performance. In most cases, optimum nano-particle filler contents could be identified at which the highest wear resistance of these polymers occurred. The optimum filler content of small particles was mostly in a range between 1 and 6 vol.%. However, in comparison to micro-fillers such as short fibers, the improvement in wear resistance obtained by the use of nano-particles is modest. On the other hand, the critical volume contents of nano-fillers are significantly lower than those of micro-fillers, and therefore, nano-composites can produce improved wear performance while retaining or even improving other mechanical properties of the polymer matrix.

To achieve high wear resistant polymer composites, it is a traditional route to integrate various functional fillers (see Fig. 6.6) [43]. To date, however, little effort has been directed toward the development of hybrid composites by combining inorganic nano-particles with traditional fillers. Wetzel et al. [39] found that the combination of nano-Al_2O_3 (13 nm) and micro-$CaSiO_3$ (4–15 μm) induced some kind of synergistic effect and improved both the wear resistance and the stiffness of epoxy. Cho and Bahadur [44] reported a synergistic action in the tribological behavior of polyphenylene sulfide composites made with nano-CuO and short fibers. The lowest steady state wear rate was obtained with hybrid composites containing both nano-sized CuO particles and fiber reinforcements. Zhang et al. [45–47] indicated that the incorporation of nano-particles with optimized contents could further increase the wear resistance of carbon fabric composites. The beneficial effect of additional nano-particles on wear performance of the composites could be caused by increased mechanical strength of the fabric composites and better bonding strength of the transfer film developed on the metallic counterfaces. It is thus obvious that the incorporation of nano-size inorganic particles together with traditional tribo-fillers into a polymer can provide synergy in terms of an improved wear resistance.

To fully promote the effect of nano-particles, systematic studies of their combinative effect with traditional fillers have been recently carried out by Zhang et al. [24, 48–51]. Various polymers were chosen as matrices, e.g., epoxy, polyamide 66 (PA 66) and polyetherimide (PEI). SCF and two solid lubricants, graphite and PTFE, were used as traditional tribo-fillers. The average diameter of the SCF was ~14.5 μm, with an average fiber length of ~90 μm. The graphite flakes and the PTFE powders were ~20 and ~4 μm, respectively. Nano-sized TiO_2-inorganic particles were applied as additional fillers. The average diameter of these particles was 300 nm.

The tribological performance of a series of epoxy-based composites was preliminarily investigated at a pressure of 1 MPa and a sliding speed of 1 m/s [24, 50].

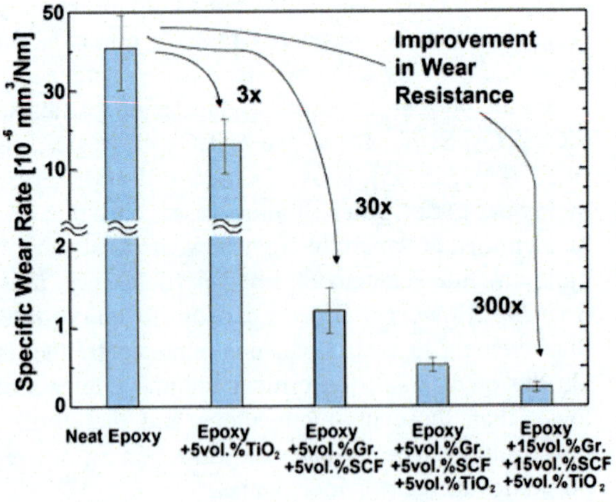

Fig. 6.15 Various degrees of improvement in wear resistance, depending on micro- and nano-filler combination (nano-TiO_2; *Gr.* Graphite, *SCF* short carbon fibers)

The results in Fig. 6.15 exhibit the synergistic effect of nano-TiO_2 particles and traditional tribo-filler on the wear resistance of epoxy-based composites. The wear rate of the hybrid composites filled with both nano-particles and traditional fillers was significantly lower than the values linearly interpolated between those of the composites filled only with nano-TiO_2 or traditional fillers. Moreover, the addition of nano-particles could further reduce the coefficient of friction and the wear rate of the epoxy composites filled with traditional fillers, especially under extreme sliding conditions. The interrelationship between the time-related depth wear rate (calculated with Eq. 6.3), the wear factor (specific wear rate), and the load-carrying capacity (*pv*) for two epoxy composites (one filled only with traditional fillers and the other with both nano-particles and traditional fillers) is shown in Fig. 6.16. It was found that the wear factor of the composite only filled with traditional fillers was clearly enhanced with an increase of *pv*, due to changes in the dominant wear mechanisms. For the composite with both nano-particles and traditional fillers, however, the wear factor of the nano-composite was relatively stable at $\sim 1 \times 10^{-6}$ $mm^3/(Nm)$ even under high *pv* conditions. The slope indicates that the time-related depth wear rate of the nano-composite was much lower than that of the composite filled only with traditional fillers under the same sliding conditions. Therefore, the limiting *pv* of the nano-composite was remarkably improved, which would favor the use of this material for tribo-applications with more severe wear conditions.

The wear synergy detected in epoxy composites has also been found in further investigations of thermoplastic composites, i.e., with PA6.6 [52] or PEI matrices [53]. The composition of these two polymers filled with only conventional fillers, i.e., 5 vol.% graphite and 15 vol.% SCF, was used as a benchmark. It was selected as the optimum content of conventional fillers, based on work previously carried out for evaluating of the wear performance of a series of epoxy-based composites. Nano-TiO_2 particles served as additional fillers, at a content of 5 vol.%.

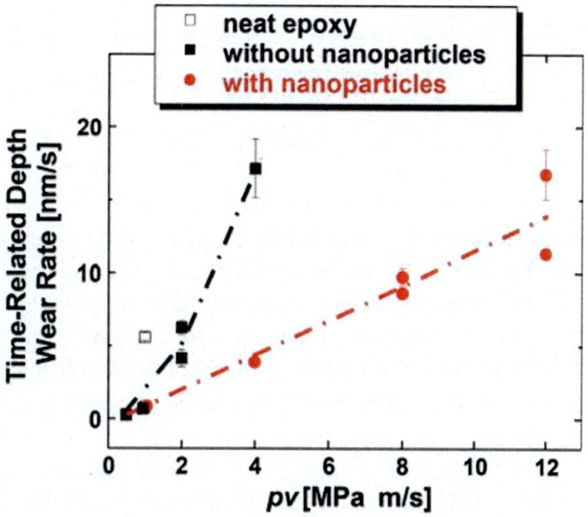

Fig. 6.16 Improvement of the load bearing capacity of a tribo-compound (EP with 5 vol.% PTFE, 5 vol.% Gr and 15 vol.% SCF) by the additional use of 5 vol.% TiO_2-nano-particles [24]

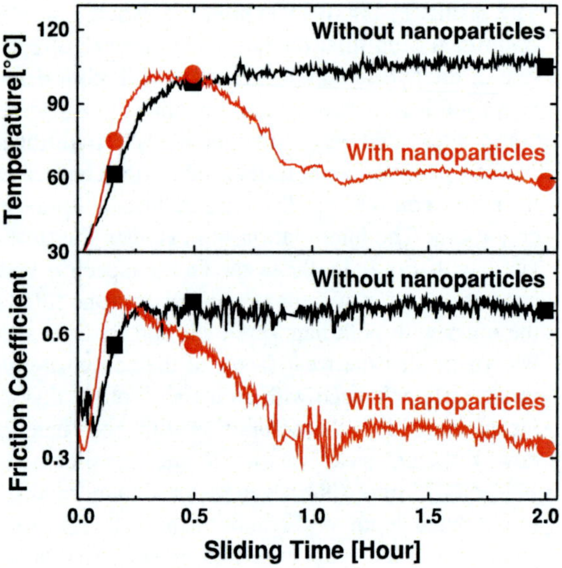

Fig. 6.17 Comparisons of the sliding process of two PA 66 composites with and without nano-particles tested at 2 MPa and 1 m/s, with different durations, i.e., 10, 30, and 120 min

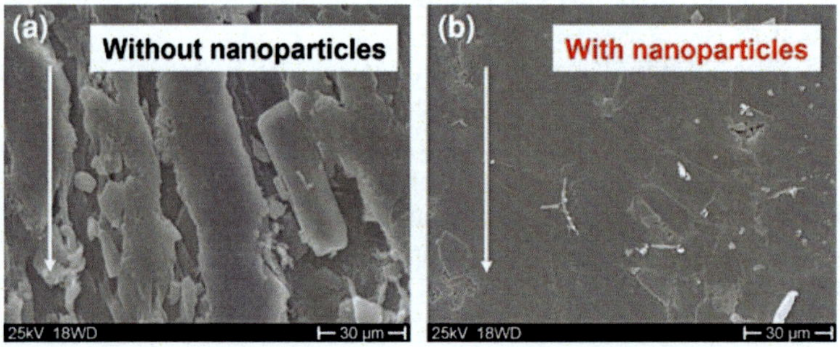

Fig. 6.18 Worn surfaces of PA66 composites **a** without and **b** with nano-particles after 2 h

As expected, the coefficient of friction of both fiber-reinforced thermoplastic composites was remarkably reduced by the addition of nano-TiO_2, associated with a decrease in the contact temperature under all test conditions. This means, the wear resistance of the composites was improved through the incorporation of nano-particles, especially under high contact pressure and high sliding speed conditions. Typical courses of the coefficient of friction and the contact temperature as a function of time are illustrated in Fig. 6.17 for two PA6.6 composites, with and without nano-particles, tested at 2 MPa and 1 m/s. It is clear that at the beginning of the running-in stage, sliding performance was similar for the two composites. However, after about an hour the coefficient of friction of the nano-composite was significantly reduced. The surface of the composites with additional nano-particles became much smoother (Fig. 6.18b) than in the one without nano-particles (Fig. 6.18a).

6.4 Development of Polymer Composites for Tribological Loadings in Various Industries

6.4.1 Mechanical Engineering

6.4.1.1 Sliding Elements in Textile Drying Machines

Textile drying machines consist of a big oven system, which is designed for drying and thermal treatment of flat textile structures with definite width, e.g., after being printed. For this purpose, the printed textiles are fixed by a number of needle clamps, which are attached to a chain system, which transports the stretched textile through the oven. Due to the fact that no external oil or grease lubrication is acceptable in the oven (fire hazard) and before the textile is entering the oven (contamination of the textiles), the individual elements of the chain need to be equipped with sliding shoes, made of self-lubricating polymer composites (Figs. 6.19 and 6.20) [54].

The classical approach for the development of such materials was partly illustrated in Fig. 6.6, i.e., the use of a high temperature resistant polymer matrix, filled with internal lubricants and reinforced with additional fibers. As an alternative, three different matrices were under consideration, i.e., PEEK, polybenzimidazol (PBI), and polyimide (PI). Their physical properties are illustrated in Table 6.1, and their friction and wear properties at room temperature are given in Fig. 6.21. It turns out that the two thermosets are superior to PEEK, when the tribological properties of the polymeric materials are considered only. On the other hand, PEEK has two advantages, which are finally determining its selection for being the matrix material for the sliding shoes: (a) PEEK is injection moldable into

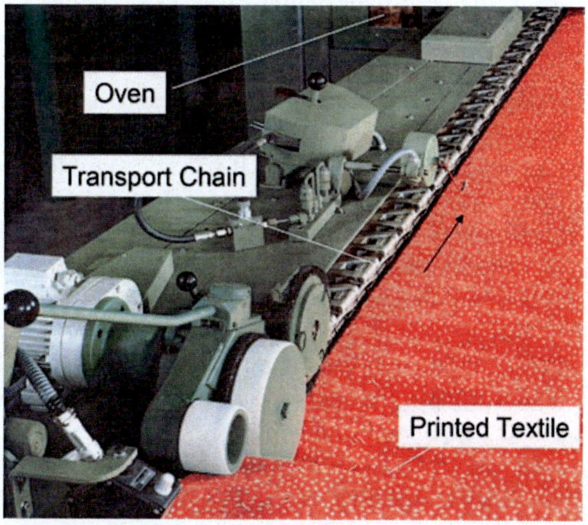

Fig. 6.19 Principle structure of a textile drying machine (*Source*: http://www.babcock-textilmaschinen.de)

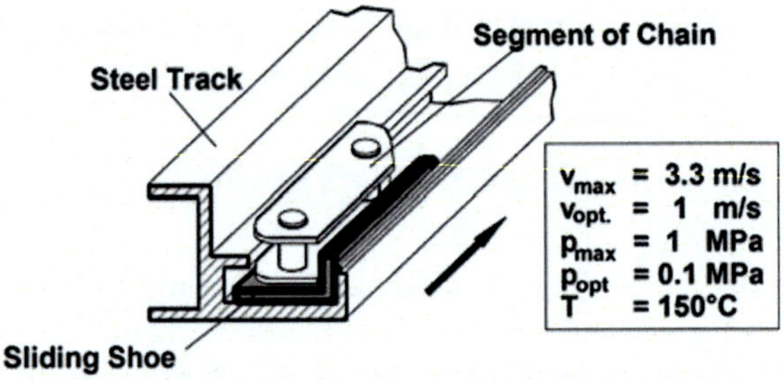

Fig. 6.20 Schematic position of a polymer composite sliding shoe in the chain system of a textile drying machine (*left*), and range of operating parameters (*right*)

Table 6.1 Physical and mechanical properties of two thermoplastic (TP) PEEK-versions and two other high temperature resistant polymers, i.e., PBI and PI

Materials	PEEK	PEEK-CF/Gr/TF	PBI	PI
Type of polymer	Semicrystal. TP	Semicrystal. TP	Semicrystal. TS	Crosslinked TS
Density [g/cm^3]	1.32	1.45	1.30	1.34
Glass transition temperature [°C]	143	143	399	315
Melting temperature [°C]	334	334	427(HDT)	–
Tensile strength [MPa]	92	147	159	140
Tensile E-modulus [GPa]	3.6	15	5.9	2.8
Izod impact energy [J/m]	83	66	28	46
Vickers hardness	26	35	42	16
Processability	Injection moulding	Injection moulding	Sintering	Casting, curing

PEEK Polyether-ether-ketone, *PBI* Polybenzi-midazole, *PI* Polyimide, *TP* Thermoplastic, *TS* Thermoset, *HDT* Heat Deflection Temperature

many of these parts within a very short time, and (b) it has a much higher toughness, which is important for the sliding shoes because they experience a lot of impacts during the movements of the transport chains through the steel tracks [55]. Besides, the tribological behavior of the PEEK can be further improved by the addition of 10% of each, PTFE particles (TF), graphite flakes (Gr), and SCFs (Table 6.2). It becomes visible that at both testing temperatures (room temperature RT, and 150°C) the internal lubricants mainly affect the coefficient of friction, whereas the fibers alone mainly affect the specific wear rate. In combination, however, both tribological characteristics are reduced at the same time in a synergistic fashion.

Making use of 6.3, and assuming that the allowable height reduction of the sliding shoes is 2 mm, their maintenance interval can be calculated as being 5005 h (under the standard operating conditions of $T = 150°C$, a pressure of $p = 0.1$ MPa, and a sliding speed of $v = 1$ m/s), based on the material's specific wear rate of 1.11×10^{-6} mm^3/(Nm). If the machine operates ca. 40 h per week, this leads to a service life of the sliding shoes of ca. 2.5 years.

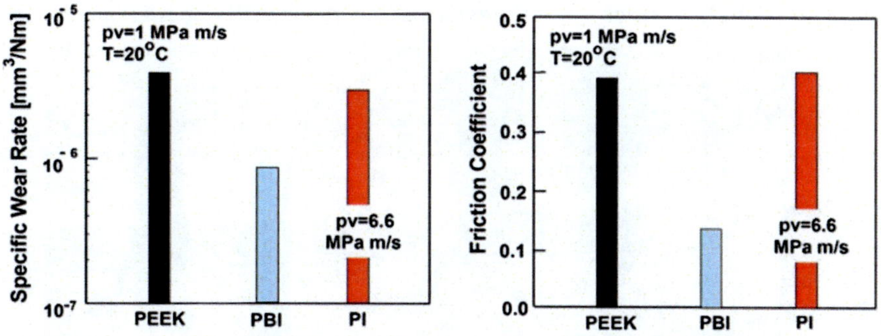

Fig. 6.21 Specific wear rate and friction coefficient of three high temperature resistant polymers tested at room temperature [55]

6.4.1.2 Filament Wound Bushings for Harsh Environments

There are many mechanical engineering applications where high loads, strong vibrations and corrosive elements can act on the bushings of movable joints. Such applications include, e.g., the lifting devices of refuse trucks, components of agriculture and forestry machines and equipment, packaging machines, or cranes on off-shore platforms. In recent years, it has been found out that under these conditions, filament wound, polymer composite bushings can bring a beneficial solution (Fig. 6.22) [56].

Such bushings, which are commercially available in different diameters and widths, are manufactured using a complex fiber winding technique. Figure 6.23 indicates that they are composed of two distinct layers. The high strength backing layer consists of a high volume fraction of glass fibers, and the sliding surface is made of PTFE- and other polymer fibers. Both layers are embedded in an epoxy resin matrix. This material selection combines the special mechanical properties of glass fibers with the outstanding tribological properties of PTFE- and high strength polymer fibers. In this way, these bushings bring together also other benefits and features, including: (a) good impact resistance, (b) insensitivity to edge loading and misalignment, (c) good noise and vibration damping, (d) excellent resistance to corrosive media, even to salt water, and other chemicals, and (e) good insulation

Table 6.2 Specific wear rate (w_s) and coefficient of friction (μ) of various PEEK-compounds at room temperature (RT) and at $T = 150°C$; CF mainly reduces the wear rate, while TF and Gr mainly reduce μ [55]

PEEK-composites vs. steel	RT		150°C	
	w_s (mm³/Nm)	μ (1)	w_s (mm³/Nm)	μ (1)
PEEK	8×10^{-6}	0.45	1.9×10^{-5}	0.46
PEEK + TF + Gr	9×10^{-7}	0.21	2.5×10^{-6}	0.18
PEEK + CF	2.5×10^{-7}	0.29	8.5×10^{-7}	0.35
PEEK + CF + TF + Gr	7.5×10^{-8}	0.17	8.7×10^{-7}	0.13

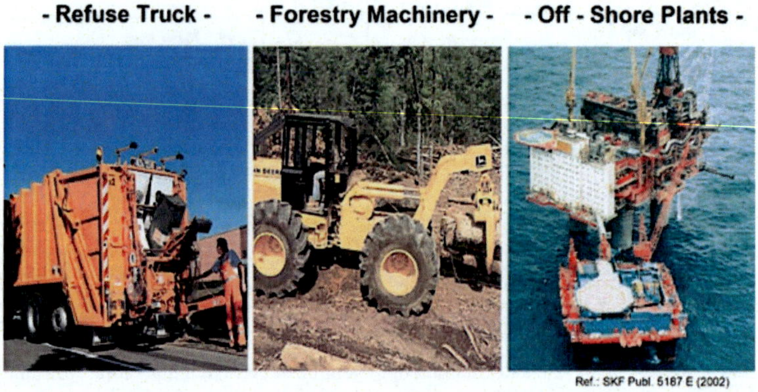

Fig. 6.22 Three examples in which filament wound bushings have to operate under harsh environmental conditions

Fig. 6.23 FW bushings with different diameters and widths

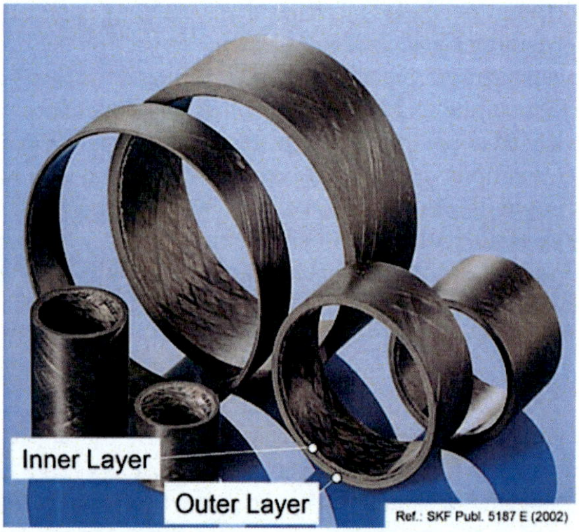

preventing passage of electric current. Their load bearing capacity under low sliding speeds (less than 0.01 m/s) can be up to 150 MPa.

A new way to produce such bearings involves a thermoplastic solution. This brings about further benefits, such as higher impact toughness, a greater flexibility in the design of the final components, and faster processing cycles. Figure 6.24 illustrates schematically the individual processing steps:

(a) starting with a pre-designed commingled yarn, consisting of reinforcing fibers (e.g., aramid fibers), self-lubricating PTFE-fibers, and, e.g., polyamide (PA) fibers, of which the latter are transferred during the thermoplastic filament winding process into the final matrix of the composite;

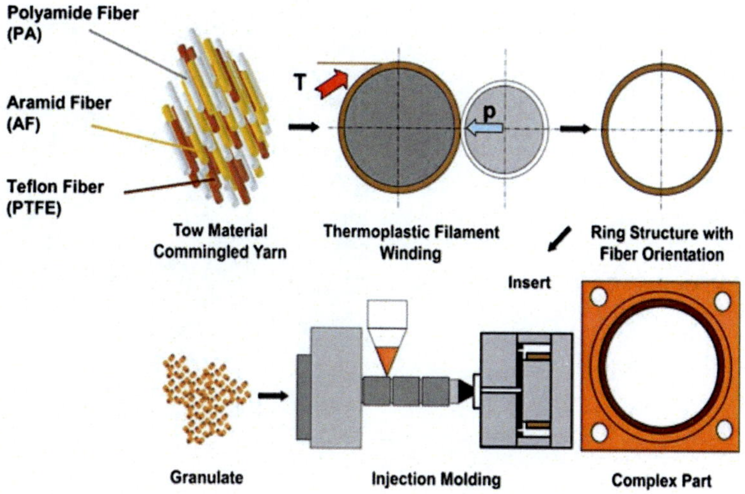

Fig. 6.24 Principle processing steps for producing filament wound thermoplastic bushings or flange bearings

(b) filament winding of the tribologically loaded, inner layer of the composite bushing by using a certain steel mandrel, a heating device (e.g., hot air gun; *T*) and a compaction roller (*p*) [57];
(c) over-winding of the inner layer with a backing layer, using another commingled yarn which consists of the same matrix fibers and a high volume fraction of glass fibers, in order to provide the bushing with a high load bearing capacity;
(d) alternatively, the filament wound inner layer can be used as an insert in an injection molding tool, around which a short glass fiber-reinforced thermoplastic (usually being the same as the matrix fibers in the commingled yarn) can be injection molded in order to create a more complex end-geometry, such as a full flange bearing.

That such products can be produced in this way, is shown in Fig. 6.25. The left part represents the wound structure of the inner layer, in the lower right a simple ring represents an inner layer with an injection molded (white looking) outer layer around, and in the inserted picture, a cross-section through the inner layer can be seen. The latter represents in yellow the aramid fiber bundles, in black the PTFE-fiber bundles, both impregnated with and embedded in the PA-matrix (as a result of the molten PA-fibers). Prior to the injection molding process the insert was preheated in order to guarantee a strong bonding between the wound insert and the surrounding polymer. A very important parameter was the hot air temperature used for preheating. Air temperatures of about 400°C led to the desired shear strength values of about 18 MPa between the two layers. Testing of this final component in a journal bearing tester indicated its good performance in terms of coefficient of friction, wear resistance and high thermal stability, in relation to a competitive

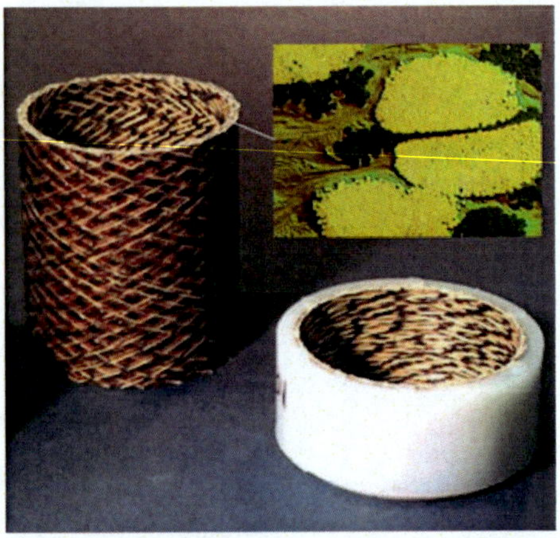

Fig. 6.25 Real bushings made by thermoplastic filament winding, without or in combination with injection molding

commercial material under comparable pressure, temperature and velocity conditions. In fact, the commercially available thermosetting composite bearing resulted in higher values of the coefficient of friction than the thermoplastic filament wound bearing [58].

6.4.1.3 Cages of High-Precision Ball Bearings in Dental Turbines

A thermosetting prepreg winding process is used to produce phenolic (PF) resin matrix-based composite tubes, which are afterward machined into small cages for high precision, miniature ball bearings. The latter are used in dental turbines that operate under water lubrication at a speed of 400,000 rpm (Fig. 6.26) [59]. At first, cotton fiber-based fabrics are impregnated with liquid phenolic resin, in order to achieve textile fiber-based prepregs, which are then wound on a steel mandrel in order to achieve a small tube. After curing, the tubes are cut into rings, from which the cage geometry is machined (Fig. 6.27).

6.4.1.4 Pumps for Aggressive Media

Tribotechnical systems, in which abrasive wear cannot be avoided, are for instance pumps used for the transport of abrasive fluids, as they can be found in chemical factories, on- and off-shore conveyor systems, or in the mining industry. Is the abrasive fluid also chemically aggressive, so that no leakage during the fluid transport is acceptable, hermetically sealed pumps must be used (Fig. 6.28), in which the medium to be conveyed simultaneously acts as a lubricant for the various bearing positions in the pump [60]. Important for such pumps is a high reliability, long maintenance intervals, and good emergency running properties during malfunctions in operation. The use of ceramic bearings is in this respect a

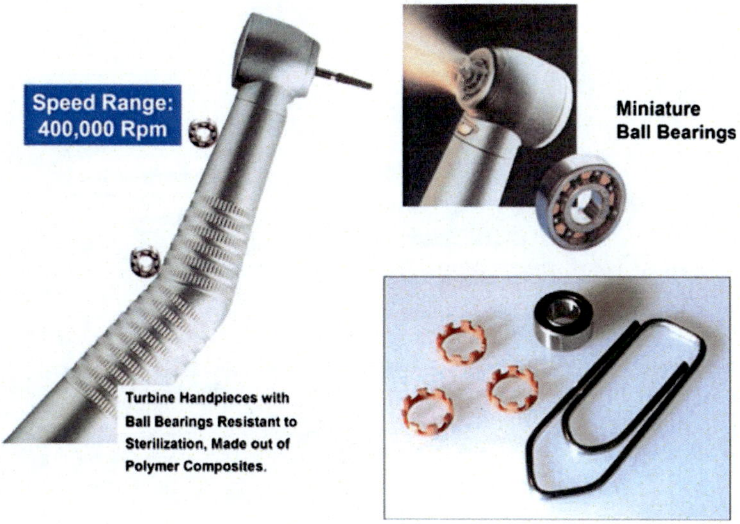

Fig. 6.26 Polymer composite cages in dental turbine handpieces [59]

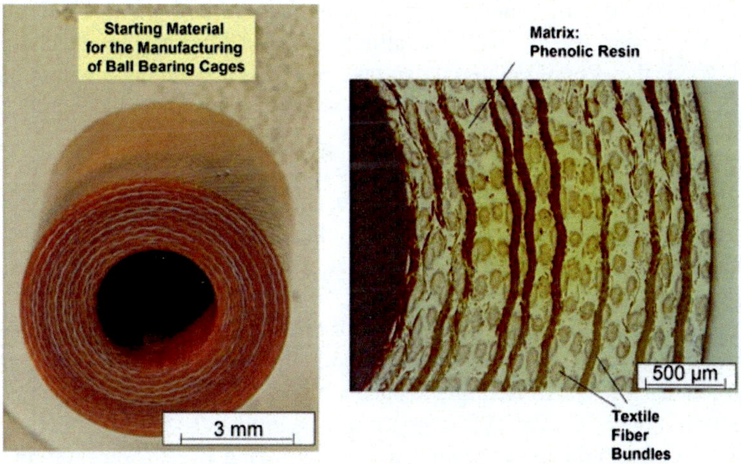

Fig. 6.27 Textile wound tube (*left*), and enlargement of its cross-section, showing axial and tangential cotton fiber bundles, embedded in a phenolic resin matrix (*right*)

good material selection, since they possess under lubricated, abrasive and corrosive conditions an excellent tribological potential, which cannot be beaten by polymeric composite solutions. However, an important drawback of the currently used monolithic silicon carbide (SiC) ceramic bearings is based on their brittleness and therefore their low tolerance against impact loadings (e.g., during cavitation effects in the pumps). Besides, this material is very expensive, hard to machine

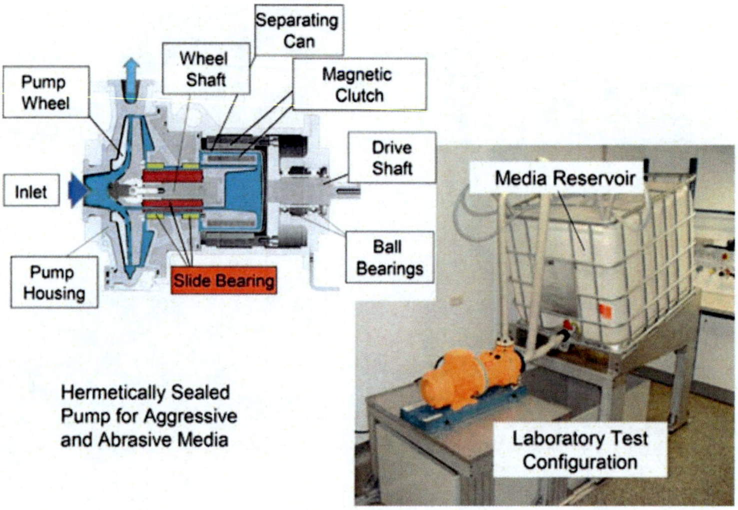

Fig. 6.28 Cross-section of hermetically sealed pump (*left*), and setup for testing the wear behavior of slide bearing inside the pump under realistic conditions (*right*)

into desired geometries, and it does not allow any kind of geometrical tolerances. The latter results in the fact that already by small misalignment chippings or spallings of the ceramic material can take place. The resulting ceramic pieces, in turn, can act very severely as third body abrasives and may cause a catastrophic failure of the whole pump. By the use of polymeric composites, these disadvantages could be reduced or even eliminated, especially they can be designed for better emergency running properties, also under unlubricated operational conditions. In addition, polymer composites offer, due to their higher ductility in comparison to SiC, a higher damage tolerance in the case of edge pressures or impact loadings.

An approach to replace SiC-bearings for this application in the future is to use a thermosetting or thermoplastic resin, highly filled with fibrous and particulate reinforcements [61]. An example of such a highly filled epoxy matrix composite is shown in Fig. 6.29. The SCFs contribute significantly to the strength of the material, the graphite flakes provide a self-lubricating effect (especially in the case of dry operational conditions), the hard SiC-filler particles result in a higher hardness of the composite (since the hardness of the abrasive particles in the fluid is usually lower), and the nano-sized TiO_2-particles fill the gaps between the other micro-sized fillers and provide, therefore, a more uniform overall mechanical and tribological behavior of the composite system.

For the development and testing of these materials on a laboratory level, a new wear testing device had to be built in which the block on ring-configuration could be operated under the presence of a fluid, containing additional abrasive particles (Fig. 6.30). Using this device, with wollastonite abrasive particles in water as the abrasive fluid, it could be shown that a replacement of wollastonite filler particles

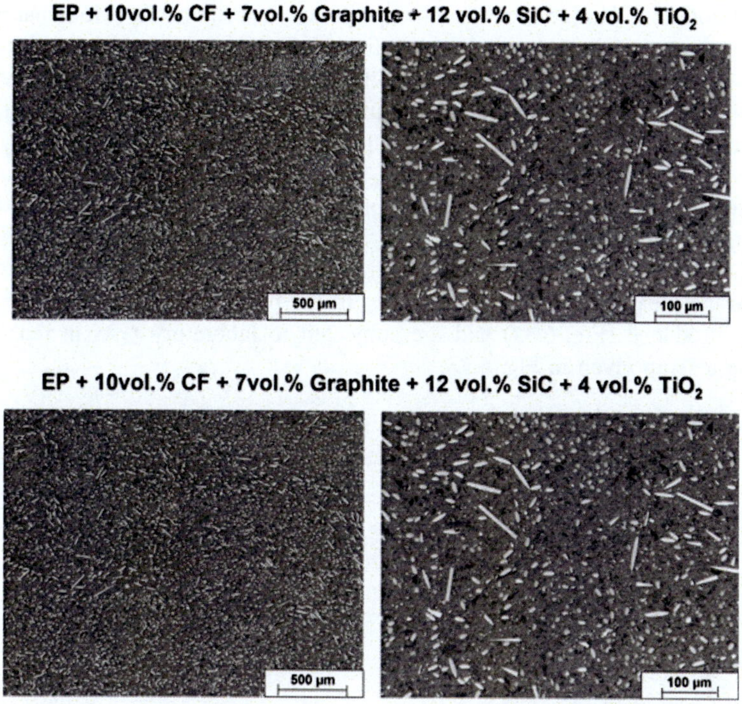

Fig. 6.29 Low (*left*) and high magnification (*right*) of a highly filled epoxy-based composite

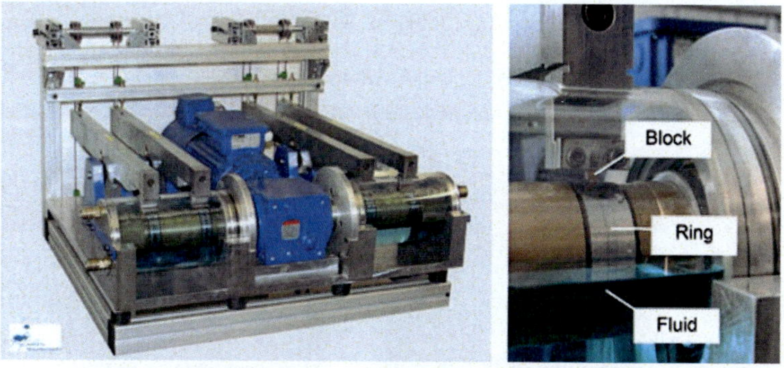

Fig. 6.30 Newly designed four stations-block on ring-testing facility, operating in a fluid medium

in the composite by harder SiC-particles of equivalent amounts (keeping the other types of fillers constant) resulted in a better wear resistance of the composites (Fig. 6.31). If one compares, for example, 8 vol.% wollastonite filler in the composite with 8 vol.% SiC-filler in the composite, the improvement in wear resistance is more than a factor of 10. This confirms that for abrasive loading conditions, the hardness of the filler plays an important role (Mohs hardness of wollastonite is 4.8; Mohs hardness of SiC is 9.5). It should also be mentioned here that the composites with the best compromise in the filler composition (10% carbon fibers, 10% graphite, 12% of 9 μm-sized SiC-particles) resulted in a similar wear behavior as the monolithic SiC when tested against diamond grinding wheels (Mohs hardness of diamond is 10, i.e., harder than SiC). Only when the abrasive counterpart was softer than SiC, e.g., corundum polishing paper (Mohs hardness of corundum is 9), the pure SiC was superior to the composites in its wear resistance [62].

In the meantime, the first prototypes of the polymer composite bearings have been produced (Fig. 6.32) and are subjected to laboratory tests in real pumps, using a setup given in Fig. 6.28.

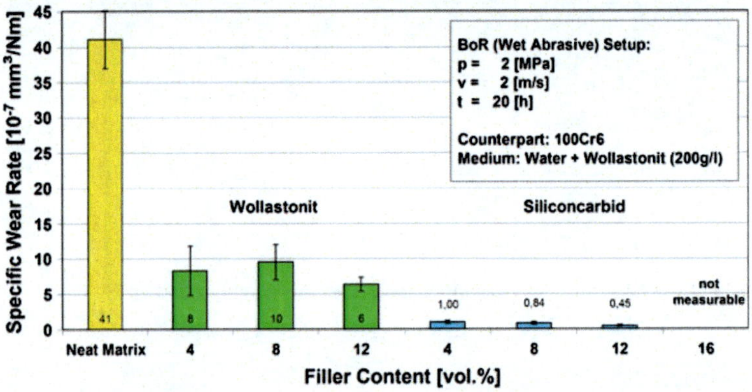

Fig. 6.31 Specific wear rate of various highly filled epoxies under wet/abrasive conditions

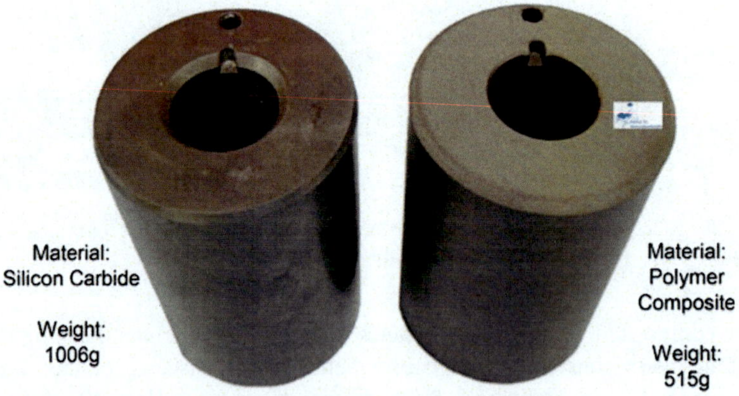

Fig. 6.32 Comparison of the new composite bearing (*right*) with the existing one made of monolithic SiC (*left*)

6.4.2 Paper Making Industry

6.4.2.1 Calender Roller Covers

Huge machines with numerous calender rollers are usually used to produce paper from cellulose slurry (Fig. 6.33). In certain sectors of these machines, some calender rollers have a thick polymer composite layer on their surface. These calender roller "covers" must possess a wide mechanical property profile, i.e., being stiff, strong, and hard, on the one side, and impact resistant, on the other. In addition, their sliding and abrasive wear resistance should be high, in order to prevent short maintenance intervals of the huge production machines (high economical factor). The composition of currently used calender roller covers is based on an epoxy resin matrix, filled with μm-sized ceramic particles. The amount of the compounds used for covering one roller only can range up to 500 kg, depending on the roller's length and diameter (Fig. 6.34) [63].

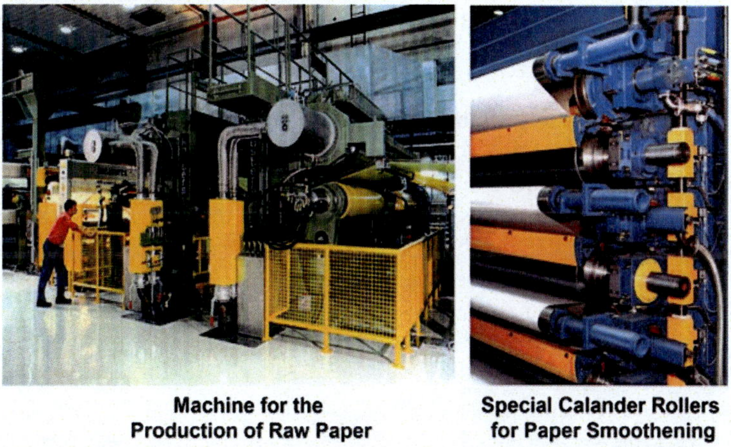

Fig. 6.33 Numerous calender rollers in a huge paper making machine

Fig. 6.34 A large calender roller, freshly covered with a newly designed nano-compound

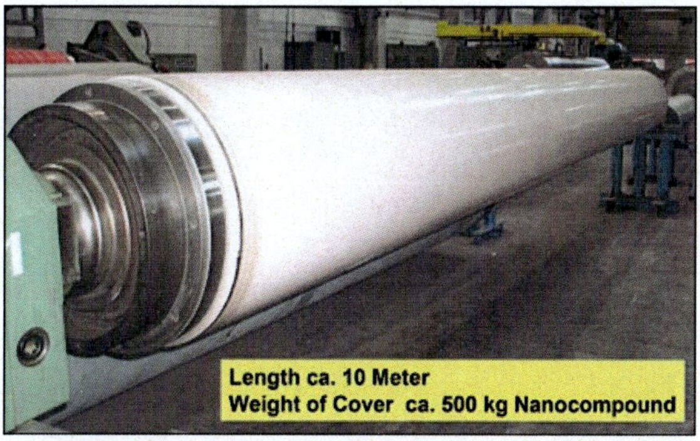

Recent developments have shown that for the future generation of these covers, the use of additional nano-particles can further improve their property profile. In fact, in laboratory experiments it could be verified that the use of nano-sized alumina particles in combination with classical µm-sized silicon carbide particles improves the bending strength, the elongation to break, the impact energy, and the abrasive wear resistance simultaneously, when compared to the standard grade (Fig. 6.35). These improvements are also reflected in the life cycle of the roller covers, when tested under very severe (therefore less time consuming) rolling conditions. Here, a small steel roller (diameter 100 mm; width 15 mm) rotated under line contact load against the cover of a calender roller specimen (external diameter ca. 100 mm). The damage development in the nip point region was observed by the use of a thermocamera. Developments of local hot spots indicated the failure initiation, before finally real chunks of the composite material broke out of the contact track. Measuring the time to this catastrophic failure resulted in a clearly better performance of the new, nano-modified cover materials relative to the commercial standards (Fig. 6.36) [64]. In the meantime, field tests with real rollers in paper machines have also proved to perform better when the nano-compounds were applied, and also the quality of the paper seemed to be higher.

6.4.2.2 Roller Cleaning Blades

Another important application of polymer composites in the paper making industry are the so-called doctor blades that are used to clean the surfaces of rotating rollers from remains of the cellulose slurry or other obstacles (Fig. 6.37) [65]. Also here, some kind of sliding/abrasive type wear takes place at the sharp edges of the blades, and improving their wear resistance also contributes to longer maintenance

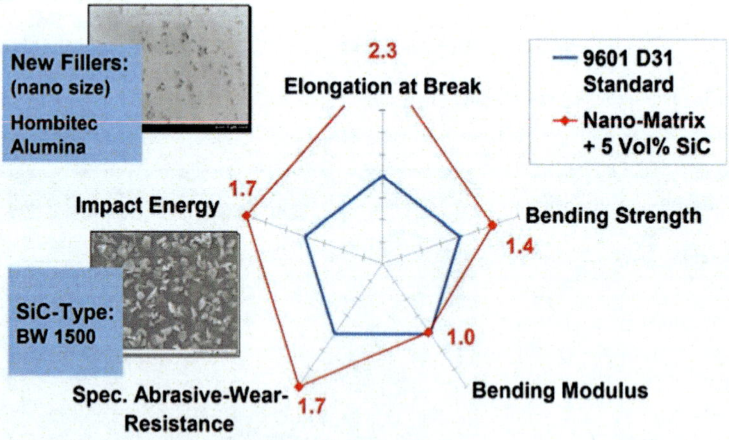

Fig. 6.35 Comparison of various properties of a standard cover material and a new nano-compound (including micro-SiC and nano-alumina particles)

intervals of the paper production lines. The classical blades are composed of a glass or carbon fiber fabric reinforcement, embedded in an epoxy matrix. The fabric reinforcement is necessary to give the blades a sufficient bending stiffness during handling and operation in the machine. For improving their wear resistance, one way is to increase the wear resistance of the matrix material by the use of additional fillers. The other way is to replace the epoxy matrix by a more wear resistant polymer (using, e.g., PEEK, if the higher cost can be justified), also in combination with additional particulate fillers. First attempts in this direction seem to be promising, even when replacing the epoxy matrix not by the more expensive

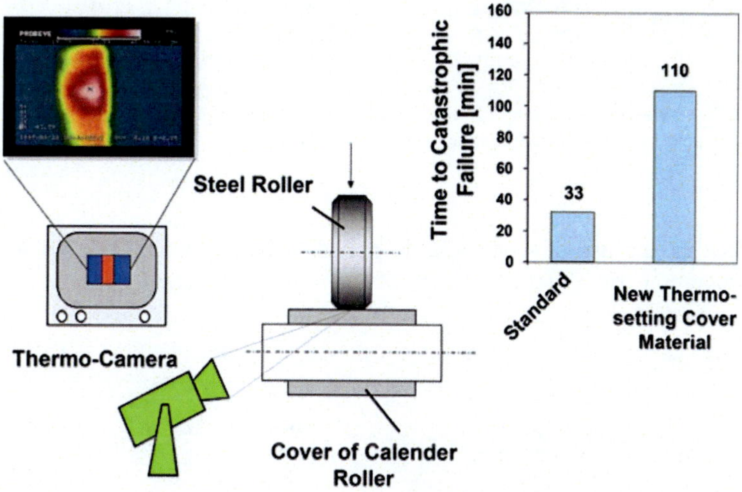

Fig. 6.36 Accelerated rolling wear test of two different materials for calender roller covers

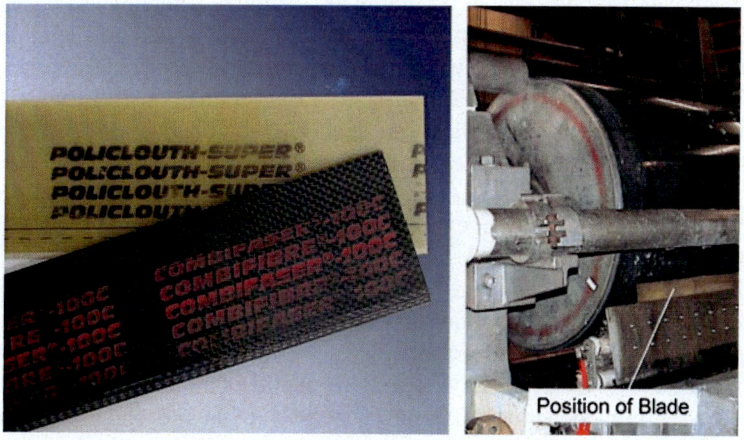

Fig. 6.37 Doctor blades with glass or carbon fiber reinforcements (*left*), and their position for cleaning the surface of rotating calender rollers (*right*) (*Source*: http://www.clouth.com)

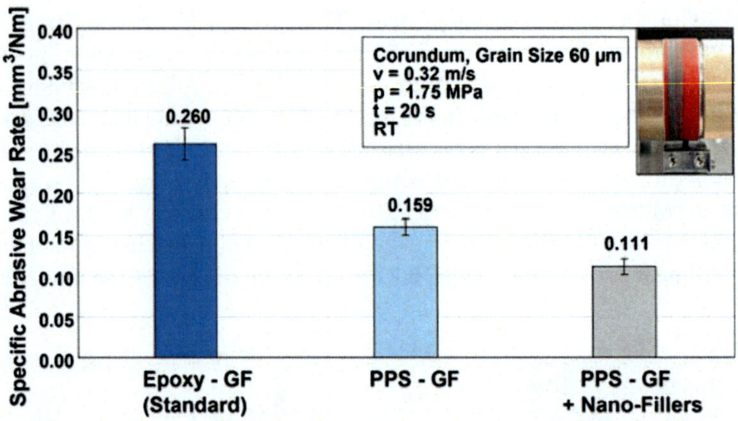

Fig. 6.38 Abrasive wear rate of a standard doctor blade against corundum paper and its improvement by various modifications (GF = glass fiber)

PEEK, but the use of thermoplastic polyphenylenesulfide (PPS). An additional incorporation of different types of nano-particles results even in further improvements (Fig. 6.38).

6.4.3 Automotive Components

6.4.3.1 Hybrid Bushings in Under-the-Hood-Aggregates

There are many applications in the automotive industry where hybrid bushings are needed to guarantee the function of different car components over a long period of time. The components include windshield wiper motors, shock absorbers, steering shaft joints, door hinges, etc. (Fig. 6.39). By incorporating a plastic material into a porous bronze sinter layer applied to a steel or aluminum back (hybrid structure), a low friction matrix that unites favorable tribological properties with the load-carrying properties and thermal conductivity of metals is obtained. The use of solid lubricants in the plastic matrix produces a film between the sliding surfaces and makes it possible to use such bearings in applications without oil- and grease lubrication. It also attributes to low-noise operation at constant speeds and low coefficients of friction throughout the entire service life of the component [66].

In recent years, the requirements on the performance of such bushings have been increased toward higher temperature applications and higher (pressure × velocity)—loading conditions. The new generation of these bushings is supposed to be used as camshaft bearings in high pressure, diesel fuel injection pumps (Fig. 6.40), or even in the engine of the cars. One way to fulfill these extremely high requirements, was to formulate and apply a PEEK plastic matrix compounded with special nano-scaled fillers to improve its tribological properties (Table 6.3) [67].

During the development phase of this, now commercially available product (Permaglide®, KS Gleitlager, Germany), the compounding of the composites and

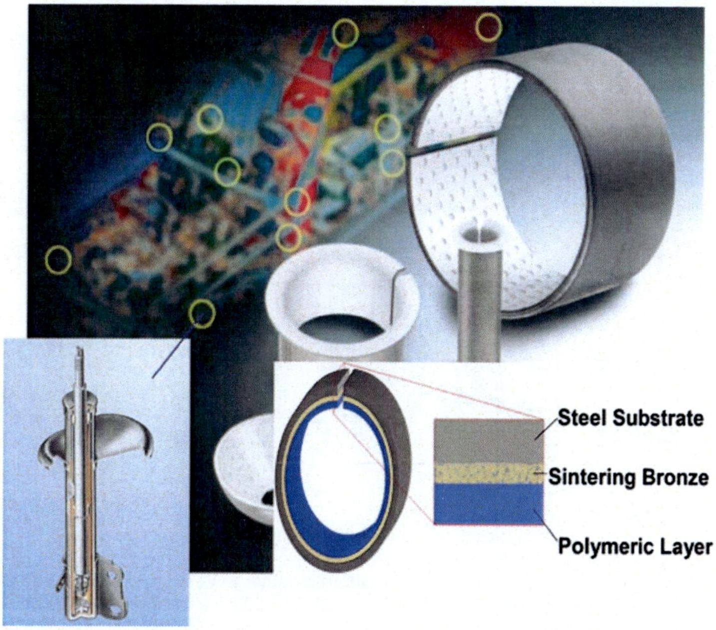

Fig. 6.39 Schematic structure of hybrid bushings (*lower right*) and their use in various automotive locations, including shock absorbers (*lower left*)

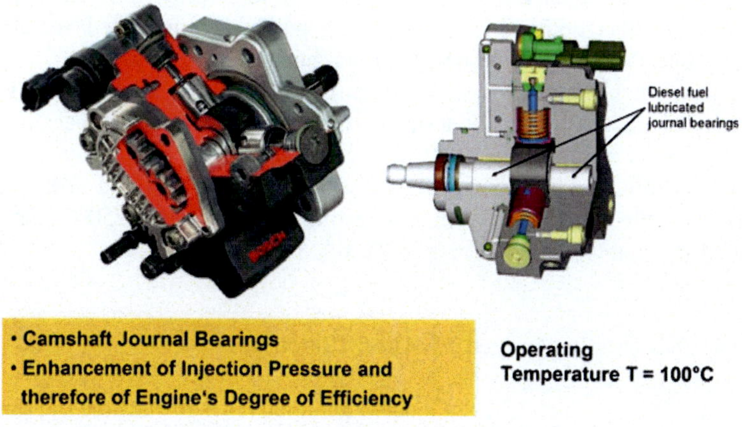

Fig. 6.40 Camshaft journal bearings in a diesel fuel injection pump (*upper left*: view into a real pump; *upper right*: schematic, three dimensional drawing of the bearings' position); Courtesy of Robert Bosch GmbH, Stuttgart, Germany (modified)

Table 6.3 Compositions of two PEEK-composites investigated

PEEK compound no.	Code name	C-fibers	PTFE	Graphite	Nano 1	Nano 2
4	CPZ	x	x	x	–	–
6	CGZT	x	–	x	x	x

Nano 1 = TiO_2, *Nano 2* = ZnS

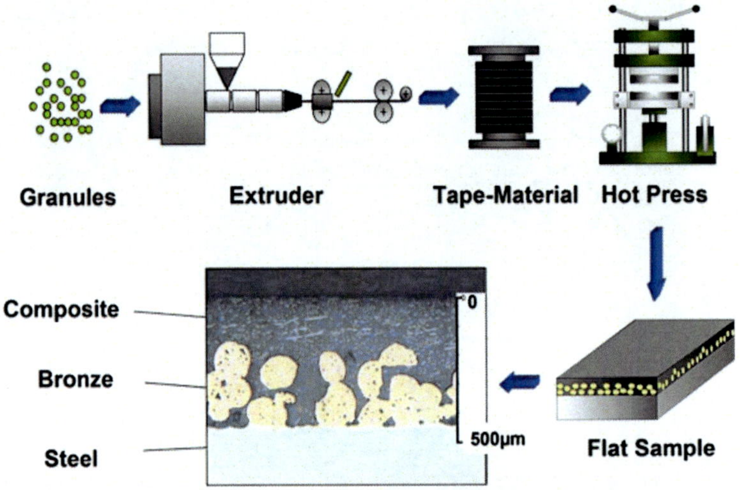

Fig. 6.41 Laboratory production steps for impregnating a PEEK-composite into the porous bronze layer on top of the steel substrate

their extrusion into flat tapes had to be studied on a laboratory scale. The same was true for the incorporation of the tape material into the sinter bronze modified steel substrates, using a laboratory hot press. A good impregnation as well as the achievement of a uniform thickness of the polymer composite layer above the porous sinter bronze scaffold needed to be guaranteed (Fig. 6.41)

In fact, when comparing the two PEEK-compounds with regard to their tribological characteristics (using a ring on flat test configuration), it became evident that, especially at higher loading conditions and elevated temperatures, the nano-modified PEEK was superior to the classical PEEK variant and other, commercially available references. Even at a testing temperature of 250°C, the PEEK6 resulted in reliable test data (Fig. 6.42) [68, 69].

6.4.3.2 Elements in Damped Flywheel Clutches

The function of such clutches in modern automotives is to shift the transmission's resonance frequency below the engines initial running frequency. In this way it shall reduce gear rattles and prevent the transfer of vibrations from the engine to the vehicle's chassis. This, in turn, improves the driving comfort.

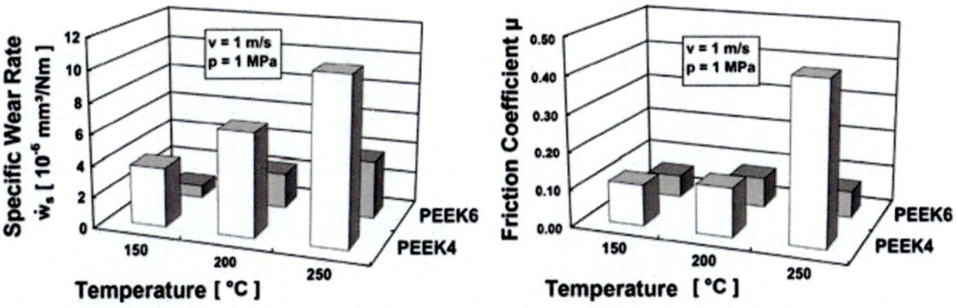

Fig. 6.42 Specific wear and coefficient of friction of two PEEK-composites in a temperature range between 150 and 250°C

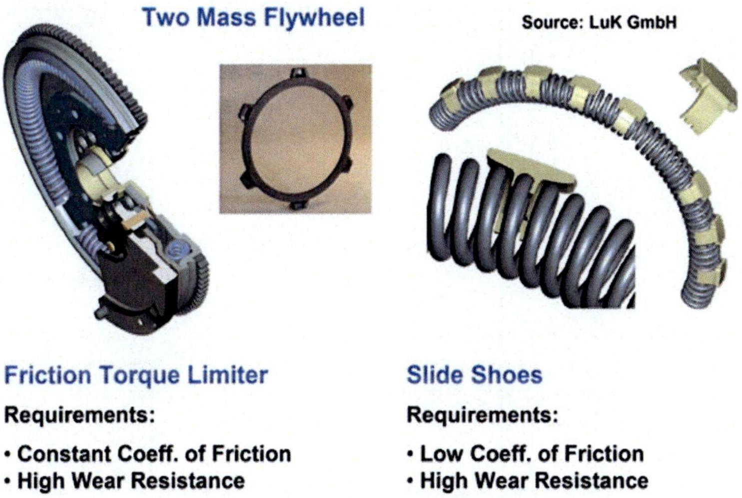

Fig. 6.43 Polymeric components in an automotive damped flywheel clutch

Polymer components within this complicated system are sliding shoes attached to the coils springs within the dual mass flywheel of the clutch, and friction torque limiters (Fig. 6.43). The requirements to the latter are to protect both the engine and the transmission from torque peaks. For this to happen, the coefficient of friction must not change during the entire lifetime, there should not be any or at least only a very short running-in behavior, and the material must have a high sliding wear resistance [70].

As a matrix for this application, a high temperature resistant polyamide (PA 4.6) was chosen. In a comprehensive study of this polymer it was found out that a good combination of SCFs with PTFE-particles as internal lubricants systematically improves its friction and wear properties [71]. The data have also been analyzed by the use of an artificial neural network (ANN) approach, a mathematical tool to empirically evaluate highly non-linear, multi-parametric relationships [72, 73]. In order to train such an ANN, enough experimental data must be

Table 6.4 Set of input data for the training of an artificial neural network

Material composition		Material data				Test parameters					Test result	
Nr.	Material	$\bar{\sigma}$ (MPa)	E (MPa)	ε (%)	a_k (J/mm^2)	T (°C)	F (N)	f (Hz)	A (mm)	v (m/s)	μ (1)	ΔV (mm^3)
1	PA46	76	2650	3.8	9.8	20	5	40	0.5	0.04	0.89	0.3917
2	PA46	76	2650	3.8	9.8	20	22	40	0.5	0.04	0.93	1.8755
3	PA46-GF	201	7090	4.5	4.88	20	8	20	0.5	0.02	0.38	0.0301
9	PA46-GF	201	7090	4.5	4.88	20	22	40	2.5	0.2	0.67	0.8704
10	PA46-GF-PTFE	193	7058	4.2	4.85	20	9	20	0.5	0.02	0.14	0.0075
16	PA46-GF-PTFE	193	7058	4.2	4.85	20	23	40	2.5	0.2	0.53	0.4925
17	PA46-CF	100	3848	3.4	1.27	20	7	20	0.5	0.02	0.27	0.0428
23	PA46-CF-PTFE	95	3674	3.3	1.29	20	23	40	2.5	0.2	0.56	1.4281
24	PA46-CF-PTFE	95	3674	3.3	1.29	20	9	20	0.5	0.02	0.16	0.0129
30	PA46-CF-PTFE	95	3674	3.3	1.29	20	20	40	2.5	0.2	0.53	0.9857
72	PA46-GF-PTFE-Gr	53	2039	2.9	4.2	150	6	40	2.5	0.2	0.35	0.2060

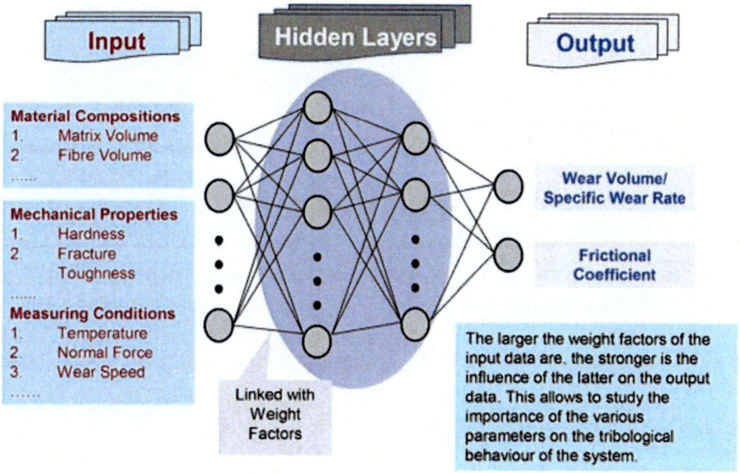

Fig. 6.44 Input data, output data, and schematic construction of an artificial neural network for correlating tribological properties with testing and material parameter [43]

available, so as to achieve reliable prediction results at the end. In the case of the PA 4.6-composites, the total data set of 72 measurements was randomly subdivided into 69 training data and three test data (Table 6.4). The training data set is used to obtain the coefficients of the neural network equation so that the mean squared error of the predicted wear volume is minimized (Fig. 6.44). The test data set is used to compare the ANN predictions with the experimental results.

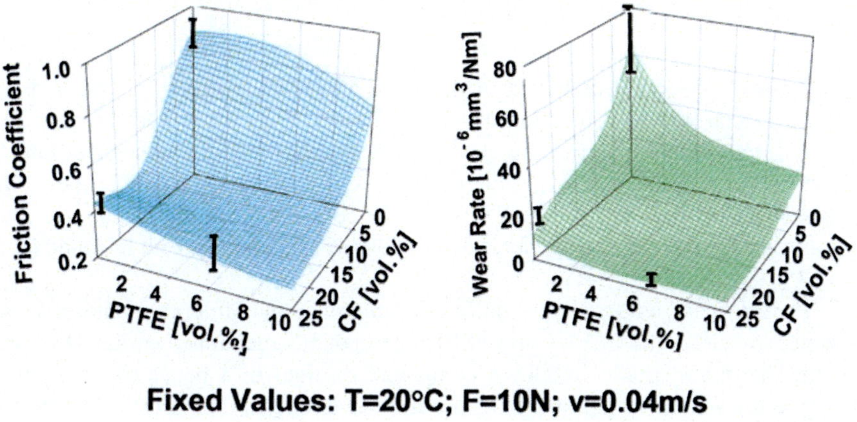

Fig. 6.45 The coefficient of friction (*left*) and specific wear rate (*right*) of a polyamide 4,6 (PA4,6) composite as a function of PTFE- and short CF-volume content. The experimental data points and their scatters are given by the *black bars*, whereas the rest of the 3D-grid was calculated by an artificial neural network approach

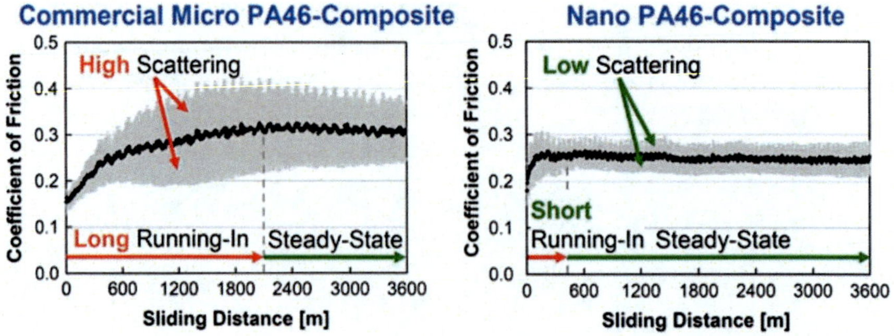

Fig. 6.46 Coefficient of friction of PA4,6 composites without (*left*) and with (*right*) additional nano-particles

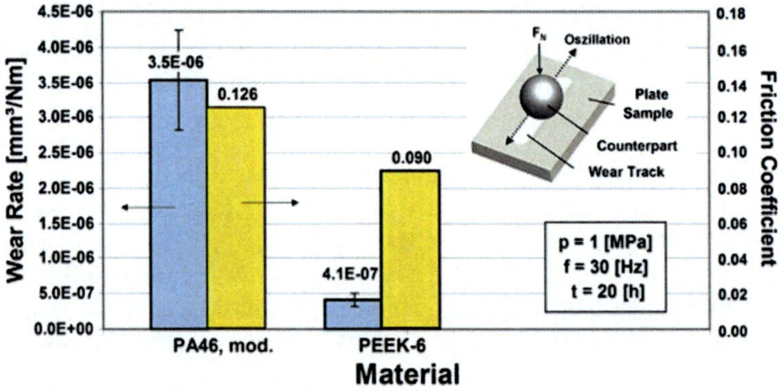

Fig. 6.47 Comparison between the tribological properties of a modified PA4,6-compound with the newly developed PEEK 6–composite under dry oscillatory wearing conditions

Figure 6.45 demonstrates the changes in the coefficient of friction and the specific wear rate as a function of PTFE particle- and carbon fiber-content. The grids refer to the predictions by the well trained ANN, and the three error bars in each diagram represent experimental values for testing the predictions. The agreement between the two data sets is quite convincing. In the meantime, other polymeric composite systems have been analyzed successfully with this method as well [74].

For the final friction torque limiters, the combination of fillers was chosen in the same way as for the PEEK4 and PEEK6 compounds mentioned earlier. And also here, the nano-particles modified compound resulted in a better overall performance toward the requirements of the friction torque limiter (Fig. 6.46). In particular, (a) a shorter running-in period resulted in more uniform clutching characteristics, (b) the same is true for the better time stability of the coefficient of friction in the steady state range, and (c) less scattering of the data (achieved in various tests) indicated a higher production uniformity of the individual parts [75].

With regard to the sliding shoes attached to the coil springs, these elements are subjected to an oscillatory motion against the surrounding metallic frame, since the springs are loaded under tension and compression in a reciprocating fashion. In order to find out, which potential is available in reducing both, friction coefficient and specific wear rate under these conditions, the reference material (a PA 4.6 compound containing a high amount of PTFE filler) was compared to one of the best PEEK—compounds, so far available on the market (PEEK6). Tests were carried out under external initiation lubrication, using a special kind of grease. As expected, compared to the reference material (which has already a good tribological performance under these conditions), the use of the PEEK6-nanocomposite can even top this behavior, especially with regard to the specific wear resistance (inverse of the specific wear rate) (Fig. 6.47).

6.5 Conclusions

In conclusion, it can be stated that the use of polymer-based composites for tribological applications is very widespread, but their structural design depends highly on the engineering system in which these materials have to operate. In most of the cases discussed here, they had to slide against a metallic counterpart, using their self-lubricating function to reduce the coefficient of friction. Special reinforcements helped to make them also quite wear-resistant. New developments in this respect use additional nano-particles that incorporate further, wear reducing mechanisms into the tribo-system. This has not only been shown on a laboratory scale, but also in various applications, such as in paper making machines, automotive components or other mechanical engineering facilities. But there is still enough room for further, future developments. These include also the use of carbon nano-tubes or nano-fibers, as it was highlighted by some recent publications in this field [e.g., 76, 77].

Acknowledgments The authors are grateful to the IVW GmbH, Technical University Kaiserslautern where most of the results were generated. One of us, Dr.-Ing. L. Chang greatly appreciates the support of the Alexander von Humboldt-Foundation for his research stay at IVW during the year 2008.

References

1. Fischer S, Marom G (1987) The flexural behaviour of aramid fibre hybrid composite materials. Compos Sci Technol 28:291–314
2. Hofer K Jr, Stander M, Bennett L (1978) Degradation and enhancement of the fatigue behavior of glass/graphite/epoxy hybrid composites after accelerated aging. Polym Eng Sci 18:120–127
3. Schulte K, Reese E, Chou TW (1987) Fatigue behaviour and damage development in woven fabric and hybrid fabric composites. In: Mathews FL et al (eds) Proceedings of ICCM-VI/ECCM-11, 4th edn. Elsevier, London

4. Marom G, Harel H, Friedrich K, Schulte K, Wagner HD (1989) Fatigue behaviour and rate-dependent properties of aramid fibre/carbon fibre hybrid composites. Compos A 6:537–544
5. Nalwa HS (2003) Handbook of organic–inorganic hybrid materials and nanocomposites, vol 2. American Scientific Publishers, Stevenson Ranch
6. Wetzel B, Haupert F, Zhang MQ (2003) Epoxy nanocomposites with high mechanical and tribological performance. Compos Sci Technol 63:2055–2067
7. Wetzel B (2006) Mechanische Eigenschaften von Nanokompositen aus Epoxydharz und keramischen Nanopartikeln. Dissertation Technische Universität Kaiserslautern. In: Schlarb AK (ed) IVW-Schriftenreihe, Band 69, Kaiserslautern, Germany
8. Zhang MQ, Rong MZ, Friedrich K (2003) Processing and properties of non-layered nanoparticle reinforced thermoplastic composites. In: Nalwa HS (ed) Handbook of organic–inorganic hybrid materials and nanocomposites. American Scientific Publishers, Los Angeles
9. Chow TS (1980) Review: the effect of particle shape on the mechanical properties of filled polymers. J Mater Sci 15:1873–1888
10. Coleman JN, Khan U, Blau WJ, Gun'ko YK (2006) Small but strong: a review of the mechanical properties of carbon nanotube-polymer composites. Carbon 44:1624–1652
11. Sullivan JL, Blais EJ, Houston D (1993) Physical aging in the creep behavior of thermosetting and thermoplastic composites. Compos Sci Technol 47:389–403
12. Zhang Z, Yang JL, Friedrich K (2004) Creep resistant polymeric nanocomposites. Polymer 45:3481–3485
13. Giltrow JP, Lancaster JK (1970) The role of the counterface in the friction and wear of carbon fibre reinforced thermosetting resins. Wear 16:359–374
14. Lancaster JK (1972) Polymer-based bearing materials, the role of fillers and fibre reinforcement. Tribology 5:249–255
15. Albert K, Schledjewski R, Harbaugh M, Bleser S, Jamison R, Friedrich K (1994) Characterization of wear in composite material orthopaedic implants. Part II: the implant/bone interface. Biomed Mater Eng 4:199–211
16. Czichos H, Habig KH (1992) Tribologie Handbuch Reibung und Verschleiss. Vieweg, Braunschweig
17. Friedrich K (1997) Wear performance of high temperature polymers and their composites. In: Luise RR (ed) Application of high temperature polymers. CRC Press, Boca Raton
18. Reinicke R, Haupert F, Friedrich K (1998) On the tribological behaviour of selected, injection moulded thermoplastic composites. Compos A 29:763–771
19. Häger AM, Davies M (1993) Short-fiber reinforced, high temperature resistant polymers for a wide field of tribological applications. In: Friedrich K (ed) Advances in composite tribology. Elsevier, Amsterdam
20. Schwartz CJ, Bahadur S (2000) Studies on the tribological behavior and transfer film-counterface bond strength for polyphenylene sulfide filled with nanoscale alumina particles. Wear 237:261–273
21. Zhang LC, Zarudi I, Xiao KQ (2006) Novel behaviour of friction and wear of epoxy composites reinforced by carbon nanotubes. Wear 261:806–811
22. Haupert F, Xian G, Oster F, Walter R, Friedrich K (2004) Tribological behaviour of nano-particle reinforced polymeric coatings. In: Bartz WJ (ed) Proceedings of 14th International Colloquium Tribology, Stuttgart
23. Werner P, Altstädt V, Jaskulka R, Jacobs O, Sandler JKW, Shaffer MSP, Windle A (2004) Tribological behaviour of carbon-nanofiber-reinforced poly(ether ether ketone). Wear 257:1006–1014
24. Zhang Z, Breidt C, Chang L, Haupert F, Friedrich K (2004) Enhancement of the wear resistance of epoxy: short carbon fibre, graphite, PTFE and nano-TiO_2. Compos A 35:1385–1392
25. Friedrich K, Reinicke R, Zhang Z (2002) Wear of polymer composites. J Eng Tribol 216:415–426
26. Cirino M, Friedrich K, Pipes RB (1988) Evaluation of polymer composites for sliding and abrasive wear applications. Compos A 19:383–392

27. Friedrich K, Theiler G, Klein P (2008) Polymer composites for tribological applications in a range between liquid helium and room temperature. In: Sinha SK, Briscoe BJ (eds) Polymer tribology. Imperial College Press, London
28. Gebhard A, Knör N, Haupert F, Schlarb AK (2007) Nanopartikelverstärkte Hochleistungsthermoplaste für extreme tribologische Belastungen im Automobilbau. In: Proceedings of 48. Tribologie-Fachtagung, GfT, Göttingen I:22/1–22/11
29. Zhang Z, Friedrich K (2005) Tribological characteristics of micro- and nanoparticle filled polymer composites. In: Friedrich K, Fakirov S, Zhang Z (eds) Polymer composite—from nano- to macro-scale. Springer, New York
30. Chang L, Zhang Z, Ye L, Friedrich K (2008) Synergistic effects of nanoparticles and traditional tribo-fillers on sliding wear of polymeric hybrid composites. In: Friedrich K, Schlarb AK (eds) Tribology of polymer nanocomposites. Elsevier, Amsterdam
31. Xue Q, Wang Q (1997) Wear mechanisms of polyetheretherketone composites filled with various kinds of SiC. Wear 213:54–58
32. Wang Q, Xue Q, Liu H, Shen W, Xu J (1996) The effect of particle size of nanometer ZrO_2 on the tribological behavior of PEEK. Wear 198:216–219
33. Xing XS, Li RKY (2004) Wear behavior of epoxy matrix composites filled with uniform sized sub-micron spherical silica particles. Wear 256:21–26
34. Bahadur S, Sunkara C (2005) Effect of transfer film structure, composition and bonding on the tribological behavior of polyphenylene sulfide filled with nano particles of TiO_2, ZnO, CuO and SiC. Wear 258:1411–1421
35. Friedrich K (1986) Wear of reinforced polymers by different abrasive counterparts. In: Friedrich K (ed) Friction and wear of polymer composites. Elsevier, Amsterdam
36. Zhang MQ, Rong MZ, Yu S, Wetzel B, Friedrich K (2002) Improvement of tribological performance of epoxy by the addition of irradiation grafted nano-inorganic particles. Macromol Mater Eng 287:111–115
37. Shi G, Zhang MQ, Rong MZ, Wetzel B, Friedrich K (2003) Friction and wear of low nanometer Si_3N_4 filled epoxy composites. Wear 254:784–796
38. Shi G, Zhang M, Rong M, Wetzel B, Friedrich K (2003) Sliding wear behavior of epoxy containing nano-Al_2O_3 particles with different pretreatments. Wear 256:1072–1081
39. Wetzel B, Haupert F, Friedrich K, Zhang MQ, Rong MZ (2002) Impact and wear resistance of polymer nanocomposites at low filler content. Polym Eng Sci 42:1919–1927
40. Sreekala MS, Eger C (2005) Property improvements of an epoxy resin by nanosilica particle reinforcement. In: Friedrich K, Fakirov S, Zhang Z (eds) Polymer composites—from nano- to macro-scale. Springer, New York
41. Li F, Hu K, Li J, Zhao B (2002) The friction and wear characteristics of nanometer ZnO filled polytetrafluoroethylene. Wear 249:877–882
42. Sawyer WG, Freudenberg KD, Bhimaraj P, Schadler LS (2003) A study on the friction and wear behavior of PTFE filled with alumina nanoparticles. Wear 254:573–580
43. Friedrich K, Zhang Z, Klein P (2005) Wear of polymer composites. In: Stachowiak GW (ed) Wear—materials, mechanisms and practice. Wiley, Chichester
44. Cho MH, Bahadur S (2005) Study of the tribological synergistic effects in CuO-filled and fiber-reinforced polyphenylene sulfide composites. Wear 258:835–845
45. Zhang ZZ, Su FH, Wang K, Jiang W, Men XH, Liu WM (2005) Study on the friction and wear properties of carbon fabric composites reinforced with micro- and nano-particles. Mater Sci Eng 404:251–258
46. Su FH, Zhang ZZ, Wang K, Jiang W, Men XH, Liu WM (2006) Friction and wear properties of carbon fabric composites filled with nano-Al_2O_3 and nano-Si_3N_4. Compos A 37:1351–1357
47. Su FH, Zhang ZZ, Liu WM (2006) Mechanical and tribological properties of carbon fabric composites filled with several nano-particulates. Wear 260:861–868
48. Zhang Z, Haupert F, Friedrich K (2005) Enhancement of the wear resistance of polymer composites by nano-fillers. German Patent Appl. 103 29 228.4-43

49. Jiang Z, Gyurova LA, Schlarb AK, Friedrich K, Zhang Z (2008) Study on friction and wear behavior of polyphenylene sulfide composites reinforced by short carbon fibers and sub-micro TiO_2 particles. Compos Sci Technol 68:734–742
50. Chang L, Zhang Z, Breidt C, Friedrich K (2005) Tribological properties of epoxy nanocomposites: I. Enhancement of the wear resistance by nano-TiO_2 particles. Wear 258:141–148
51. Chang L, Zhang Z (2006) Tribological properties of epoxy nanocomposites: II. A combinative effect of short carbon fiber and nano-TiO_2. Wear 260:869–878
52. Chang L, Zhang Z, Zhang H, Schlarb AK (2006) On the sliding wear of nanoparticles filled polyamide 6,6. Compos Sci Technol 66:3188–3198
53. Chang L, Zhang Z, Zhang H, Friedrich K (2005) Effect of nanoparticles on the tribological behavior of short carbon fiber reinforced poly(etherimide) composites. Tribol Int 38:966–973
54. NN (1989) Die Spannmaschine mit horizontaler Kettenrückführung für Artos: Famatex Spannrahmen der Typenreihe btm 5300. http://www.babcock-textilmaschinen.de
55. Lu Z, Friedrich K (1997) Polymere Hochtemperatur-Verbundwerkstoffe für Anwendungen als Gleitelemente. Mater Wiss Werkst Tech 28:116–123
56. NN (2002) The maintenance-free heavy duty bushing, no. 5187 E. http://www.skf.com
57. Haupert F, Chen C, Friedrich K (1995) Manufacturing of thermoplastic composite parts by combined filament winding and injection molding. In: Proceedings of international conference on composite materials ICCM-10, Whistler, Canada, August 13–18, vol. III. Woodhead Publ. Ltd, Cambridge, pp 381–388
58. Friedrich K, Haupert F, Chen C, Flöck J (1996) New manufacturing techniques for thermoplastic composite bearings. In: Wang TC, Chou TW (eds) Progress in advanced materials and mechanics. Proceedings of ICAM '96. Peking University Press, Beijing
59. NN (2004) Hochpräzisionskugellager für den Dentalbereich. http://www.grw.de
60. NN (2006) Chemiepumpen mit Magnetkupplung. http://www.munsch-chemie-pumpen.de
61. Prehn R (2007) Tribologisch optimierte Hochleistungsverbundwerkstoffe für den Einsatz unter abrasiven Bedingungen. Dissertation Technische Universität Kaiserslautern, June 6. http://kluedo.ub.uni-kl.de/volltexte/2007/2099/index.html
62. Prehn R, Haupert F, Friedrich K (2005) Sliding wear performance of polymer composites under abrasive and water lubricated conditions for pump applications. Wear 259:693–696
63. NN (2002) Ivory and Ivory Xtreme, first commercial covers to bring the exponential benefits of nanoparticle technology to supercalender applications. http://www.xerium.com/stoweWoodwardEurope
64. Haupert F, Paasonen J, Schwambach D, Löhnert K (1999) Optimierung von Hochleistungs-Verbundwerkstoff-Beschichtungen für Kalanderwalzen in der Papierindustrie. Wochenbl Pap Fabr 8:519–521
65. NN (2008) Schaberklingen aus Kunststoff/Verbundfasermaterial. http://www.clouth.com
66. NN (2008) Bleifreier Stahl-Kunststoff-Verbundwerkstoff KS P212. http://www.kspg-ag.de
67. Oster F, Haupert F, Friedrich K, Bickle W, Müller M (2004) Tribologische Hochleistungsbeschichtungen aus neuartigen Polyetheretherketon (PEEK)-Compounds. Tribol Schmiertech 51(3):17–24
68. Oster F, Haupert F, Friedrich K, Müller M, Bickle W (2004) Neuartige Polyetheretherketon (PEEK)-Beschichtungen für hohe tribologische Beanspruchungen. Mater Wiss Werkst Tech 35:690–695
69. Oster F (2005) Hochtemperaturbeständige Polymer-Beschichtungen für tribologische Anwendungen. Dissertation Technische Universität Kaiserslautern. In: Schlarb AK (ed) IVW-Schriftenreihe, Band 53, Kaiserslautern, Germany
70. Gebhard A, Englert M, Bittmann B, Haupert F, Schlarb AK (2007) Nanoparticle reinforced polymeric composites for tribological applications in the automotive industry. In: Proceedings of 2nd international conference on micro- and nano-technology, Vienna
71. Reinicke R (2000) Eigenschaftsprofil neuer Verbundwerkstoffe für tribologische Anwendungen im Automobilbau. Dissertation Technische Universität Kaiserslautern. In: Neitzel M (ed) IVW-Schriftenreihe, Band 21, Kaiserslautern, Germany

72. Velten K, Reinicke R, Friedrich K (2000) Wear volume prediction with artificial neural networks. Tribol Int 33:731–736
73. Zhang Z, Friedrich K, Velten K (2002) Prediction on tribological properties of short fibre composites using artificial neural networks. Wear 252:668–675
74. Jiang Z, Gyurova L, Zhang Z, Friedrich K, Schlarb AK (2008) Neural network based prediction on mechanical and wear properties of short fiber reinforced polyamide composites. Mater Des 29:628–637
75. Gebhard A, Haupert F, Schlarb AK (2008) Development of nanostructured slide coatings for automotive components. In: Friedrich K, Schlarb AK (eds) Tribology of polymeric nanocomposites. Elsevier, Amsterdam
76. Ruckdäschel H, Sandler JKW, Altstädt V (2008) On the friction and wear of carbon nanofiber-reinforced PEEK-based polymer composites. In: Friedrich K, Schlarb AK (eds) Tribology of polymeric nanocomposites. Elsevier, Amsterdam
77. Jacobs O, Schädel B (2008) Wear behavior of carbon nanotube-reinforced polyethylene and epoxy composites. In: Friedrich K, Schlarb AK (eds) Tribology of polymeric nanocomposites. Elsevier, Amsterdam

Chapter 7
Graphite Nanoplatelet Composites and Their Applications

H. T. Hahn and O. Choi

7.1 Introduction

Carbon materials are widely used in various forms, such as fibers and flakes, as reinforcements and additives to improve properties of polymers. The use of carbon fiber composites in 50% of Boeing 787's structural weight is a crowning achievement of composites research over the past 5 decades. During the last decade new forms of carbon have become available, including carbon nanotubes, carbon nanofibers, and graphite nanoplatelets (GNPs).

Much research has been done on carbon nanotubes to fully exploit their excellent properties in structural composites. However, expected benefits still appear to remain somewhat elusive [1]. Some of the properties which make carbon materials attractive are their high stiffness and strength, high electrical and thermal conductivities, and chemical inertness, while being light-weight. One of the new promising carbon reinforcements is graphite nanoplatelet [2–7]. A graphite nanoplatelet consists of lesser than 300 graphene layers bound by weak van der Waals forces with their planar dimensions ranging from a micrometer to a few micrometers. Full exfoliation of micron-size GNPs can thus result in individual graphene sheets with a large aspect ratio easily exceeding 1000.

The benefits of two dimensional (2D) reinforcements via exfoliation have been demonstrated by organoclay nanoplatelets. Compared with clay, graphite has much more attractive properties [8, 9] in many aspects while they both share the

H. T. Hahn (✉) · O. Choi
Mechanical and Aerospace Engineering Department, University of California, Los Angeles, CA 90095, USA
e-mail: hahn@seas.ucla.edu

H. T. Hahn
Materials Science and Engineering Department, California NanoSystems Institute, UCLA, Los Angeles, CA 90095, USA

L. Nicolais et al. (eds.), *Composite Materials*,
DOI: 10.1007/978-0-85729-166-0_7, © Springer-Verlag London Limited 2011

Table 7.1 Approximate ratios of composite modulus to matrix modulus for large aspect ratio and $E_r/E_m \gg 1$

	1D Aligned	2D Random	3D Random
	N/A	N/A	$1 + 3Vr$
Fiber	$1 + V_rE_r/E_m$	$1 + 1/3\ V_rE_r/E_m$	$1 + 1/6\ V_rE_r/E_m$
Platelet	$1 + V_rE_r/E_m$	$1 + V_rE_r/E_m$	$1 + 1/2V_rE_r/E_m$
	V_r: Reinforcement volume fraction	E_r: Reinforcement modulus	E_m: Matrix modulus

same layered structure. Therefore, given proper functionalization, graphite nanoplatelets are expected to yield much better reinforcement effects.

The effect of reinforcement morphology on composite modulus is represented in Table 7.1, which follows from a simplified mechanics analysis under the assumption of high aspect ratio and high modulus ratio. When the reinforcements are randomly distributed in a three dimensional (3D) space, the plate geometry yields three times as high, an improvement in modulus, as the fiber geometry does.

The full utilization of nanoscale reinforcements is contingent upon uniform dispersion of reinforcement phase and good interfacial bonding between the reinforcements and the matrix.

To improve interfacial bonding, a number of methods are used to treat the surface of carbon fibers [10]. Finally, much more work has been done on functionalizing carbon nanotubes and nanofibers [11–13]. One facile method of functionalization is oxidation with nitric acid treatment. The nitric acid oxidation leaves the carboxyl group, among other oxygenated groups such as ketone, alcohol, and ester groups, on the surface that can improve interfacial bonding to the surrounding matrix. A variety of other functional groups can also be attached to the GNP via the carboxyl group. Furthermore, when an amine curing agent is used, the carboxyl group on GNP can react with the amino group on the curing agent, thereby forming an amide linkage. The resulting chemical bonding between the GNPs and the amine-cured epoxy resin yields excellent properties for the resulting composite.

The present chapter shows that a good quality GNP/epoxy composite can be produced by a combination of proper nitric acid treatment and intense sonication. The importance of processing sequence and surface functionalization is demonstrated using amine- and epoxy-functionalized GNPs. A significant amount of strength improvement is shown to be possible through prolonged sonication.

7.2 Materials

7.2.1 Graphite Nanoplatelets

There are a large variety of graphite powders commercially available. A preliminary study with a few different grades of flake graphite has led to the selection

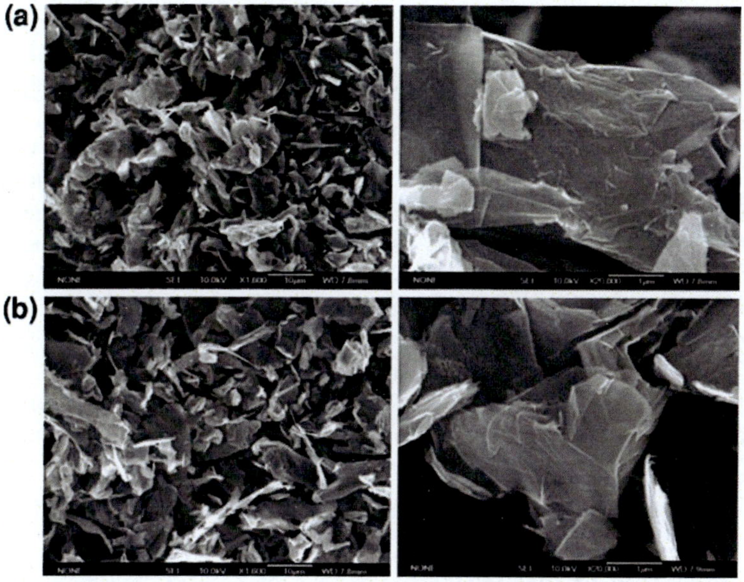

Fig. 7.1 Graphite nanoplatelets (GNPs): **a** as received and **b** nitric acid treated for 30 min

of Asbury 3775 which is described as surface-enhanced natural flake graphite (Fig. 7.1) [14]. It has a nominal carbon content of 98% with 24 m^2/g of surface area. Asbury 3775 has been expanded and milled from larger natural graphite flakes using a fluid energy milling technology to average dimensions of 5–10 μm in plane and about 100 nm in thickness.

7.2.2 Epoxy Resin

The epoxy resin used is a diglycidyl ether of bisphenol F (DGEBF) under the name of Epon 862 combined with a diethyltoluenediamine (DETDA) curing agent called Epicure-W. The mix ratio is maintained at 100:26.5 in favor of Epon 862 [15].

7.3 Nitric Acid Oxidation

7.3.1 Processing

Wet oxidation of GNPs is performed with a 67% nitric acid (HNO_3) solution. GNPs are immersed in the nitric acid solution and heated to 100°C for 30 min with a 200:1 volume ratio of nitric acid to graphite. The GNPs are washed in deionized water and separated out via centrifugation until pH becomes neutral. The nitric acid treated (AT) GNPs are then dried in a vacuum oven at 200°C for 24 h. The AT GNPs are compared with the as-received (AR) GNPs in Fig. 7.1. No discernible differences are seen with the exception of somewhat cleaner appearance on the surfaces of AT GNPs.

Nanocomposites are fabricated using Epon 862 epoxy resin and Epicure-W curing agent. The desired amount of GNPs are mixed with Epon and Epicure (100:26.5 ratio), stirred first by hand, and then for 10 min by a shear mixer. A high-power ultrasonic horn is used for 20 min to achieve a more uniform dispersion of GNPs in the epoxy resin. The well dispersed mixture of epoxy and GNPs is then poured into silicone rubber molds having appropriate geometries for different types of tests in conformance with the applicable ASTM (American Society for Testing and Materials) standards.

For comparison purposes, AR GNPs are also used to fabricate the same type of specimens. These specimens provide the baseline data to show the effect of nitric acid treatment on nanocomposite properties.

7.3.2 Tensile Properties

Tensile properties have been measured using dog-bone shaped specimens having nominal dimensions of 1.2 mm thickness and 8.2 mm gage length in accordance with ASTM D-882. The test results are shown in Fig. 7.2 for both AT and AR GNPs. Regardless of the surface treatment, both strength and modulus increase with increasing GNP loading. The increases are rather rapid up to the GNP loading of 1 vol% and then slow down thereafter. The benefits of the acid treatment are obvious: the modulus and strength of the AT composite are much higher than those of the AR composite at each of the same GNP loadings.

With addition of just 1 vol% of AT GNPs the composite can be made more than 70% stiffer than the resin. Without the acid treatment, however, the increase is much smaller. At the maximum particle loading of 4 vol% studied, the AT

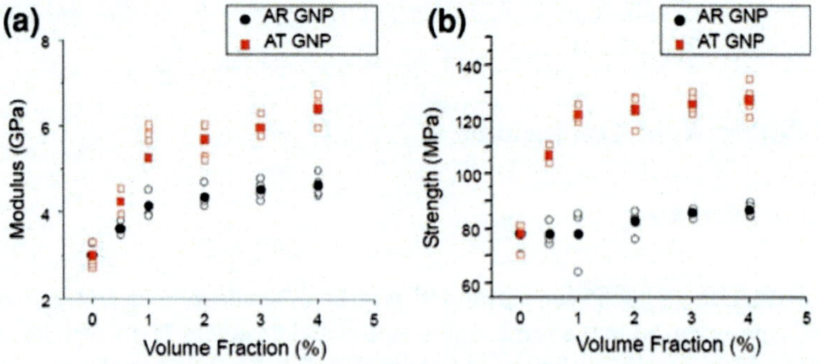

Fig. 7.2 Tensile properties of AR and AT GNP nanocomposites: **a** modulus and **b** strength

composite modulus is 6.4 GPa whereas the corresponding AR composite modulus is only 4.6 GPa.

The increase in strength shows the same trend as that in modulus. One major difference is that the strength does not increase much after 1 vol% GNP loading even for the AT composite. Furthermore, there is only a small strength increase for the AR composite—the maximum strength increase at 4 vol% is only 20% compared to 60% for the AT composite. The slowing down of strength increase for the AT composite is believed to be the difficulty of obtaining good GNP dispersion with increasing particle loading. The poor strength improvement in the AR composite is the result of poor interfacial bonding. However, the composite modulus is not as sensitive to the interfacial bonding as the strength is, and hence much higher increase in modulus is observed even for the AR composite.

Nitric acid treatment introduces carboxyl groups (–COOH) on the GNP surface which can form an amide bonding with the amine curing agent. However, an excessive oxidation may damage the GNP surface. An optimum process is thus to produce the right amount of carboxyl groups without damaging GNPs. A carboxyl group can then react with an amino group on the curing agent to produce an ammonium carboxylate salt. Subsequent heating well above 100°C removes the water byproduct and yields an amide linkage.

The same reaction can occur under sonication without heating as the sonication can locally provide the necessary energy required for the reaction [16]. Figure 7.3a shows that an optimum acid treatment time exists to yield optimum property improvement. For the amount of materials used, the optimum treatment time appears to be 30 min. The FTIR spectra in Fig. 7.3b show the presence of the carboxyl group on the GNP surfaces [16–18]. The peaks are seen to grow with increasing treatment time up to 30 min and then remain almost the same thereafter.

7.3.3 Compressive Properties

Compressive properties have been measured using cylindrical specimens 12.7 mm in diameter and 40 mm long in accordance with ASTM D695-02. The GNP

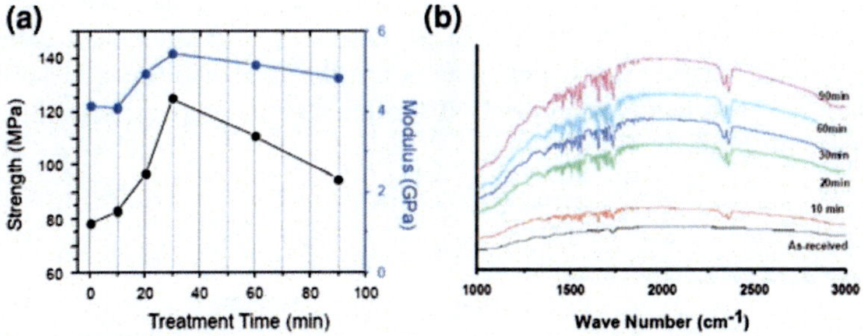

Fig. 7.3 Effects of nitric acid treatment time (1 vol% GNP): **a** tensile properties and **b** fourier transform infrared (FTIR) spectra

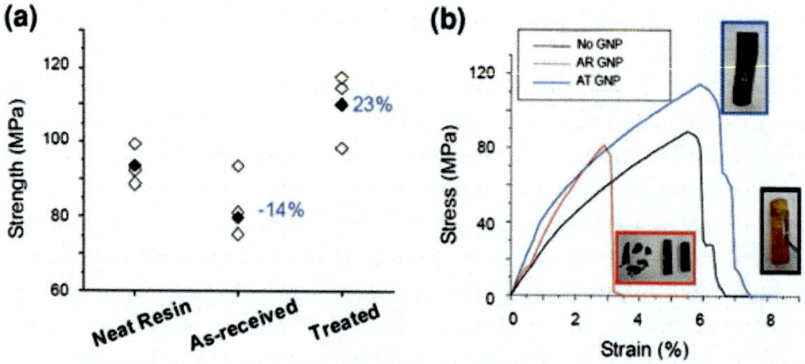

Fig. 7.4 Compressive properties (1 vol% GNP): **a** strengths and **b** stress–strain relations

loading is fixed at 1 vol%. The compressive strength rather decreases, 14%, upon the addition of AR GNPs while it increases 23% when AT GNPs are used. AR GNPs appear to render the composite more brittle, as exhibited by failed specimens (Fig. 7.4). However, the AT composite retains the same ductility while exhibiting a higher strength.

7.3.4 Fracture Toughness

Fracture toughness has been measured (following ASTM D5045) using single-edge-notch specimens in bending. The notch was introduced into the specimen and sharpened using a razor blade. The AT composite shows a higher plane-strain fracture toughness KIC than either of the neat resin and the AR composite (Fig. 7.5). However, the corresponding critical strain energy release rate G_{IC} calculated from K_{IC} is lower for the AT composite. The reason is that although K_{IC} is higher, so is the corresponding modulus and hence the resulting GIC could be lower. The fracture surface of the AR composite in Fig. 7.6 shows the imprint of a GNP that has been pulled out. However, there is no sign of any GNP debonding on the fracture surface of the AT composite. Although a poor interface may lead to a higher toughness especially in brittle matrix composites, e.g., ceramic matrix composites, that is not the case with epoxy matrix composites. A strong interface allows GNPs to resist crack propagation and can yield a higher toughness.

7.3.5 Adhesive Properties

Adhesive properties have been measured using single-lap joints with graphite/epoxy laminates as adherends in accordance with ASTM D3163-01.

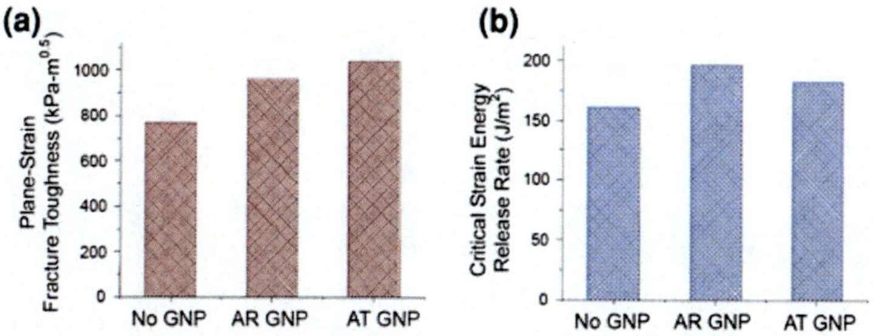

Fig. 7.5 Fracture properties (1 vol% GNP): **a** plane-strain fracture toughness and **b** critical energy release rate

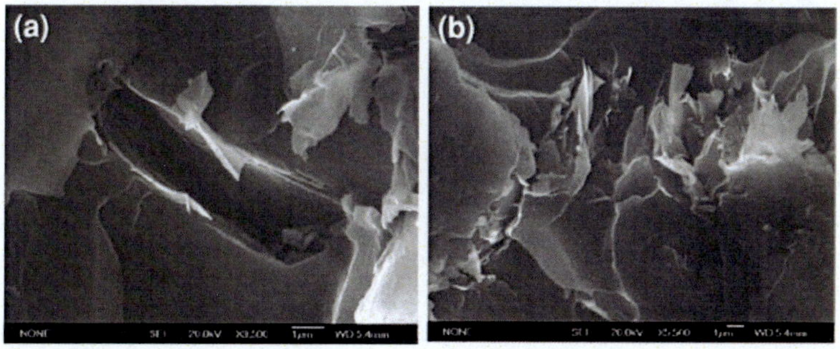

Fig. 7.6 Fracture surfaces (1 vol% GNP): **a** AR composite and **b** AT composite

The adherend laminate has eight layers of AS4 carbon fabric impregnated with Epon 862.

Two types of resins are used as adhesives: Epon 862 and a commercial epoxy glue based on a combination of bisphenol A-epichlorohydrin and a mercaptan curing agent. The commercial glue is included for comparison purposes. As for compressive strength, the addition of AR GNPs does not improve the adhesive strength of Epon 862 although it is effective somewhat for the commercial glue (Fig. 7.7). However, the acid treatment increases the reinforcement effectiveness of GNPs for both adhesives. The improvement is much more for Epon 862 than for the commercial glue. The reason may be the amide bond that forms between the carboxyl group on the GNP surface and the amino group in the Epicure-W curing agent.

The higher composite modulus induced by the addition of AT GNPs manifests itself in a stiffer joint. Figure 7.7b plots the applied stress as a function of the average strain between grips. The AT GNP/Epon 862 composite shows the stiffest joint behavior followed by the AT GNP/commercial glue composite. AR GNPs do not appear to increase the joint stiffness significantly.

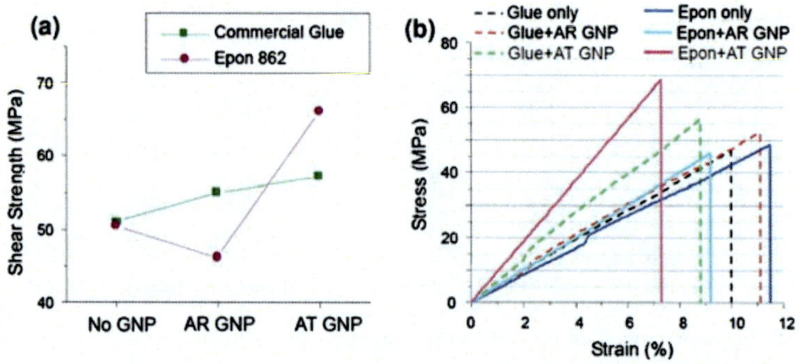

Fig. 7.7 Adhesive properties (1 vol% GNP): **a** single-lap shear strength and **b** stress–strain relations

7.3.6 *Thermal Conductivity*

The transient hot-wire method has been used to measure the thermal conductivity of the polymer nanocomposites [19]. Figure 7.8 shows the thermal conductivities of the neat resin and the two types of nanocomposites monotonically increased with increasing temperature. This trend is typical of highly disordered dielectric materials. Compared with the neat resin, the improvement in thermal conductivity is approximately 2–3% for the AR composite and 3–6% for the AT composite. The modest improvement in thermal conductivity is rather surprising since the thermal conductivity of graphite ($\sim$3000 W/mK) is orders of magnitude higher than that of the matrix resin. It appears that the large resistance to heat conduction across interfaces between the GNPs and the polymer matrix strongly impedes heat conduction in the nanocomposites. Nevertheless, the stronger interfacial bonding enabled by the acid treatment leads to a slightly higher thermal conductivity.

7.3.7 *Electrical and Dielectric Properties*

Similarly to thermal conductivity, electrical conductivity increases as more GNPs are added (Fig. 7.9).

The increase in electrical conductivity accelerates with increasing GNP loading, which is contrary to the increase in strength. As more GNPs are added to the matrix, the chances of their coming into contact with one another increase and hence the resulting conductivity increases. The results in Fig. 7.9 show that AT GNPs yield higher composite conductivity than AR GNPs as the former allows for better interfacial bonding.

Figures 7.10 and 7.11 show the real and imaginary permittivities, respectively, of the nanocomposites [20]. Both permittivities increase with increasing GNP loading regardless of the surface treatment. Similar trends are observed for

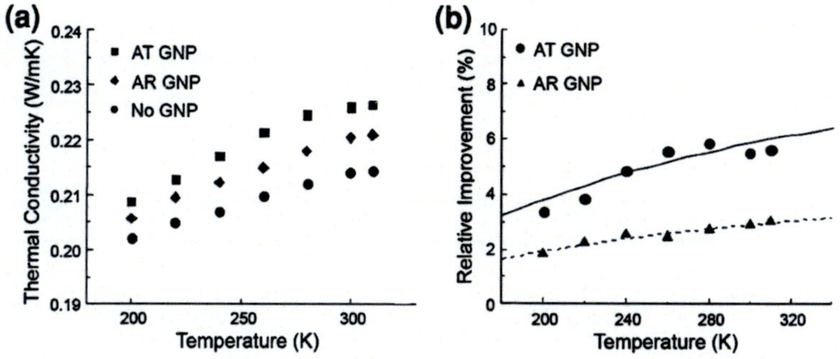

Fig. 7.8 Thermal conductivity (1 vol% GNP): **a** thermal conductivity increasing with temperature and **b** thermal conductivity improvement increasing with temperature

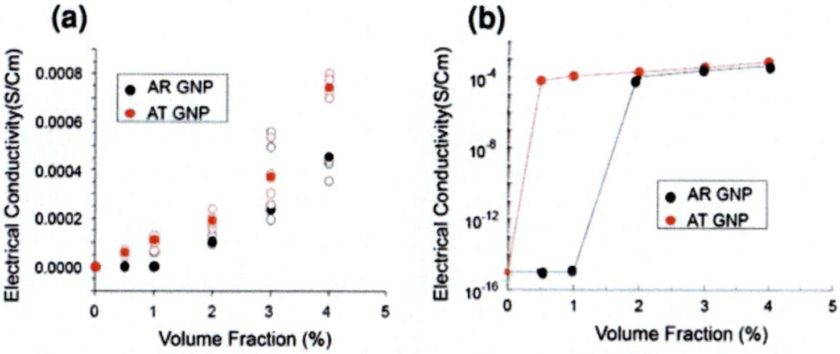

Fig. 7.9 Electrical conductivity: **a** absolute scale and **b** logarithmic scale

composites reinforced with carbon nanotubes and carbon blacks when the particle loading is low [21, 22] (Wang Z, Wang DH, Tan L-S, Hahn HT, unpublished work).

A GNP/epoxy composite is a mixture of insulating regions and a conducting network. The electron conduction between conductive particles occurs via a combination of direct contact, electron tunneling through gaps and dielectric breakdown of the matrix in gaps. The effective scale of gaps is dependent on the electromagnetic frequency and is related to the distance of electron movement in the alternating electric field. The gaps that are smaller than electron displacements act as insulators and contribute to the real part of permittivity, i.e., the dielectric constant of the composite. The remaining parts can be treated as part of the conducting network and contribute to the imaginary permittivity.

Figure 7.10 shows the real permittivities of the composites increasing slightly after the additional nitric acid treatment. The surface treatment may reduce pores and unbonded interfaces between the conductive GNPs and the insulating epoxy, and remove contaminants from the GNP surfaces, thereby improving the real permittivity. Also, better dispersion in the AT GNP composite may facilitate the

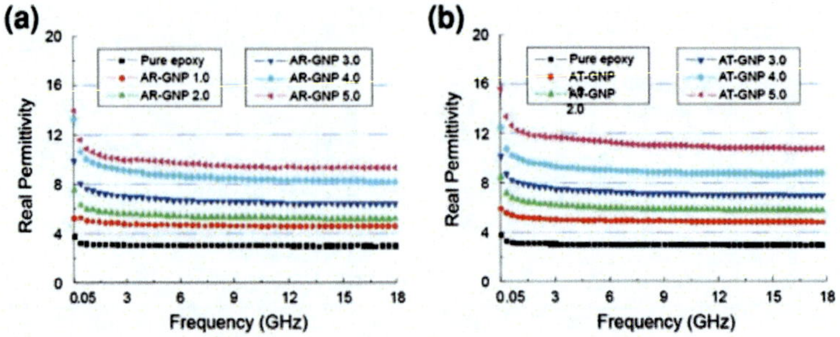

Fig. 7.10 Real permittivity: **a** AR composite and **b** AT composite

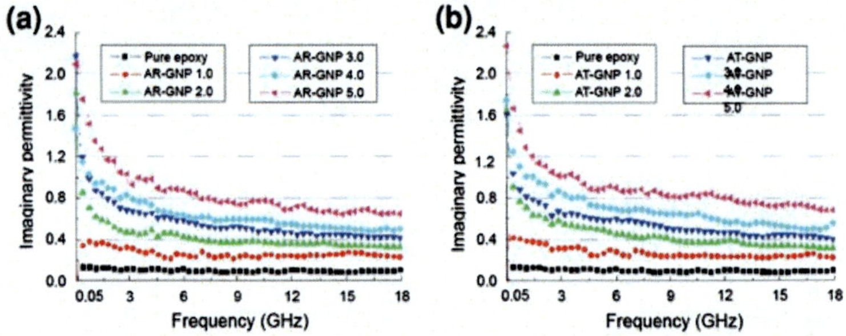

Fig. 7.11 Imaginary permittivity: **a** AR composite and **b** AT composite

electrical isolation of individual GNPs. Contrary to the real permittivity, the imaginary permittivity shows little change after the nitric acid treatment, Fig. 7.11.

7.4 Effect of GNP Dispersion

Sonication at an ultrasonic frequency is an effective means of achieving good dispersion of nanoparticles while promoting the formation of amide linkage between the carboxyl group and the amino group. However, it is not clear how much sonication is needed to yield optimum results. Therefore, two sets of experiments have been carried out to answer this question.

In the first set of experiments a mixture of AR GNPs, Epon 862, and Epicure W is sonicated in an ice bath using an ultrasonic horn for various periods of time. The mixture is then degassed, poured into molds and cured at 120°C for 4 h. In the second set of experiments, Epon 862 is left out during the initial sonication. It is later added to the mixture of AR GNPs dispersed in Epicure W. The final three component mixture is mechanically stirred briefly for 20 min and then sonicated further for 30 min. The final cure procedure is the same as in the first set of experiments.

The quality of GNP dispersion as seen on an optical microscope is shown in Fig. 7.12 for the first experiments. After 6 h, there is no more discernible improvement in dispersion quality. Similar results are obtained for the second experiments.

The effect of sonication time on tensile strength is shown in Fig. 7.13a for the two sets of experiments. In both cases, the strength increases initially with increasing sonication time. However, after 4–6 h, there is no more strength increase, indicating probably no further improvement in particle dispersion. In the first experiments where both Epon 862 and Epicure W are sonicated together, the local heating induced by sonication is large enough to cure the resin at the tip of the horn after 4 h of sonication. This is believed to explain a slight decrease in strength observed after thereafter. In the second set of experiments where only the curing agent is sonicated initially and Epon 862 is added later, there is no decrease in strength. Rather the strength increases slightly even after 4 h of sonication. Nevertheless, for the amount of materials used, the optimum sonication time is seen to be 6 h.

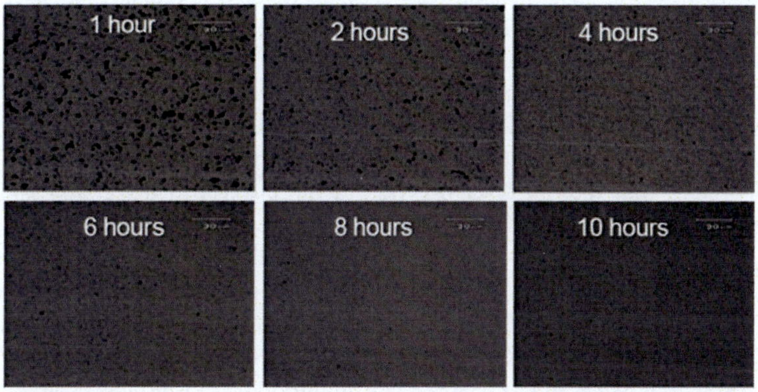

Fig. 7.12 GNP dispersion quality as a function of sonication time (0.25 vol% AR GNP in Epon and Epicure)

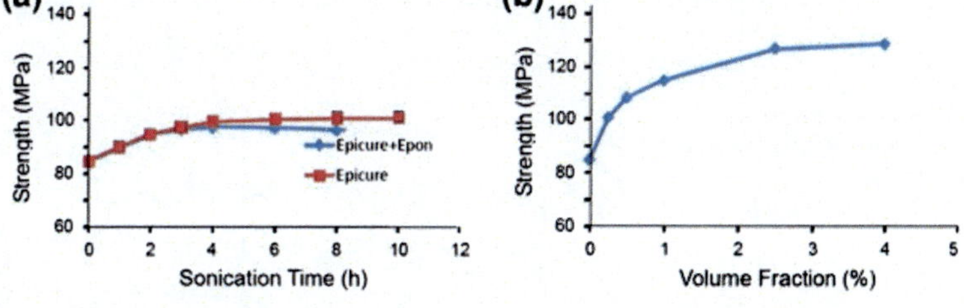

Fig. 7.13 Variation of tensile strength with **a** sonication time (0.25 vol% AR GNP) and **b** AR GNP loading (6-h sonication)

The effect of higher GNP loading on tensile strength is shown in Fig. 7.13b where a fixed sonication time of 6 h is used. The strength increases with GNP loading is asymptotic as in Fig. 7.2, with a maximum strength of almost 130 MPa reached at 4 vol%. It is interesting to note that this AR composite strength obtained after 6 h of sonication is almost the same as the AT composite strength which is realized with only 20 min of sonication.

7.5 Chemical Functionalization

Functional groups chemically bonded on graphite surfaces that are compatible with the matrix resin are expected to lead to improved interfacial bonding and hence higher composite strength. The two types of functional groups chosen to study this effect are an epoxy-based group and an amine-based group, Fig. 7.14 (Wang Z, Wang DH, Tan L-S, Hahn HT, unpublished work). Both types have been synthesized and provided by Dr. Loon-Seng Tan's group at AFRL/RXBP. Three different processes have been used to disperse the functionalized GNPs (f-GNPs) in the resin using an ultrasonic bath [23]. In process E (Epon first), f-GNPs are sonicated in Epon for 1 h. The curing agent is then added, mechanically stirred for 30 min and finally sonicated again for 1 h. The final step is to degas, mold, and cure at 120°C for 4 h. In process C (curing agent first), the sequence of adding Epon and Epicure is reversed while the rest of the steps remain the same.

Optical micrographs of the mixtures before curing are shown in Fig. 7.15. It is clearly seen that the amine-GNPs yield a more uniform dispersion and higher strengths than the epoxy-GNPs in both processes E and C. The same trend is observed when Epicure is added before Epon: that is, process C yields better dispersion and higher strengths than process E. These results indicate that Epicure has more affinity to both types of GNPs and that amine-GNPs have better bonding to the matrix resin. In order to improve the GNP dispersion, a mixed solvent consisting of ethanol and THF (tetrahydrofuran) in a 2:1 ratio has been used in the last process S (solvent). This mixed solvent has been found to work well after a few trials. In this process, f-GNPs are sonicated in the mixed solvent for 3 h, followed by addition of Epicure and 3 h of sonication. In light of the better results from process C, Epicure is added first. One-fourth of the required Epon is then added, mechanically stirred for 30 min and sonicated for 1 h. The solvent is

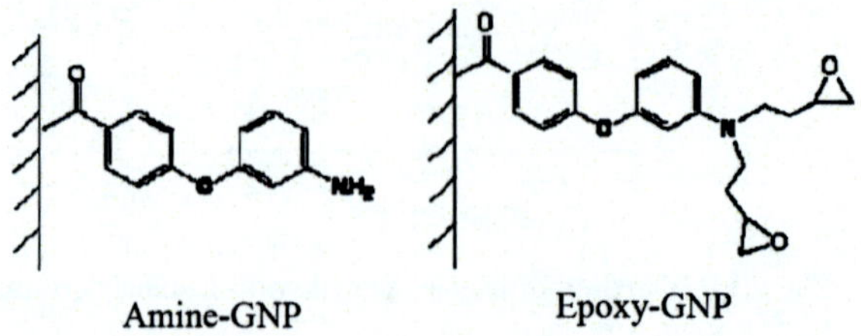

Fig. 7.14 Two types of chemical functionalization on GNP surface

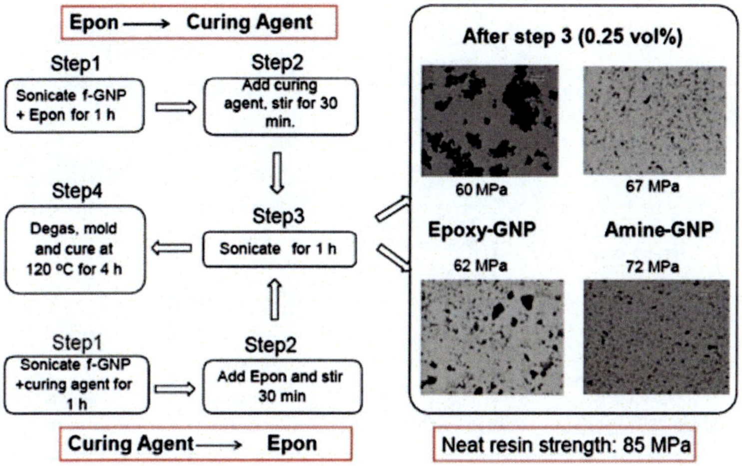

Fig. 7.15 Processes E and C for f-GNPs: amine-GNPs (*right*) and curing-agent-first mixing (*bottom*), respectively, showing better dispersion and higher strengths

evaporated in a vacuum oven, and the remaining Epon is added, mechanically stirred for 30 min and finally sonicated for 1 h. The entire mixture is then cured by following the same procedure as in the other processes. Again, amine-GNPs show better dispersion and higher strength compared with epoxy-GNPs. Also, a better dispersion resulting from the use of the solvent appears to yield a higher strength, 90 vs. 72 MPa. There is a clear correlation between the dispersion quality and the composite strength—a better dispersion yields a higher strength. (Fig. 7.16)

Process S has been used to further study the effect of higher amine-GNP loading on the composite properties. The results show that further increase in strength with increasing particle loading are possible if the dispersion is good (Fig. 7.17).

7.6 Intercalation, Expansion, and Exfoliation

The reinforcement efficiency of GNPs depends on the aspect ratio so that thinner GNPs would be more desirable for the same planar dimension. Because of the layered nature of their microstructure, GNPs can be made thinner through intercalation, expansion, and exfoliation.

Much research has been done on intercalation of various elements into graphite [24, 25]. Improvements in strength, electrical conductivity, and thermal conductivity are reported in the Literature [26–28].

Potassium (K) has been intercalated into AR GNPs to produce the first (KC_8) and fourth (KC_{48}) stage compounds using two different C/K stoichiometric ratios of 1.534 and 9.202, respectively [29, 30]. The first stage graphite intercalation

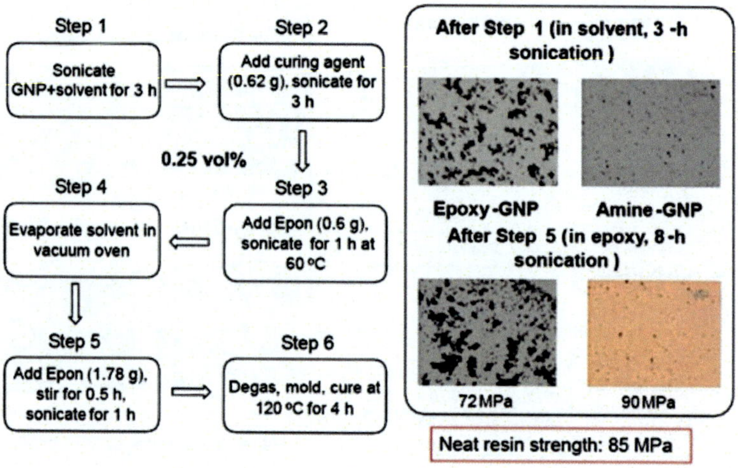

Fig. 7.16 Process S using a mixed solvent: amine-GNPs showing better dispersion and higher strengths

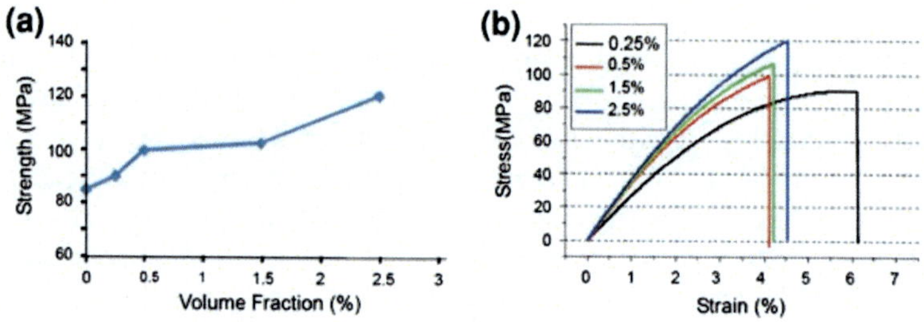

Fig. 7.17 Effect of amine-GNP loading on composite properties: **a** strength and **b** stress/strain relations

compound (GIC) consists of graphite and potassium layers alternating with each other and appears gold. The fourth stage GIC with blue color has 4 graphite layers sandwiched between two potassium layers. For expansion, these two GICs are further reacted with dehydrated benzene to produce ternary GICs: KC_8-B and KC_{48}-B.

The final treatment involves the usual nitric acid treatment. Scanning electron microscopy (SEM) micrographs of KC_{48}-B GICs are shown in Fig. 7.18. As with AR GNPs, no discernible differences are seen on the surfaces after the acid treatment.

The processing of composites using GICs is the same as for GNPs. The GICs exfoliate during this phase as a result of sonication and polymerization. Contrary to the expectation, however, the GICs do not appear to improve the composite strength much (Fig. 7.19). Rather, the effect of acid treatment is more conspicuous.

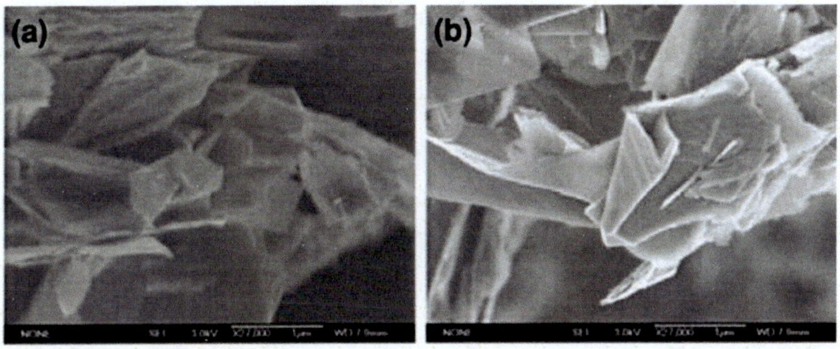

Fig. 7.18 SEM micrographs of KC48-benzene graphite intercalation compound: **a** before acid treatment and **b** after acid treatment

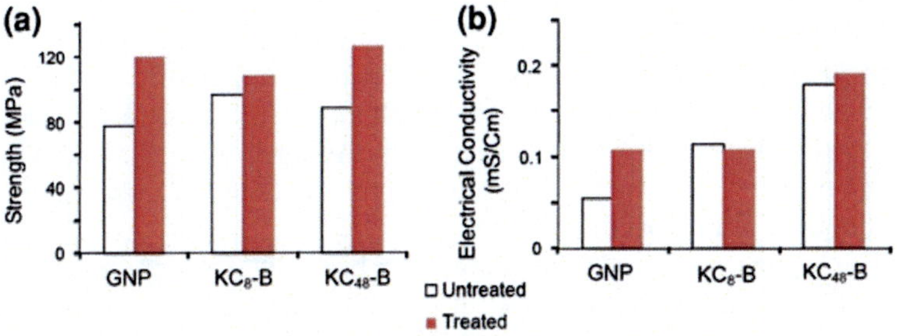

Fig. 7.19 Effects of intercalation (1 vol% GNP) on: **a** tensile strength and **b** electrical conductivity

The potassium intercalation definitely improves the electrical conductivity. This is believed to be due to the increased conductivity of potassium GICs themselves [31]. Compared with untreated AR GNPs, KC_{48}-B GIC yields almost four times as high as an electrical conductivity. The lower conductivity of KC_8-B composite is the result of KC_8 having a lower conductivity than KC_{48}. The conductivity of K-GIC reaches a maximum around 5th stage and then increases as the stage number increases or decreases [31].

7.7 Potential Applications

With their ready availability, GNPs offer a cost-effective alternative to carbon nanotubes in many applications as they share almost the same properties. With a 2D structure, GNPs are more efficient as a reinforcement phase. Thus they can be used to reinforce polymers, ceramics, and metals.

Their platelet geometry makes GNPs ideally suited for application in diffusion barrier films and coatings, similarly to organoclays. They are not photo reactive and can protect the matrix polymer from ultraviolet light. Their high electrical conductivity can be used to provide protection from electromagnetic interference.

Graphite fiber composites are finding ever increasing applications as demonstrated by the new Boeing 787. GNPs can be added to the matrix of these composites to improve the matrix-controlled properties, such as matrix cracking. At present, the biggest advantage of GNPs is their cost effectiveness compared with carbon nanotubes.

7.8 Conclusions

GNPs possess many desirable properties such as those carbon nanotubes and fibers offer. Thus they can be used in many applications where a platelet geometry is needed or as a complement to carbon nanotubes and fibers. They are readily available and cost effective.

The key to the full utilization of GNP properties in composites is their uniform dispersion in and strong interfacial bond with the matrix. These are essentially the same requirements as for carbon nanotubes. As much effort has been spent on meeting these requirements for carbon nanotubes, results of these efforts can no doubt be used to improve the properties of GNP composites.

When a proper grade of flake graphite (Asbury 3775) is used together with an epoxy (Epon 862 with Epicure W), the required processing to produce a good quality composite is rather simple. Oxidation of GNPs with nitric acid followed by their thorough dispersion via intense sonication can yield composites of high quality. The sonication appears to help the carboxyl group on the GNP surface react with the amino group on the curing agent to form an amide linkage. The best composite strength obtained this way is as high as 1.7 times the neat resin strength with just 1-vol% addition of AT GNPs. The corresponding electrical conductivity is about 0.1 mS/cm. Intercalation of potassium and benzene into GNPs can further increase the electrical conductivity.

Further improvements in composite properties appear possible when AT GNPs are sonicated longer in the amine curing agent to allow the full formation of amide linkage. The GNP-coupled amine curing agent can then be used together with a base epoxy resin to fabricate GNP composites. However, further research is needed to find the optimum sonication time. Full exfoliation of GNPs followed by optimum acid treatment and sonication is another area of promising research to improve GNP composites.

Acknowledgments This chapter is based on work supported by the U.S. Air Force Office of Scientific Research under Grant F9550-05-1-0138 with Dr. B. Les Lee as the Program Manager. Appreciation is extended to the Department of Mechanical, Aerospace and Systems Engineering, Korea Advanced Institute of Science and Technology for an invited professorship, to Mr. Albert Tamashausky, Asbury Carbons for providing graphite nanoplatelets, and to Dr. Loon-Seng Tan, Air Force Research Laboratory for providing functionalized graphite nanoplatelets.

References

1. Dzenis Y (2008) Structural nanocomposites. Science 319:419–420
2. Delhaes P (ed) (2001) Graphite and precursors. CRC Press, Amsterdam
3. Choi O, Gilje S, Hahn HT, Kaner RB (2005) Graphite nanoplatelet reiforced epoxy composites: the effect of exfoliated and surface treatment. Proc 2005 SAMPE ISSE, SAMPE, Covina, CA
4. Li J, Kim J-K, Sham ML (2005) Conductive graphite nanoplatelet/epoxy nanocomposites: effects of exfoliation and UV/ozone treatment of graphite. Scr Mater 53:235–240
5. Li J, Sham ML, Kim J-K, Marom G (2007) Morphology and properties of UV/ozone treated graphite nanoplatelet/epoxy nanocomposites. Compos Sci Technol 67:296–305
6. Drzal LT, Fukushima H (2003) Proc SAMPE
7. Drzal LT, Fukushima H (2004) Proceedings of the American Society for Composites 19th Technical Conference
8. Vaia RA, Giannelis EP (2001) Polymer nanocomposites: status and opportunities. MRS Bull 26(5):394–401
9. Ray SS, Okamoto M (2003) Polymer/layered silicate nanocomposites: a review from preparation to processing. Prog Polym Sci 28:1539–1641
10. Riggs DM, Shuford RJ, Lewis RW (1982) Graphite fibers and composites. In: Lubin G (ed) Handbook of composites. van Nostrand Reinhold Company, New York, pp 196–271
11. Banerjee S, Hemraj-Benny T, Wong SS (2005) Covalent surface chemistry of single-walled carbon nanotubes. Adv Mater 17:17–29
12. Hirsch A (2002) In: Angew Chem Int (ed) 1853
13. Lakshminayaranan PV, Toghiani H, Pittman CW (2004) Carbon 42, 2433 Asbury Carbons, www.asbury.com
14. Hexion Specialty Chemicals, http://www.resins.com/resins/am/pdf/SC1183.pdf
15. Ramanathan T, Fisher FT, Ruoff RS, Brinson LC (2005) Amino-functionalized carbon nanotubes for binding to polymers and biological systems. Chem Mater 17:1290–1295
16. Peng H, Alemany LB, Margrave JL, Khabashesku VN (2001) Noncovalent sidewall functionalization of single-walled carbon nanotubes for protein immobilization. J Am Chem Soc 125:3838–3839
17. Wang Y, Iqbal Z, Malhotra SV (2005) Electrochemical nitration of single-wall carbon nanotubes. Chem Phys Lett 402:96
18. Hung MT, Choi MT, Ju YSO, Hahn HT (2006) Heat conduction in graphite-nanoplatelet-reinforced polymer nanocomposites. Appl Phys Lett 89:023117
19. Lee SE, Choi O, Hahn HT (2008) Microwave properties of graphite nanoplatelet/epoxy composites. Appl Phys Lett 104:1063
20. Lee SE, Kang J-H, Kim V-G (2006) Fabrication and design of multi-layered radar absorbing structures of MWNT-filled glass/epoxy plain-weave composites. Compos Struct 76:397–405
21. Oh J-H, Oh S, Kim C-G, Hong CS (2004) Design of radar absorbing structures using glass/epoxy composite containing carbon black in X-band frequency ranges. Compos Part B: Eng 35:49–56
22. Wang DH, Arlen MJ, Baek J-B, Vaia RA, Tan L-S (2007) Nanocomposites derived from a low-color aromatic polyimide (CP2) and amine-functionalized vapor-grown carbon nanofibers: in situ polymerization and characterization. Macromolecules 40:6100–6111
23. Dresselhaus MS, Dresselhaus G (2002) Intercalation compounds of graphite. Adv Phys 51:1–5
24. Enoki T, Suzuki M, Endo M (2003) Graphite intercalation compounds and applications. Oxford University Press, New York
25. Stankovich S, Dikin DA, Dommett DHB, Kohlhaas KH, Zimney EJ, Stach EA, Piner RD, Nguyen ST, Ruoff RS (2006) Graphene-based composite materials. Nature 442:282–286
26. Fukushima H, Kalaitzidou K, Drzal LT (2007) In: Proceedings of the 16th international conference on composite materials

27. Yu A, Ramesh P, Itkis ME, Bekyarova E, Haddon RC (2007) Graphite nanoplatelet–epoxy composite thermal interface materials. J Phys Chem C 111:7565–7569
28. Viculis LM, Mack JJ, Mayer OM, Hahn HT, Kaner RB (2005) Intercalation and exfoliation routes to graphite nanoplatelets. J Mat Chem 15:974–978
29. Mack JJ, Viculis LM, Ali A, Luoh R, Yang G, Hahn HT, Ko FK, Kaner RB (2005) Graphite nanoplatelet reinforcement of electrospun polyacrylonitrile nanofibers. Adv Mat 17:77–80
30. McRae E, Billaud D, Mareche JF, Herold A (1980) Basal plane resistivity of alkali metal-graphite compounds. Physica B 99:489–493
31. Kim H, Hahn HT, Viculis LM, Gilje S, Kaner RB (2007) Electrical conductivity of graphite/polystyrene composites made from potassium intercalated graphite. Carbon 47:1578–1582

Chapter 8
Developments in Characterising the Structural Behaviour of Composites in Fire

A. G. Gibson, S. Feih and A. P. Mouritz

8.1 Introduction

Large-scale structural fire resistance tests have always been available for the purposes of verifying the suitability of particular designs and materials combinations. Such tests, whilst serving the important purpose of ensuring fire-safe structures are often expensive due to their scale, and deliberately non-material specific. As a result, they have not been useful in promoting the competitive development of composite structures with improved fire safety, which is unfortunate because fire performance can be said to be the single most significant factor that is currently delaying the much wider use of composites in engineering structures [1].

It is interesting to note the significant differences in engineering approach, requirements and test regimes between different composite product fields of application including, for instance, the marine [2–5], rail transport [5, 6] and aerospace [7–9] sectors. Here the time requirements for the survival of a structure in fire can range from the order of 1 h for the marine sector, down to minutes for the case of aircraft fuselages in a post-crash situation. Heat release and smoke toxicity requirements also vary considerably across these areas.

Test procedures for quantifying fire reaction behaviour, the response of a material when exposed to fire, have achieved greater convergence, the most significant advance being the development of the cone calorimeter [10–14], which

A. G. Gibson (✉)
Centre for Composite Materials Engineering, Stephenson Building, University of Newcastle upon Tyne, Newcastle upon Tyne, NE1 7RU, UK
e-mail: a.g.gibson@ncl.ac.uk

S. Feih and A. P. Mouritz
School of Aerospace, Mechanical and Manufacturing Engineering, RMIT University, GPO Box 2476V, Melbourne 3001, Australia

L. Nicolais et al. (eds.), *Composite Materials*,
DOI: 10.1007/978-0-85729-166-0_8, © Springer-Verlag London Limited 2011

has resulted in a single small-scale reproducible test, being accepted as the basis for standards by several industry sectors.

Fire scenarios are complex and all are different. The situation in the case of organic matrix composites, as shown in Fig. 8.1, is especially complex, as the material can be affected by as well as contributing to the development of the fire [1]. In this respect the quantity of composite material present, relative to other possible sources of heat release, is important. In some scenarios the composite material may be a minor component of the system with the fire established from another fuel source such as fuel or other flammable material. In others the composite material itself may be the main flammable component present. Either way, the heat release from the fire drives the onset of decomposition of the polymer matrix present in the composite, producing flammable volatiles which may contribute to a greater or lesser extent to the overall heat release from the fire.

Figure 8.2 shows the processes occurring in a relatively thick composite laminate subject to fire.

The material receives radiant heat, which causes a 'front' of heated material to pass through the thickness of the structure. The first significant event is when the resin reaches its glass transition temperature (in the case of a thermosetting resin, or softening point in the case of a thermoplastic matrix). This causes the resin phase to lose much of its mechanical integrity, which can have a serious effect if the structure is under load. In tensile loading the effect may not initially be significant, but if there is an element of compression, such as in compressive or flexural loading, there is likely to be a considerable reduction in load-bearing capability, due to the resin-dependent nature of compressive strength. Up to this

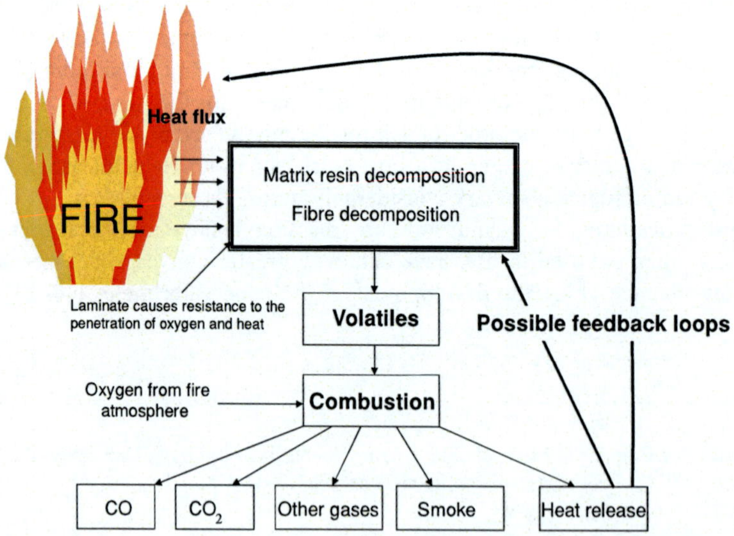

Fig. 8.1 General mechanisms involved in the thermal decomposition of a polymer matrix composite in fire, showing possible feedback loops involving heat flux [1]

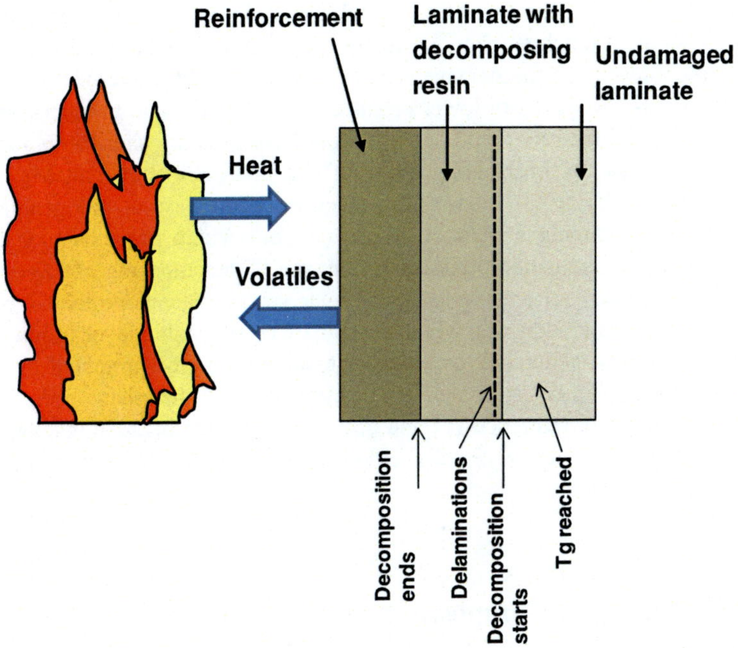

Fig. 8.2 Processes of heat and mass transfer at the laminate surface in fire, as well as the decomposition and other processes occurring through the thickness of the laminate [1]

point, if no collapse takes place, there may be no permanent damage, as occasional excursions above Tg are not necessarily damaging. Next, however, the matrix material begins to decompose, which occurs about 100–150°C above the glass transition temperature. Decomposition generates volatiles within the resin phase at a temperature where it has little strength, so this produces microvoids which grow into small delaminations, as shown schematically in Fig. 8.2. These delaminations constitute the first permanent damage to the structure. Decomposition continues, with volatiles migrating through the laminate towards the hot surface. Ignition often occurs at some point, as a result of the combination of hot face temperature and volatile production rate. After ignition the heat flux onto the laminate surface is no longer determined solely by the incoming flux from the fire, but is augmented by heat transfer from the burning decomposition products, a fundamental problem which occurs in many fire characterisation procedures for flammable materials.

Depending on the heat flux level and the laminate thickness the resin in the surface layers may become entirely depleted, with a front of decomposing material passing through the thickness of the laminate. As indicated in Fig. 8.1, the burning volatiles contribute to heat release, as well as resulting in smoke and a range of toxic products that enter the fire atmosphere.

Depending on the nature of the resin chemistry, decomposition can result in two further products not indicated in Figs. 8.1 and 8.2. These are liquid by-products, which are hazardous and which can take the form of flaming droplets, as well as carbonaceous char. Char formation, which occurs in some thermosets with a high aromatic content (such as phenolic resins), is desirable because the char contributes some integrity to the damaged material. It is also desirable because material remaining as char results in lower production of smoke, toxic products, and heat. Some successful fire retardant additives work by promoting char formation. Other additives operate by obstructing some of the pathways shown in Fig. 8.1, for instance by hindering the combustion reaction, in the case of halogenated additives, or by producing a blanket of inert vapour which prevents oxygen from mixing with decomposition products (in the case of decomposing additives such as alumina trihydrate). Alternatively the laminate surface may be protected from heat flux by intumescent additives, which cause a thermally stable layer of low thermal conductivity to be generated, or indeed the surface may be protected by an inorganic fire protection layer. The effects mentioned briefly here have been discussed at greater length in reference [1] and elsewhere. It must be acknowledged, however, that there is no universally effective solution for the fire protection of composite structures.

8.2 Modelling of Composite Fire Behaviour

8.2.1 Thermal Response to Fire

The research in this area has been recently reviewed [1]. Several studies, including going back to early work on the behaviour of wood and ablative materials for re-entry vehicles, have been used to model and interpret the physical response of composites to fire [15–26]. The key achievement in this area is Henderson Equation [18, 19], which accurately describes the thermal and decomposition effects during exposure to heat flux. The improved understanding that derived from these modelling studies has led to several useful works on the characterisation and modelling of composite structures under load in fire [27–55].

8.2.2 Behaviour under Load

The mechanical properties of composites can be modelled in terms of the properties of the constituent materials: the fibre and matrix, as described in many standard texts, including [56–58]. For modelling behaviour in fire it is necessary to extend these ideas to account for the effects of varying temperature and decomposition, as shown in Fig. 8.2.

It is useful to discuss how the modelling approach can be adapted to consider thermal effects and ultimately the fire behaviour of composites under load. In some cases, when all the necessary properties of a particular composite material are known as a function of temperature, this approach may not be required. More often, however, the full range of information will not be available and it will be necessary to use models for the temperature dependence of composite properties to calculate and model behaviour.

8.3 Response of Composite Laminates to One-Sided Heat Flux under Load

The simplest method of characterising the fire resistance of a composite system under load is to carry out small-scale tests similar to stress–rupture tests [1, 29, 33–45, 49–55]. Of course, for the qualification of full-scale composite structures larger scale testing is needed, but this is generally carried out as a final design check, rather than as a method of obtaining primary data. Small-scale fire tests under load have only been investigated relatively recently, but they have been shown to be reproducible and to produce useful indications of the probable failure mode and whether some form of structural fire protection will be needed. Small-scale tests are best carried out under conditions of constant heat flux, rather than one of the 'standard' time–temperature profiles, for reasons of scale, and because times to failure of unprotected samples are often quite short.

Two methods have been found convenient for heating the samples in tests of this type: electrical radiant heating sources, similar to that used in the cone calorimeter [33, 35, 37, 38, 43, 45, 48, 49], and gas burners [36, 37, 51, 54, 55].

A propane burner, Fig. 8.3, has been used successfully for this purpose [54, 55]. This involves low cost, but offers the possibility of achieving heat flux values approaching 200 kWm^{-2}. Testing can be carried out with a conventional mechanical testing machine, albeit with added safety and extraction facilities.

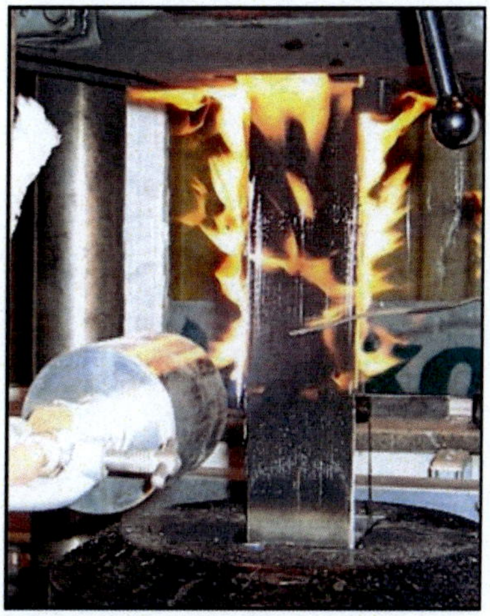

Fig. 8.3 Propane burner test on a glass/vinyl ester laminate under tension [54]

Figure 8.4 shows examples of the results obtained on glass/polyester, glass/vinyl ester and glass/polypropylene laminates, which are described in Table 8.1. It is informative to correlate and plot test results under load in fire as 'stress rupture' curves, in other words, as plots of time-to-failure under constant heat flux are shown on the horizontal axis against the constant applied stress on the vertical axis. This, in effect, treats fire exposure as being similar to other types of environmental effect.

One aspect of the test procedure that affects the reproducibility of the results is the thermal boundary conditions. It has been found possible, with both radiant electrical means and with gas burners, to achieve a near constant incoming heat flux to the exposed face of the sample. It is also desirable to have a quantifiable boundary condition for the rear (cold) face of the sample. One possibility is to insulate the rear face with a material such as mineral wool or kaowool. This provides an approximation to the fully insulated condition. An alternative is to leave the cold face open to air, which, when modelling, would require an air convective boundary condition to be applied.

Figure 8.4 shows that tensile load-bearing capability falls off rapidly under the effect of one-sided heat flux. Nevertheless, in the case of thermosetting materials containing continuous fibres, a reasonable residual level of strength is maintained. It should be noted that, using the setup shown in Fig. 8.3, it is desirable to thermally insulate the upper grips to prevent premature failure due to softening and pull-out of the material in the grips, arising from convective heating.

For measurements under compressive load the key problem is to achieve high constant compressive stresses, without the problem of Euler buckling, i.e. global buckling, affecting the results. Some workers have successfully taken the approach

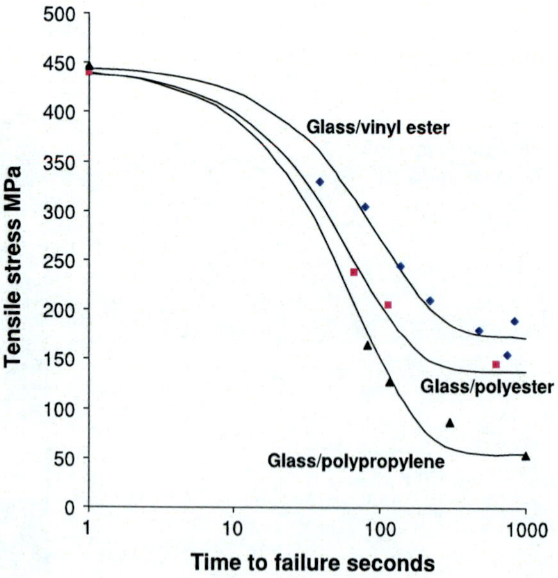

Fig. 8.4 Fire test results under tensile load [54], at a constant propane burner heat flux of 50 kWm^{-2}, on 12 mm thick glass/vinyl ester, glass/polyester and glass/polypropylene composites, as described in Table 8.1

Table 8.1 Details of polyester, vinyl ester and polypropylene E-glass fibre laminates, employed in some of the work reported here [54]

Laminate	E-glass fabric type	Resin type	Fibre mass fraction	Fibre volume fraction	Void volume fraction	Fabrication process
Glass/ polyester	Biaxial 0/90	Scott Bader Crystic 489 isophthalic polyester	0.62	0.44	0.026	Contact moulding
Glass/ vinyl ester	Biaxial 0/90	Dow 411 45 epoxy vinyl ester	0.64	0.46	0.046	Contact moulding
Glass/ polypropylene	Twintex Balanced 0/90 twill weave	TR pp 60B 1870	0.60	0.35	0.023	Oven vacuum bag moulding

of using short samples in the form of panels or plates [33, 35, 37, 38, 43, 45]. An alternative method of suppressing local buckling is to restrain the edges of the specimen, usually a ‘picture frame’ test jig, as in Fig. 8.5 [51, 54, 55]. This configuration is similar in principle to the well-known Boeing compression-after-impact test [59]. The edge restraint raises the load required for buckling failure, enabling laminate specimens of reasonable size to be placed under significant compressive stress during fire testing. Figure 8.6 shows compressive failure results for 12 mm thick laminates under a heat flux of 50 kWm^{-2}, in

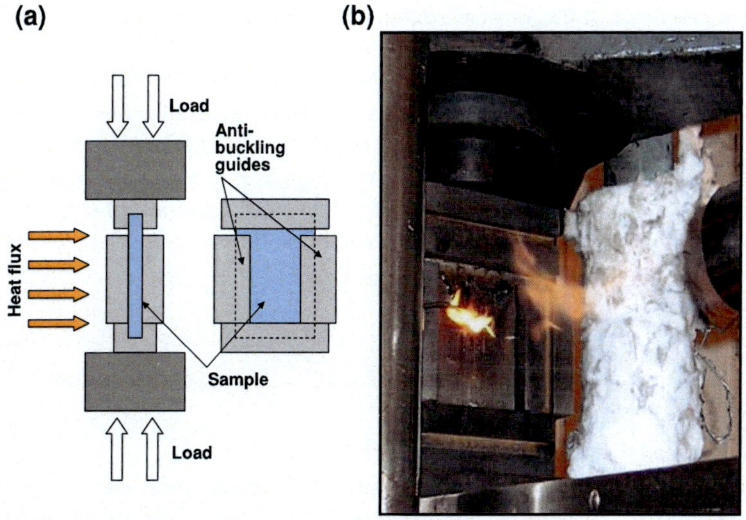

Fig. 8.5 Restrained compression test [54, 55]. **a** Schematic of picture frame restraint jig, and **b** propane burner test on a glass/vinyl ester laminate under compression

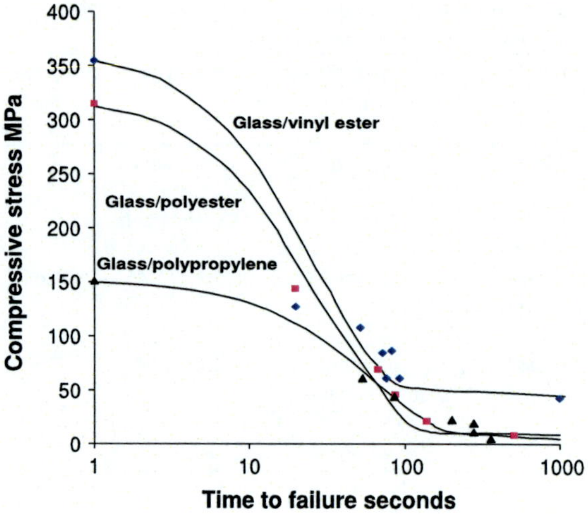

Fig. 8.6 Fire test results under compressive load [54], at a constant propane burner heat flux of 50 kWm^{-2}, on 12 mm thick glass/vinyl ester, glass/polyester and glass/polypropylene composites, as described in Table 8.1

constrained compression [54]. The rate of decline under compressive load is similar to that for behaviour in tension, Fig. 8.4, but the timescale is about an order of magnitude shorter. The residual load-bearing capability at times longer than ~100 s is very low. Behaviour in compression is acknowledged to be the Achilles' heel of composite behaviour under load in fire.

Electrical radiant heat sources, similar to that employed in the cone calorimeter, are also a convenient and easily calibrated means of applying a known heat flux. Mouritz et al. and Feih et al. [42, 49, 50] employed the radiant element from a cone calorimeter in the vertical configuration. Results were reported in both tension and compression covering a wide range of heat flux [49], as shown in Figs. 8.7 and 8.8.

The compressive failure mode under one-sided heat flux, Fig. 8.9, resembles the morphology that has been widely reported for unidirectional laminates in isothermal tests [60]. In other words, the failure is localised, involving formation of a band of sheared material. However, a separate delaminated surface layer of decomposed material is often present in addition to the band of sheared material.

8.4 Modelling Properties as a Function of Temperature

With thermally stable, post-cured thermosetting laminates, as well as thermoplastic-based ones, changes in properties with temperature can be considered reversible up to the point where decomposition of one of the phases, usually the resin, begins. With fire it is necessary to consider changes beyond this point, and a method of achieving this will also be discussed.

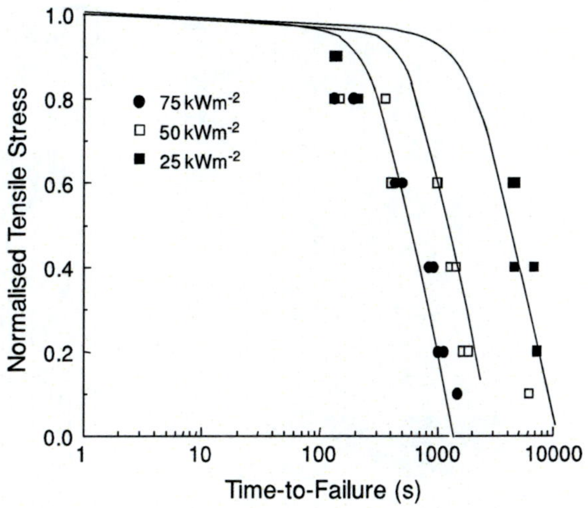

Fig. 8.7 Effect of one-sided heat flux employing a radiant electrical element on the time-to-failure of woven glass/vinyl ester laminate (0.55 fibre volume fraction) under tensile loading [49]. The tensile stress has been normalised with respect to the room temperature tensile strength of the laminate, which was 480 MPa

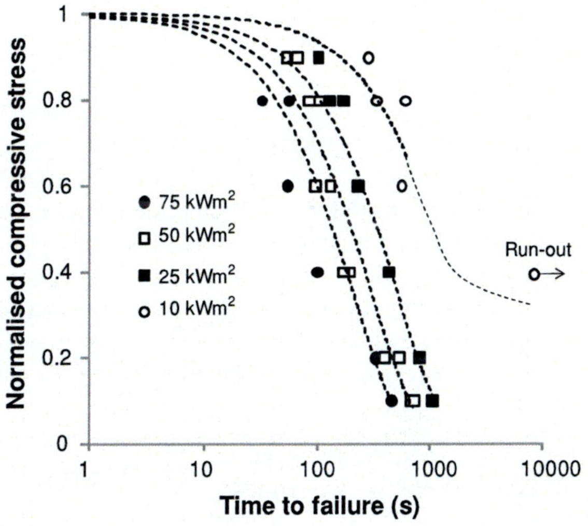

Fig. 8.8 Effect of one-sided heat flux employing a radiant electrical element on the time-to-failure of woven glass/vinyl ester laminate (0.55 fibre volume fraction) under compressive loading [49]. Stresses have been normalised with respect to the Euler buckling stress which, in this case, was 21 MPa. The room temperature compressive strength was 435 MPa

8.4.1 Property Changes up to the Onset of Decomposition

Ideally, for a particular composite system, each elastic constant or strength value would be measured and expressed as a function of temperature. However, there are few if any systems where all the data needed are available in this form. It will be assumed here, mainly for convenience, that all the mechanical properties, including strength, can be fitted to relationships similar in form to that for the modulus. This assumption appears to work well for all thermosetting resin systems, which usually happen to be amorphous. On heating an amorphous polymer from room temperature only one transition, the glass transition, occurs before

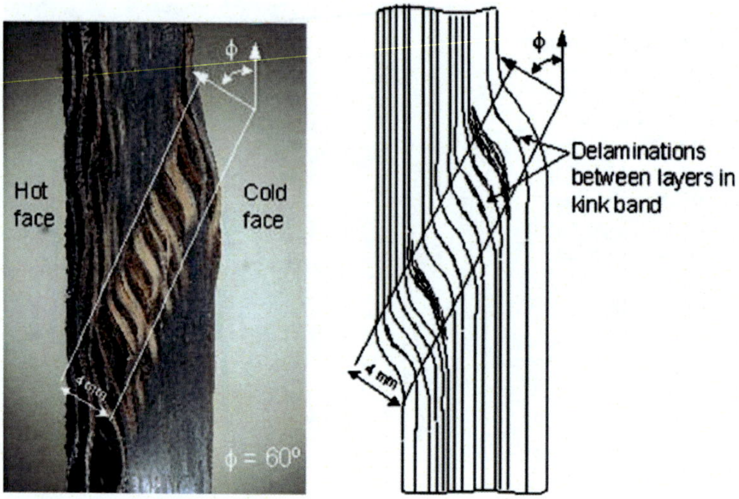

Fig. 8.9 Failure mode of a glass/vinyl ester woven laminate subject to compressive stress and a one-sided heat flux of 50 kWm^{-2}

decomposition of the resin begins, so the problem is really one of fitting a suitable relationship to the property versus temperature relationship in this region.

A polynomial in temperature is one way of describing the variation of, say Young's modulus in the transition region, but this can sometimes be inconvenient because a polynomial of order at least 6 is generally needed to describe the property–temperature relationship across the glass transition temperature region with the required accuracy. Moreover, polynomials only behave reliably within the range of the fitted data. This problem was overcome by Kulkarni and Gibson [61] who fitted a polynomial in normalised terms, to give

$$\frac{P(T)}{P_0} = 1 - a_1\left(\frac{T - T_0}{T_g - T}\right) - a_2\left(\frac{T - T_0}{T_g - T}\right)^2 - a_3\left(\frac{T - T_0}{T_g - T}\right)^3 \tag{8.1}$$

where $P(T)$ is a particular property, and P_0 is the value of that property at some low temperature, say room temperature T_0. T_g is the glass transition temperature and a_1, a_2 and a_3 are fitting constants.

Another model, according to Mahieux and Reifsnider [62, 63], assumes that increasing temperature has the effect of 'breaking' or, more accurately, relaxing increasing numbers of intermolecular bonds in the resin. The bond 'strength' was assumed to follow the cumulative Weibull distribution as a function of temperature, giving rise to a simple functional relationship of the form:

$$P(T) = P_R + (P_U - P_R)\exp\left(-\left(\frac{T}{T_0}\right)^m\right) \tag{8.2}$$

where P_U and P_R are the unrelaxed (low temperature) and relaxed (high temperature) values of that property, respectively, T_0 is the relaxation temperature and m is the Weibull exponent. For this model the temperatures are in Kelvin. Some success was achieved in fitting modulus versus temperature data for several polymers. The model works well in the present context: acceptable fitting of property data can be achieved for most thermosets with m values, in the range 9–21.

A number of empirical functions showing the required anti-symmetric behaviour as a function of temperature were examined for fitting mechanical properties [36, 37, 54, 55]. Particular success was achieved with functions based on the hyperbolic tanh function, which leads to a relationship of the following form, which describes behaviour as a function of both temperature and timescale:

$$P(T) = P_U - 0.5(P_U - P_R)\left(1 + \tanh\left(k'\left(\text{In}(a_T) + \frac{H}{R}\left(\frac{1}{T_g} - \frac{1}{T}\right)\right)\right)\right) \quad (8.3)$$

Here, P_U and P_U are the unrelaxed and relaxed property values, respectively, and k$'$ is a constant describing the breadth of the relaxation. T is the absolute temperature and T_g is the 'mechanical' glass transition temperature.

Arrhenius time–temperature dependence was assumed, from which it follows that a shift in timescale or frequency is related to an equivalent change in temperature by

$$\text{In}(a_T) = \frac{H}{R}\left(\frac{1}{T_{ref}} - \frac{1}{T}\right) \quad (8.4)$$

where T_{ref} is the original or reference temperature. Provided the relaxation process is governed by Arrhenius kinetics, this relationship applies independently of the profile of the relaxation process (i.e. the relaxation time distribution).

$a_T = \frac{t}{t_0}$ for creep measurements, where t is time and t_0 is a reference time.

Alternatively $a_T = \frac{\omega_0}{\omega}$ for DMTA measurements, where ω is the frequency and ω_0 is the reference frequency. H and R are the activation energy and the gas constant, respectively.

When the results are all generated on the same timescale, a_T is equal to one and the expression reduces to

$$P(T) = P_U - 0.5(P_U - P_R)\left(1 + \tanh\left(k'\frac{H}{R}\left(\frac{1}{T_g} - \frac{1}{T}\right)\right)\right) \quad (8.5)$$

Like Mahieux and Reifsnider expression, Eq. 8.4, this involves only four fitting constants, in this case, P_U, P_R, $k'\frac{H}{R}$ and T_G. Eq. 8.5 predicts property–temperature curves that are anti-symmetric when plotted versus reciprocal temperature. In many cases the curves are also close to being anti-symmetric against linear temperature so some simplification can be achieved:

$$P(T) = P_U - 0.5(P_U - P_R)\left(1 + \tanh\left(k(T - T_g)\right)\right) \quad (8.6)$$

Finally, the unrelaxed and relaxed quantities, P_U and P_R, may themselves vary with temperature. Treating one or both as linear functions of temperature requires one or two additional fitting constants.

There are no theoretical restrictions on the shape of the modulus temperature relationship so, in practice, the choice may be made between Eqs. 8.1, 8.2, 8.5 or 8.6 on the basis of which best fits the data.

In some composite structures the state of cure may not be complete at the start of service life. The most extreme examples are large marine craft in polyester and vinyl ester, where elevated temperature post-cure is not viable because of their size. Here, it is common for the cure state to advance during the course of any elevated temperature testing, producing apparent increases in resin glass transition temperature and strength with rising temperature. To achieve consistent results when this happens it may be necessary to post-cure the test samples, but this procedure of course changes the state of the material. In some cases it is possible to model the progression of cure during testing or fire simulation simply by shifting the glass transition temperature value in Eqs. 8.1, 8.2, 8.5 or 8.6. When high test temperatures are used the cure state probably advances significantly during testing, even when the material has been previously well-cured. Fortunately the effect is largely masked by the magnitude of other effects that take place, most notably resin decomposition, which will be discussed in the next section.

8.4.2 *Effects of Resin Decomposition*

Limited information is available on the effect of thermal decomposition on properties. Various assumptions have been made regarding the properties of the char remaining, following decomposition of the resin phase, most of which assume a very low level of residual properties. Until a more appropriate relationship can be found to describe the decay of properties, it has been proposed that each mechanical property be modified by a power law factor, R^n, in residual resin content (RRC). Equation (8.6) thus becomes

$$P(T) = \left(P_U - 0.5(P_U - P_R)\left(1 + \tanh\left(k\left(T - T_g\right)\right)\right)\right)R^n \tag{8.7}$$

The values for n reported so far range from zero [36] for tensile strength, a property not dominated by resin behaviour, through 1, for typical resin-dominated properties, such as compressive strength [36] up to a value of 3 which has been suggested recently [49].

8.5 High Temperature Strength of Composites

Again there is relatively little published work on the strength of composites at high temperature, especially in the range well above conventional design temperatures, where behaviour is influenced by the onset of decomposition. There are experimental problems in this region, and the temperatures may be outside the range achievable with standard testing equipment. In the case of tensile strength measurements, difficulties arise with grip slipping and failure, when the resin is above its glass transition temperature. Figure 8.10 shows a useful novel method [54, 55] of overcoming these problems by using a locally heated gauge length, instead of a temperature-controlled oven. Standard 'waisted' composite test-pieces and grips are used. Instead of using a conventional temperature-controlled oven, the gauge length temperature is determined locally by contact with temperature-controlled aluminium blocks, heated by cartridge heaters. The grip region can thus be kept cool, avoiding local slipping and failure. The upper grip is insulated with mineral wool to prevent warming by air convection from the parts below.

Figure 8.11 shows the tensile strength, up to 400°C, for three different types of woven E-glass composite, based on polyester, vinyl ester polypropylene [54]. With continuous fibre laminates there is some tensile strength retention at elevated temperature, due to the strength of the reinforcement. Returning to resin effects, it is useful to note that the strength reduction in many composites due to the initial softening of the resin is larger than would have been anticipated on the basis of the resin contribution to strength and micromechanics considerations. If loss of the resin modulus contribution were the only phenomenon occurring then a relatively small drop would be expected.

The cause of this larger than expected reduction is probably the loss of the 'composite action' which ensures that in a composite below its glass transition temperature all the fibres tend fail at around the same strain. Once the matrix phase loses its ability to maintain this condition the scatter in fibre strengths becomes much more important, and the overall fibre strength is effectively replaced by the Weibull 'bundle strength', as described in [49, 50, 64].

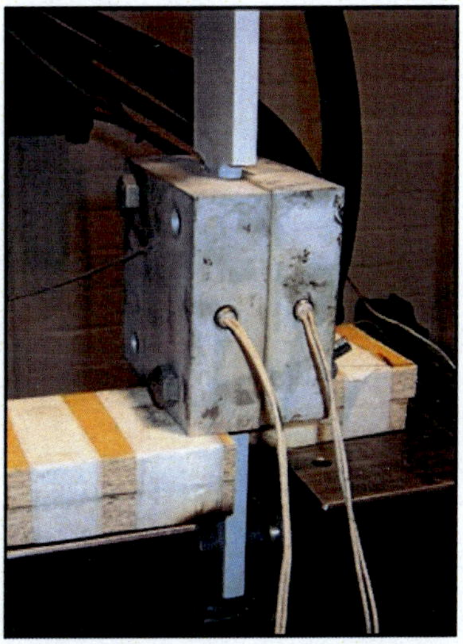

Fig. 8.10 Tensile test sample with heated gauge length to permit strength measurements at elevated temperature [54, 55]

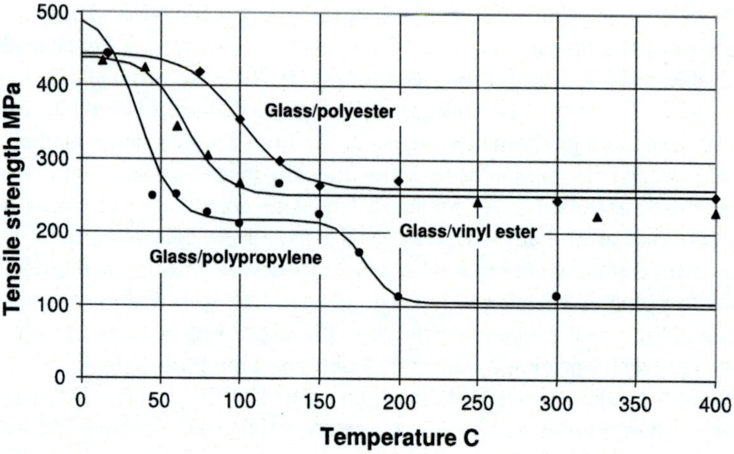

Fig. 8.11 Elevated temperature tensile strength of glass/vinyl ester, glass/polyester and glass/polypropylene laminates [54], as described in Table 8.1

Although glass fibre retains some of its room temperature strength at elevated temperature, the strength of the glass, especially when exposed to air, has been found to decay significantly with both time and temperature at 350°C and above [49, 64], as can be seen in Fig. 8.12. Various explanations have been considered for the glass fibre strength loss, including annealing of residual stress and loss of oriented network structure in the glass. Unfortunately there is no convincing evidence either for the presence of significant residual stress or for the existence of an oriented network in glass [65]. One further explanation could be a corrosive reaction at the surface of the fibre, involving a component of air, probably water vapour.

As with the elastic properties it is desirable, with strength, to have a functional relationship with temperature. The use of Eq. 8.6 has been found to be useful in

Fig. 8.12 Percentage strength decay of E-glass fibre bundles versus time in air at various temperatures [64]

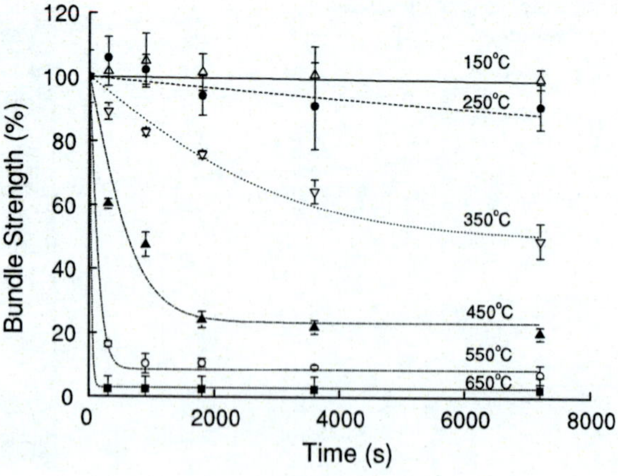

this respect and was used in the fitting of the curves in Fig. 8.11. The case of the glass-polypropylene thermoplastic laminate is rather different. Here the resin passes through not one, but two transitions in the test region, namely the glass transition (which is just below room temperature of polypropylene) and the softening transition, or α-relaxation that occurs in the crystalline region of the polymer, prior to melting. In this case an additional relaxation process was added, so that Eq. (8.8) includes a further term:

$$P(T) = P_1 - 0.5(P_1 - P_2)(1 + \tanh(k_1(T - T_1))) \\ - 0.5(P_2 - P_3)(1 + \tanh(k_2(T - T_2))) \quad (8.8)$$

Mahieux and Reifsnider [62, 63] proposed a similar method of extending their model, Eq. (8.2), to describe multiple transitions.

Determination of high temperature compressive strength also involves experimental difficulties. To overcome some of these, the test fixture shown in Fig. 8.13 was designed. Like the tensile test jig this included a set of heated close-fitting blocks. In this case they fulfilled the dual role of anti-buckling jig and heater [1, 54]. Figure 8.14 shows high temperature compressive strengths of vinyl ester, polyester and polypropylene composites. The compressive failure mode is similar to that already discussed in relation to fire tests in compression, shown in Fig. 8.9, and is very different from the tensile one, and involves the formation of a band of kinked material, probably involving the mechanism described by Budiansky and Fleck [60], in which failure initiates in a region of imperfect fibre alignment, before propagating to form the characteristic kink band. The compressive failure

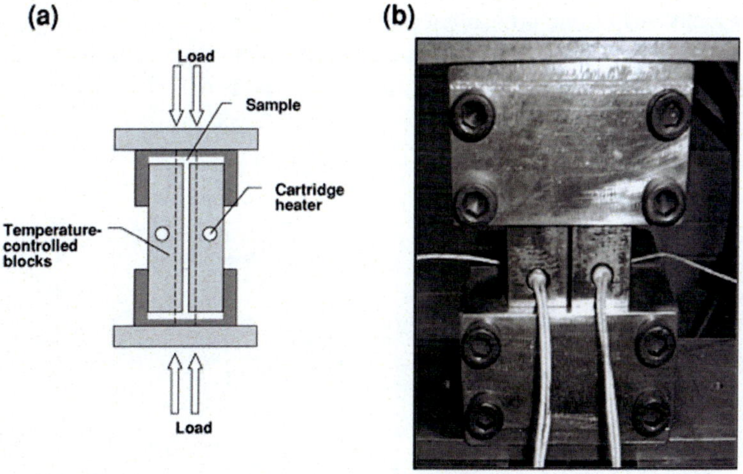

Fig. 8.13 Combined heating and anti-buckling jig used for the measurement of compressive strength at elevated temperature. **a** Schematic of jig, **b** assembly with heated blocks in place [54, 55]

mode of the laminate, therefore, reflects the shear stress–strain behaviour of planes containing the fibres and can be modelled on this basis. The key factor in compressive failure is, therefore, the softening that occurs around the glass transition temperature in the case of the thermosets. In polypropylene there are two steps in the compressive strength versus temperature relationship, corresponding first to the amorphous phase glass transition temperature and secondly to the crystalline melting point of the polymer.

The room temperature compressive strength of most thermosetting composites is only a little lower the tensile strength value, which is probably coincidental, as the failure mechanisms are radically different in each case. The same does not hold for thermoplastic composites. Figure 8.14 shows that with the glass/polypropylene system the compressive strength is substantially lower than the tensile strength. This reflects the lower fibre-matrix shear strength of the thermoplastic system—a limiting factor with many thermoplastic composites. The other key feature of the compressive behaviour is that it occurs at a generally lower temperature than the tensile failure, being a resin-dependent property. The level of compressive strength retained above the glass transition temperature for the thermosets is very low, in contrast to the tensile case. With the polypropylene composite there is zero compressive strength above the melting point of 165°C.

When modelling behaviour under load in fire it is sometimes necessary to consider and quantify the full shape of the stress–strain relationship [54]. Figure 8.15 shows the full tensile and compressive stress–strain curves obtained in the case of the glass/vinyl ester samples [54]. It is interesting to note that the tensile results show greater non-linearity than the compressive ones, which is due mainly to the effects of resin cracking. The non-linearity increases with increasing temperature. The compressive stress–strain curves are much closer to a simple 'saw-tooth' shape, due probably to the rather sudden onset of the resin-dominated compressive collapse process. A particularly convenient method of modelling slightly non-linear stress–strain curves of this type is the relationship:

Fig. 8.14 Elevated temperature compressive strength of glass/vinyl ester, glass/polyester and glass/polypropylene laminates, as described in Table 8.1 [54]

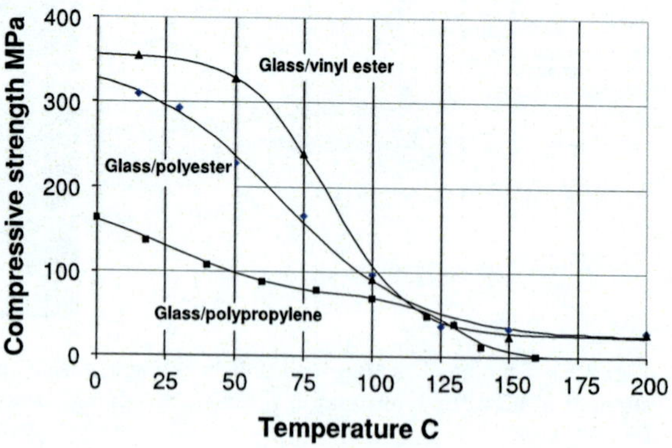

$$\sigma = \sigma_{max} \cdot \left(1 - e^{\left(\frac{-E \cdot \varepsilon}{\sigma_{max}}\right)}\right) \tag{8.9}$$

where E is the low strain Young's modulus and σ_{max} is the maximum plastic strain value. This relationship gives 'elasto-plastic' curves which are linear in the low strain region, and which go to zero slope as σ_{max} is approached. In the present case a good fit to the experimental data is obtained by setting σ_{max} to a higher value than the ultimate strength of the material, thus giving curtailed curves of the shape shown in Fig. 8.15. The stress–strain relation, therefore, requires three parameters, the modulus, the ultimate strength and σ_{max}, all of which need to be tabulated as a function of temperature. Parameterised stress–strain curves of this type were used in the modelling of tensile and compressive collapse behaviour of laminates in fire [54].

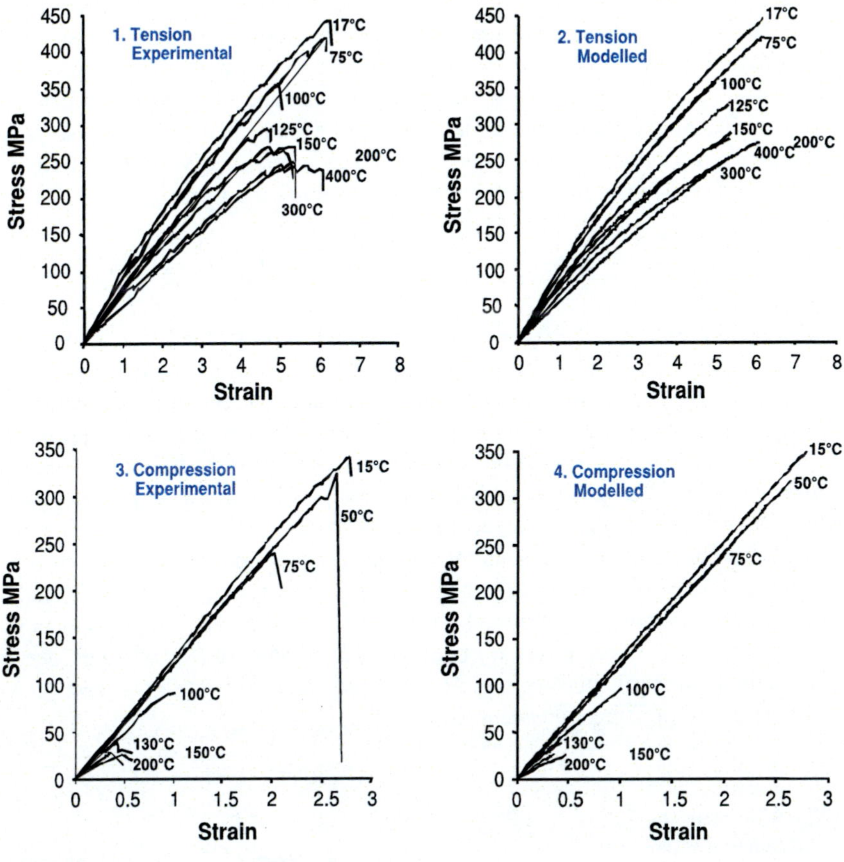

Fig. 8.15 Elevated temperature stress–strain curves for glass/vinyl ester laminate, as in Table 8.1, in tension (*upper curves*) and compression (*lower curves*). The curves on the *left* show experimental data. The curves on the *right* are modelled according to the parameters in Eq. 8.9

8.6 Modelling Fire Response

8.6.1 Thermal Equations

The phenomena taking place when an organic matrix composite laminate is exposed to fire, discussed above, are shown schematically in Figs. 8.1 and 8.2. It can be seen that several effects take place simultaneously. The laminate surface is heated by radiation, usually reaching a temperature where decomposition begins to take place. When a critical combination of surface temperature and decomposition rate are reached, flashover occurs, involving combustion of volatile laminate decomposition products. As a result of heat conduction from the hot face, a region of decomposing material passes through the thickness of the laminate, producing volatile resin decomposition products which migrate through the laminate thickness to the hot surface, where they may burn. The methodology for modelling the fire response of a laminate under load requires knowledge of the temperature distribution and the extent of resin decomposition. This is shown in Fig. 8.16.

It can be seen that fire exposure results in a number of complex effects. The most effective relationship to date for describing these phenomena is the Henderson Equation, which can be regarded as a modified version of Laplace's Equation [18, 19]. In one-dimensional form, it takes the form:

$$\rho C_P \frac{\partial T}{\partial t} = \frac{\partial}{\partial x}\left(k \frac{\partial T}{\partial x}\right) - \rho \frac{\partial M}{\partial t}(Q_P + h_C - h_G) - \dot{M}_G \frac{\partial}{\partial x} h_G \tag{8.10}$$

where T, t and x are temperature, time and through-thickness coordinates, respectively. ρ, C_P and k are the density, specific heat and conductivity of the composite. M_G is the mass flux of volatiles. h_C and h_G are the respective enthalpies of the composite and evolved gas. Q_P is the endothermic decomposition energy. The three terms on the right-hand side relate, respectively, to heat conduction, the resin decomposition process, which is endothermic and transport of heat towards the hot surface by volatile convection.

The decomposition parameters of the polymer matrix need to be taken into account. These are most conveniently determined by thermo-gravimetric analysis (TGA), which involves determining the weight loss as resin decomposes in an inert atmosphere. The decomposition of resins such as polyester, vinyl ester, acrylics and polyolefin thermoplastics can often be approximated by a single reaction with Arrhenius temperature dependence:

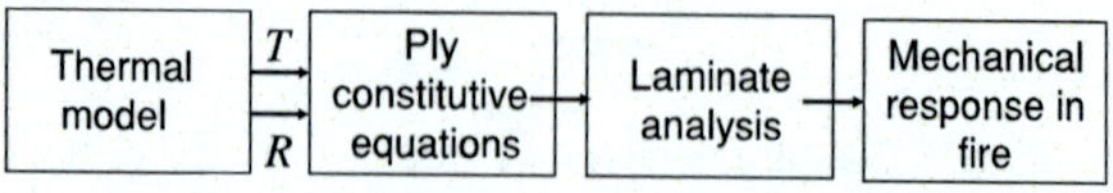

Fig. 8.16 Methodology for modelling the response of composite laminates under load, exposed to fire

$$\frac{\partial m}{\partial t} = -A\left[\frac{(m - m_f)}{m_0}\right]^n e^{(-E/RT)} \tag{8.11}$$

where m, t and T are the mass, time and temperature variables, respectively, A, E and n the rate constant, activation energy and order of the reaction and R is the gas constant. m_0 and m_f refer to the initial and final mass of the composite.

These particular resins appear to decompose in a rather simple manner, with one basic reaction which involves chain unzipping and depolymerisation, to release low molecular weight residues, including any solvent monomer that was present in the original resin. These resins decompose mainly to volatile species, leaving behind a relatively small (5–10%) proportion of solid material (char).

Other resins with a high aromatic content decompose in a more complex manner, leaving a higher proportion of carbonaceous char. These resins include phenolic, which is particularly well known for char formation, along with many epoxy resins, especially the highly cross-linked resins used in prepreg and for aerospace. In this case decomposition involves at least two stages: a primary condensation, sometimes with the evolution of small quantities of volatiles, followed at higher temperature by char formation. Decomposition modelling then requires at least two, sometimes more separate rate processes, similar in form to Eq. (8.11). The materials-related parameters in Eq. (8.10) are temperature-dependent and evolve as a result of resin decomposition.

Figures 8.17 and 8.18 show examples of the output from the COMFIRE program, in this case for glass/vinyl ester and glass/polypropylene laminates, respectively, with the rear face insulated, under a heat flux of 50 kWm^{-2} [54]. The upper graph in these figures shows the thermal profile during the fire exposure and the lower graph shows the decomposition profile. The two variables, temperature and RRC, can be regarded effectively as 'state' variables, which completely determine the resin properties at a particular point.

It is interesting to note the significant effect of the resin decomposition. As this reaction is endothermic it produces the 'plateau' that can be seen in the temperature curves, effectively by absorbing heat over the decomposition range of temperatures. This effect is very important as it lends some fire-resisting characteristics to the otherwise weak fire behaviour of the resin. The effect actually allows composite materials to be used for fire protecting steel and other structures in situations where the loss of properties of the composite and the decomposition products are unimportant. This enables composite fire protection to be employed in the oil and gas industry and in the protection of storage containers for some hazardous chemicals [66]. It is interesting to note the similar characteristics of the curves in Figs. 8.17 and 8.18, which correspond to very different thermoplastic and thermosetting resin systems. Comparing the times to reach a particular temperature or decomposition state it can be seen that these are longer in the case of the polypropylene laminate. This reflects the fact that the resin content is a little higher for this laminate and underlines the importance of the resin decomposition endotherm in delaying the passage of heat through the laminate.

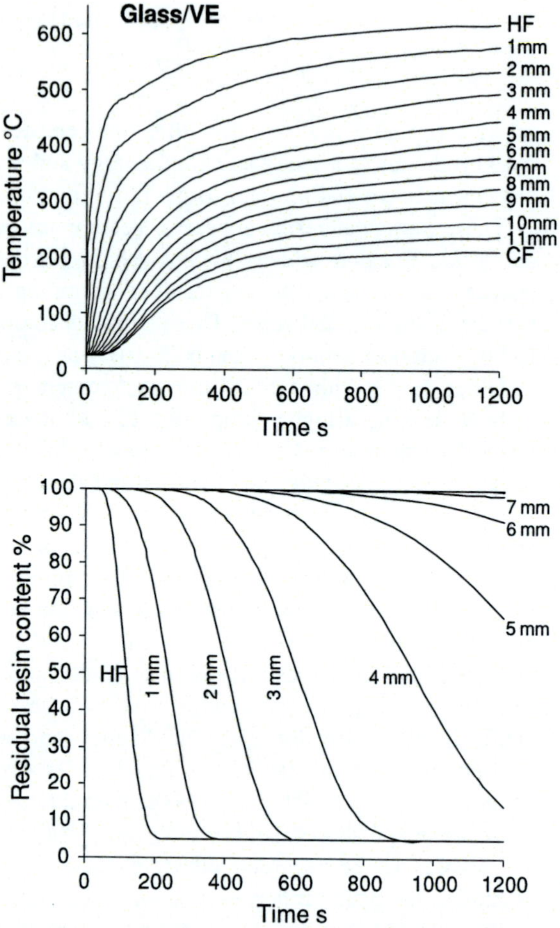

Fig. 8.17 Output from the thermal model for the case of a 12 mm thick glass/vinyl ester laminate, as in Table 8.1, subjected to a one-sided heat flux of 50 kWm^{-2}, with the rear face insulated [54]. *Upper figure* temperature field through the thickness of the laminate versus time. *Lower figure* residual resin content field through the thickness of the laminate versus time

A finite difference version of the Henderson Equation has been found to work well for different resin systems by comparing the calculated and measured thermal responses during furnace fire tests [23, 26]. This model has been developed at Newcastle University into the COMFIRE software. Finite element-based versions of the Henderson model have also been developed [25]. The one-dimensional nature of the thermal model is not a drawback for many applications involving laminated composites as these are generally shell-like in nature. However, if required, Eq. (8.10) can be extended to include two or even three-dimensional heat flow. When this is carried out, a convenient approximation involves neglecting heat transfer due to the movement of volatiles—the last term in Eq. (8.10). The effect of this term has been found to be small enough to allow it to be ignored in some cases [23, 26].

Recently, work has been carried out to further simplify the Henderson model by avoiding the use of the Arrhenius decomposition model [40, 47, 52, 67]. In the so-called 'apparent thermal diffusivity' (ATD) model [67] the rate-dependence of the decomposition behaviour is neglected, with the decomposition state at any

Fig. 8.18 Output from the thermal model for the case of a 12 mm thick glass/polypropylene laminate, as in Table 8.1, subjected to a one-sided heat flux of 50 kWm^{-2}, with the rear face insulated [54]. *Upper figure* temperature field through the thickness of the laminate versus time. *Lower figure* residual resin content field through the thickness of the laminate versus time

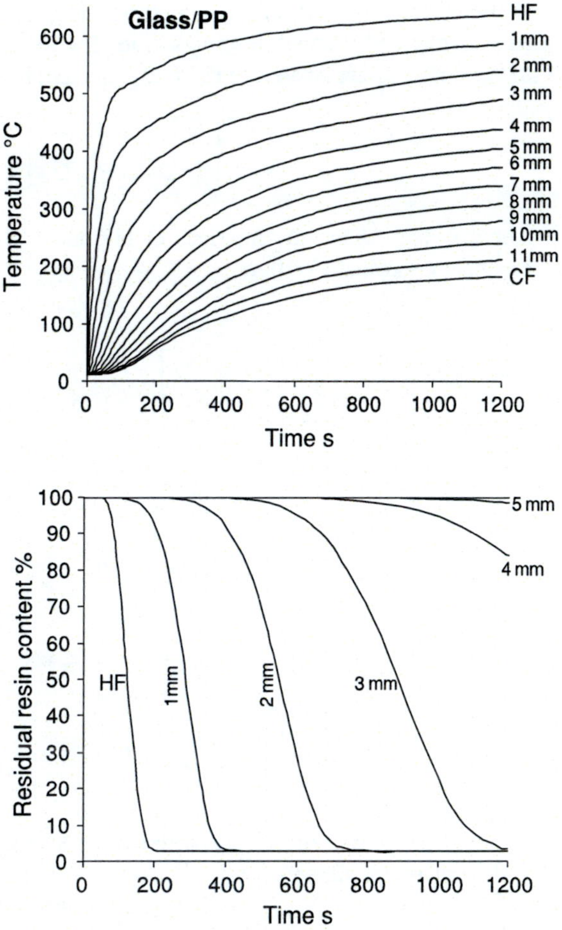

temperature being calculated directly from the TGA curve for the resin. The endothermic nature of the decomposition process is allowed for by calculating an apparent enthalpy for the resin, so the Henderson Equation (8.10) is effectively reduced to the unsteady state heat conduction Equation, albeit with a rather complex relationship between thermal diffusivity and temperature. This model has been found to work well in most circumstances relating to fire modelling. However, if heating rates are significantly different from those used in the TGA measurements, some errors can be expected.

8.6.2 Laminate Constitutive Relationship

Lamination theory, which generally applies under isothermal conditions, describes the behaviour of a multiple composites [56–58]. The theory can be readily modified to model the situation where composite properties vary as a result of increasing temperature and thermal decomposition. The forces and bending moments applied to the laminate are related to the mid-plane strains and curvatures by

$$\begin{bmatrix} \tilde{N} \\ \tilde{M} \end{bmatrix} = \begin{bmatrix} \tilde{A} & \tilde{B} \\ \tilde{B} & \tilde{D} \end{bmatrix} \begin{bmatrix} \tilde{\varepsilon}_0 \\ \tilde{k} \end{bmatrix} \tag{8.12}$$

where $\tilde{N}$ and $\tilde{M}$ are the matrices of normal loads and bending moments in the laminate coordinate system:

$$\tilde{N} = \begin{bmatrix} N_x \\ N_y \\ N_{xy} \end{bmatrix} \quad and \quad \tilde{M} = \begin{bmatrix} M_x \\ M_y \\ M_{xy} \end{bmatrix} \tag{8.13}$$

and, $\tilde{\varepsilon}_0$ and $\tilde{k}$ are the mid-plane strains and curvatures:

$$\tilde{\varepsilon}_0 = \begin{bmatrix} \varepsilon_x \\ \varepsilon_y \\ \gamma_{xy} \end{bmatrix} \quad and \quad \tilde{k} = \begin{bmatrix} k_x \\ k_y \\ k_{xy} \end{bmatrix} \tag{8.14}$$

The $\tilde{A}$, $\tilde{B}$ and $\tilde{D}$ matrices can be defined as

$$\tilde{A} = \sum_{k=1}^{n} \int_{h_{k-1}}^{h_k} \tilde{\tilde{Q}} dz \quad \tilde{B} = \sum_{k=1}^{n} \int_{h_{k-1}}^{h_k} \tilde{\tilde{Q}} z dz \quad \tilde{D} = \sum_{k=1}^{n} \int_{h_{k-1}}^{h_k} \tilde{\tilde{Q}} z^2 dz \tag{8.15}$$

where $\tilde{Q}$ is the matrix of ply stiffness constants transformed to the coordinate system of the laminate:

$$\tilde{Q} = \begin{bmatrix} \tilde{Q}_{11} & \tilde{Q}_{12} & \tilde{Q}_{16} \\ \tilde{Q}_{12} & \tilde{Q}_{22} & \tilde{Q}_{26} \\ \tilde{Q}_{16} & \tilde{Q}_{26} & \tilde{Q}_{66} \end{bmatrix} \tag{8.16}$$

These constants vary from ply to ply according to the orientation within each layer. In the present case the definitions shown in Eq. (8.15) have been modified by the addition of an integral to the summation over the plies. This is because properties can vary smoothly in the z-direction due to the effect of varying temperature and resin decomposition within the laminate. It is necessary to account for this variation in addition to the variation that would normally be expected between different plies, which is described by the summation.

For some problems it is convenient to employ a partially inverted form of Eq. (8.12):

$$\begin{bmatrix} \tilde{\varepsilon}_0 \\ \tilde{M} \end{bmatrix} = \begin{bmatrix} \tilde{A}* & \tilde{B}* \\ \tilde{B}* & \tilde{D}* \end{bmatrix} \begin{bmatrix} \tilde{N} \\ \tilde{k} \end{bmatrix} \tag{8.17}$$

This involves the following operations:

$$\tilde{A}* = \tilde{A}^{-1}$$

$$\tilde{B}* = -\tilde{A}^{-1}\tilde{B} = -\tilde{A}*\tilde{B} \quad \tilde{C}* = \tilde{B}\tilde{A}^{-1} = -\tilde{B}*^{T}$$

and

$$\tilde{D}* = \tilde{D} - \tilde{B}\tilde{A}^{-1}\tilde{B} = \tilde{D} - \tilde{C}*\tilde{B} \tag{8.18}$$

When the boundary conditions of the problem are expressed simply in terms of in-plane loads and moments it is often preferable to employ the fully inverted version:

$$\begin{bmatrix} \tilde{\varepsilon}_0 \\ \tilde{k} \end{bmatrix} = \begin{bmatrix} \tilde{A}' & \tilde{B}' \\ \tilde{B}' & \tilde{D}' \end{bmatrix} \begin{bmatrix} \tilde{N} \\ \tilde{M} \end{bmatrix} \tag{8.19}$$

This involves the following further operations:

$$\tilde{D}' = \tilde{D}*^{-1}$$

$$\tilde{B}' = \tilde{B}*\tilde{D}*^{-1} \tag{8.20}$$

$$\tilde{C}' = -\tilde{D}*^{-1}\,\tilde{C}* = \tilde{B}'^{T} = \tilde{B}'$$

and

$$\tilde{A}' = \tilde{A}* - \tilde{B}*\tilde{D}*^{-1}\,\tilde{C}* = \tilde{A}* + \tilde{B}*\tilde{D}*^{-1}\,\tilde{B}*^{T}$$

8.6.3 Thermal Expansion Effects

The laminate mechanical strain is the sum of the stress-induced and thermally induced deformations, so, modifying Eq. (8.12) to include these gives

$$\begin{bmatrix} \tilde{N} \\ \tilde{M} \end{bmatrix} = \begin{bmatrix} \tilde{A} & \tilde{B} \\ \tilde{B} & \tilde{D} \end{bmatrix} \begin{bmatrix} \tilde{\varepsilon}_0 - \tilde{\varepsilon}_0^{T} \\ \tilde{k} - \tilde{k}^{T} \end{bmatrix} \tag{8.21}$$

where $\tilde{\varepsilon}_0^{T}$ and $\tilde{k}^{T}$ are the thermally induced distortions that would occur in the absence of an externally applied load. Alternatively, it is possible to write down the matrices of thermally induced loads and moments, so that

$$\tilde{F} = \sum_{k=1}^{n} \int_{h_{k-1}}^{h_k} \tilde{\bar{Q}}\tilde{\varepsilon}^{T} dz \quad \text{and} \quad \tilde{G} = \sum_{k=1}^{n} \int_{h_{k-1}}^{h_k} \tilde{\bar{Q}}\tilde{\varepsilon}^{T} z dz \tag{8.22}$$

where $\tilde{\varepsilon}^T$ is the matrix of thermal strains for each ply. As the expansion coefficients may vary, both with temperature and $-z$ coordinate, it is preferable to formulate these matrices in terms of thermal strain, rather than products of expansion coefficient and temperature change.

The thermal loads can be added to the existing loads and moments, to give

$$\begin{bmatrix} \tilde{N} \\ \tilde{M} \end{bmatrix} = \begin{bmatrix} \tilde{A} & \tilde{B} \\ \tilde{B} & \tilde{D} \end{bmatrix} \begin{bmatrix} \tilde{\varepsilon}_0 \\ \tilde{k} \end{bmatrix} + \begin{bmatrix} \tilde{F} \\ \tilde{G} \end{bmatrix} \tag{8.23}$$

Therefore,

$$\begin{bmatrix} \tilde{N} \\ \tilde{M} \end{bmatrix} - \begin{bmatrix} \tilde{F} \\ \tilde{G} \end{bmatrix} = \begin{bmatrix} \tilde{N} - \tilde{F} \\ \tilde{M} - \tilde{G} \end{bmatrix} = \begin{bmatrix} \tilde{A} & \tilde{B} \\ \tilde{B} & \tilde{D} \end{bmatrix} \begin{bmatrix} \tilde{\varepsilon}_0 \\ \tilde{k} \end{bmatrix} \tag{8.24}$$

This can be inverted, as discussed in relation to (8.12), so the deformation with both thermal distortions and mechanical load present is given by

$$\begin{bmatrix} \tilde{\varepsilon}_0 \\ \tilde{k} \end{bmatrix} = \begin{bmatrix} \tilde{A}' & \tilde{B}' \\ \tilde{B}' & \tilde{D}' \end{bmatrix} \begin{bmatrix} \tilde{N} - \tilde{F} \\ \tilde{M} - \tilde{G} \end{bmatrix} \tag{8.25}$$

The zero-load thermal distortions can be found by putting $\tilde{N}$ and $\tilde{M}$ equal to zero, so

$$\begin{bmatrix} \tilde{\varepsilon}_0^T \\ \tilde{k}^T \end{bmatrix} = -\begin{bmatrix} \tilde{A}' & \tilde{B}' \\ \tilde{B}' & \tilde{D}' \end{bmatrix} \begin{bmatrix} \tilde{F} \\ \tilde{G} \end{bmatrix} \tag{8.26}$$

so, if required, (8.25) may alternatively be expressed as

$$\begin{bmatrix} \tilde{\varepsilon}_0 - \tilde{\varepsilon}^T \\ \tilde{k} - \tilde{k}_0^T \end{bmatrix} = \begin{bmatrix} \tilde{A}' & \tilde{B}' \\ \tilde{B}' & \tilde{D}' \end{bmatrix} \begin{bmatrix} \tilde{N} \\ \tilde{M} \end{bmatrix} \tag{8.27}$$

These relationships provide a basis for modelling thermal- and fire-induced changes in laminates under stress. They can be used, for instance, to provide the input for a finite element analysis, to model the behaviour of shell structures under load.

In most practical cases, for instance those involving bending of flat laminates and composite products of relatively simple cross-section, it is possible to make significant simplifications to the above relationships. This is useful in modelling the fire response of plates and beams under load. Modelling of the effects of fire under load can be used to compare and validate experimental results and to perform sensitivity studies to determine which material parameters are most important in influencing behaviour.

The expansion coefficients of a unidirectional ply, needed for the above calculations can be calculated from those of the fibre and matrix by an extension of micromechanics models [56–58]. However, it appears unlikely that the distortions that occur in composites during fire exposure can be described by a simple model involving single values of expansion coefficient [68], as it appears that the expansion coefficient changes significantly, first on passing the glass transition temperature and most prominently during the decomposition process. Work is currently underway to quantify these effects.

8.7 Modelling Fire Response under Load

A number of workers [29, 34, 36–39, 41, 46–55] have now successfully modelled the fire response of composites and composite structures under load.

8.7.1 Two-Layer Model

A two-layer model was successfully implemented to characterise the residual room temperature properties of composites after fire [31–33, 49, 50]. This model assumed a fire-damaged laminate to consist of: an undamaged layer having properties equal to those of the pristine material at room temperature, and a severely damaged or 'char' layer in which the mechanical properties were either negligible or a small fraction of those of the undamaged material.

The use of this approach in conjunction with simple mechanics expressions for the overall properties of the bi-layer structure was very successful in providing an interpretation of residual properties after fire [31, 37]. It is possible to combine the two-layer model with the predictions of the Henderson Equation, (8.10). This requires a criterion for the transition from undamaged material to char. The most useful practical criterion is the degree of decomposition of the resin, as described by the RRC. It has been found that an RRC value of 80% makes an effective practical distinction between undamaged and fully damaged material in many practical cases, for the purposes of the two-layer model [31, 37].

The 80% criterion applies with reasonable accuracy, independently of the resin system, this being true at least for polyester, vinyl ester, epoxy and phenolic-based glass fibre composites. It has even been found to work for the residual compressive strength of carbon fibre epoxy aerospace laminates. Figure 8.19, for instance shows the measured and modelled reductions in tensile properties for a 10 mm thick glass/polyester laminate under a heat flux of 50 kWm^{-2}.

The two-layer model was extended [34], with a small loss of accuracy, to predict the behaviour of composite structures subject to heating under load. Here, the assumption of room temperature properties for the undamaged layer allows considerable simplification of the problem and enables modelling to be carried out on systems where high temperature properties are unavailable. It was found that, for behaviour under load in fire, the effective transition from undamaged to char material occurred at a temperature of 170°C.

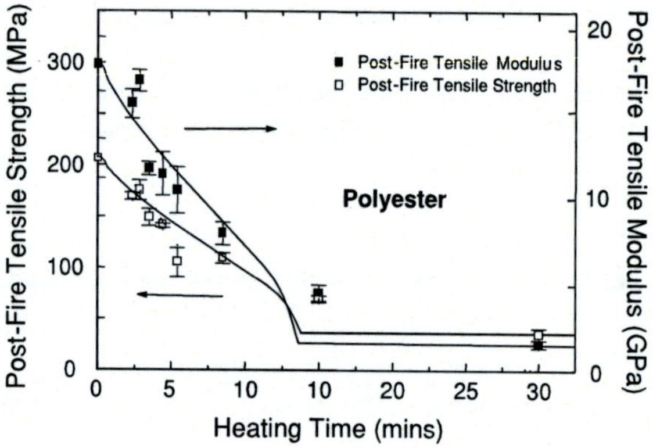

Fig. 8.19 Change in residual tensile properties of glass-polyester laminate with heating time at a heat flux of 50 kW/m^2 (experimental points). The curves show the theoretical post-fire properties determined using the two-layer model and assuming the transition between layers to occur at 80% residual resin content [31, 37]

8.7.2 Laminate Analysis Model

This provides a more accurate description of the composite structure, but requires a functional relationship for the variation of mechanical properties with temperature and resin decomposition. The Henderson model, Eq. (8.10), provides values of the temperature and RRC at all points through the depth of the laminate, as a function of time. This, along with the constitutive relationship for each ply, provides the input to the laminate analysis.

Using this approach, Fig. 8.20 shows the evolution of the *ABD* matrix components of a 12 mm thick glass/vinyl ester laminate with time, under a one-sided heat flux of 50 kWm^{-2}. The *A* matrix components, which relate in-plane loads and deformations, decline rapidly with time, over a period of about 200 s, reflecting the overall decline in the values of the elastic constants. By contrast, the *B* matrix, which describes the interaction between in-plane loads and out-of-plane bending and twisting, is zero initially, but rises to a maximum, before eventually declining over the same time period. The initial zero value of the *B* matrix reflects the symmetry of this laminate's properties about its central axis. The first effect of the heat flux is to produce an asymmetry of properties, resulting in the increase in *B* matrix values. The final fall simply reflects the ultimate decline in all the elastic constant values. It is interesting to note that the *D* matrix, which governs bending resistance, declines with time. However, the influence of the developing asymmetry can be seen from the presence of a 'shoulder' on the curve, which coincides in time with the maximum in the *B* matrix. The laminate Hook's law components in Fig. 8.19 can be used to give a straightforward prediction of the laminate response in simple loading cases, such as in-plane stress or bending. Alternatively, the *ABD* matrix data can form the input for a finite element analysis of structures with more complex geometry or loading.

Figs. 8.21 and 8.22 show measured and modelled stress rupture curves for glass/vinyl ester and glass/polypropylene laminates, respectively, in compression and tension [54]. In the compressive case, the samples were held in a constrained compression jig, as shown in Fig. 8.5, which allowed a significant compressive

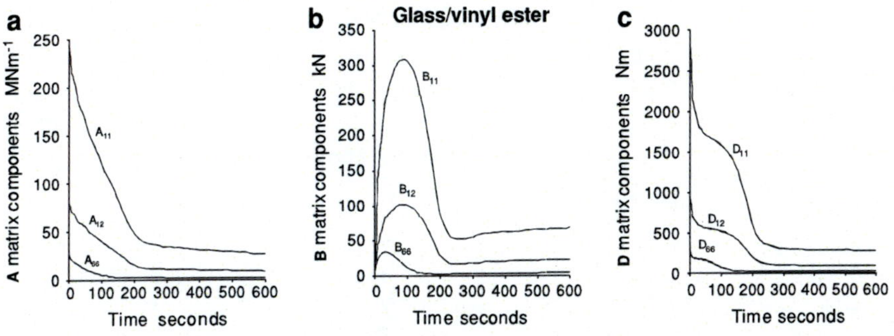

Fig. 8.20 Laminate model for a 12 mm thick glass/vinyl ester laminate, as in Table 8.1 [54]: predicted variation of the components of the laminate *ABD* matrix with time for a one-sided heat flux of 50 kWm^{-2}. **a** *A* matrix components; **b** *B* matrix components, and **c** *D* matrix components

stress to be applied to the plate without global Euler buckling occurring. The stress–rupture curves were produced by generating a laminate stress–strain curve corresponding to each time step, based on the temperature and residual resin fields shown in Figs. 8.17 and 8.18, which had been obtained by solution of Henderson Equation. The overall or average laminate tensile or compressive stress is given by

$$\bar{\sigma} = \frac{1}{t}\sum_{k=1}^{n} \int_{h_{k-1}}^{h_k} \sigma(T, R, \varepsilon) dz \tag{8.28}$$

where t is the laminate thickness and $\sigma(T,R,\varepsilon)$ is the ply stress in the loading direction, which can be seen to be a function of temperature, RRC and strain. Evaluating this function enables the average stress to be computed over a range of

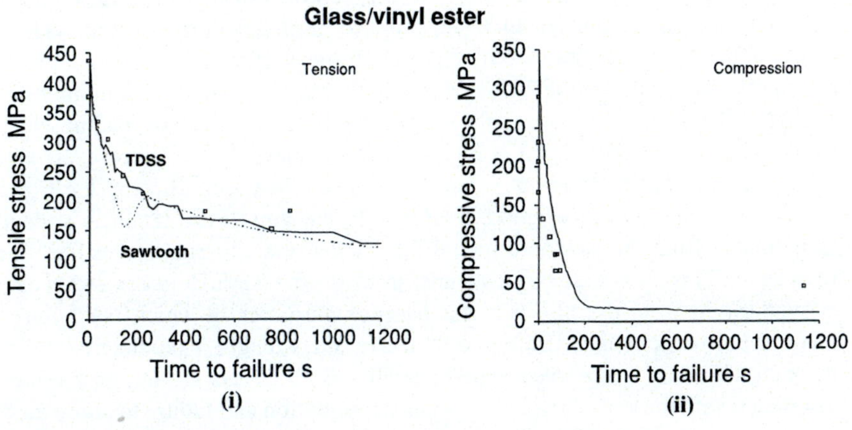

Fig. 8.21 Comparison of measured and predicted variation of lifetime under tensile and compressive load for a 12 mm thick glass/vinyl ester laminate [54], as in Table 8.1, under a heat flux of 50 kWm^{-2}. In the tensile case, the predictions of two models, the sawtooth model and the time-dependent stress–strain (TDSS) model are compared

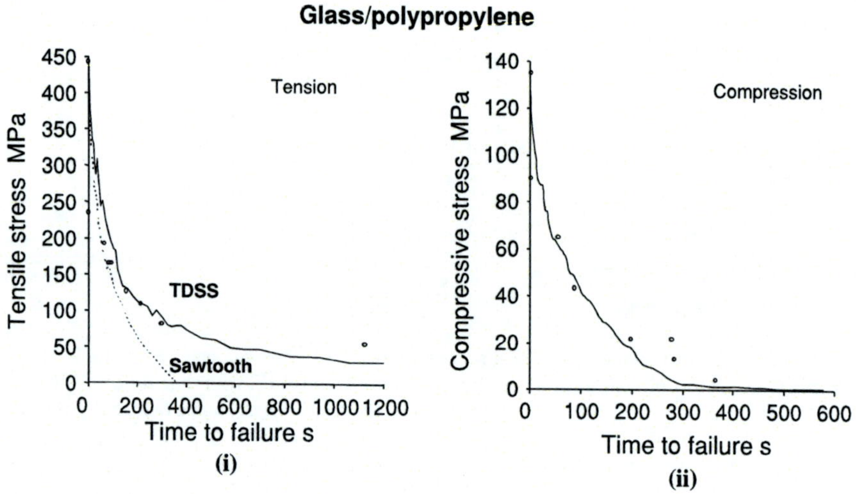

Fig. 8.22 Comparison of measured and predicted variation of lifetime under tensile and compressive load for a 12 mm thick glass/polypropylene laminate [54], as in Table 8.1, under a heat flux of 50 kWm^{-2}. In the tensile case, the predictions of two models, the sawtooth model and the time-dependent stress–strain (TDSS) model, are compared

strains, which allows the maximum stress to be found. This, in turn, enables the laminate strength to be found as a function of time, which is compared to the stress–rupture curves shown in Figs. 8.21 and 8.22. It is relevant to observe that no material time dependence or viscoelasticity was included in this model. The time evolution of the rupture stress in these figures was entirely due to the evolution of the material stress–strain curve as a function of temperature and resin decomposition. The model was evaluated for two different assumed parametric shapes of stress–strain relationship. The first, and simplest, assumed all stress strain relations to be of the triangular ‘sawtooth’ type. Here the performance was assumed to be entirely described by the Young’s modulus and by the tensile or compressive strength. The sawtooth relationship worked well for compressive loading, where the stress–strain curves, shown in Fig. 8.15 for the glass/vinyl ester case, are close to having this shape. However, it can be seen that in tensile loading the experimental agreement is not so good. In Fig. 8.21 the vinyl ester laminate strength, as predicted from the sawtooth model falls below the experimental values, then rises again. This is because of the manner in which the laminate stress–strain curve is synthesised from the ply data and because the order in which ply failure is predicted to occur changes. In Fig. 8.22 the tensile strength is predicted to fall off more rapidly than is observed experimentally. Both effects are due to the errors associated with the two-parameter sawtooth assumption and failure to allow for the non-linearity of the tensile stress–strain curves, which can be seen in Fig. 8.15.

To overcome the problems with the sawtooth model in the tensile case, the more complex three-parameter model, based on Eq. (8.11), was employed. This was referred to as the ‘temperature-dependent stress–strain’, or TDSS model.

It can be seen from Figs. 8.21 and 8.22 that the TDSS model, although requiring an extra parameter, produces a considerable improvement in the accuracy of the failure prediction. It was later found that a three-parameter model may be unnecessary. A simple averaging of the material tensile strength across the section, which greatly simplified the calculations, was found to give rather similar predictions to the TDSS model. This is, in effect, equivalent to assuming that the laminate shows a perfectly plastic stress–strain relation.

The results discussed here show that it is possible to achieve good agreement between model predictions and test data on composites under load in fire. One effect that has not yet been taken into account is viscoelastic and viscoplastic time dependence of composites at elevated temperatures. The omission of these effects is probably justified in the current models because the path followed by the material in the thermal domain is much more critical than that followed in time. The time periods covered here range from the order of 1–1000 s. The justification for omitting time dependence at this stage is one of simplification of computation requirements. Using isochronous creep data based on 1000 s, rather than on 1 s makes relatively little difference to the predictions reported here. The approach presented here will no doubt be extended to include full time-dependent analyses, of both the linear and non-linear kind: the foundations for doing this have been established by Boyd et al. [69].

8.8 Conclusions

The engineering basis for high temperature measurements of both elastic properties and the strength of composites has been briefly reviewed. Methods of characterising fire response under load by means of small-scale tests have also been discussed, and requirements for modelling fire behaviour under load in fire have been examined. It has been demonstrated that meaningful simulations can be achieved.

Acknowledgments The research reported here was carried out in research programmes at Newcastle University UK and at RMIT Australia. The authors wish to acknowledge the support of two organisations that have contributed to the advances described: the United States Office of Naval Research (under Grant Nos N00014-04-10026 and N00014-07-10514) and the European Union (Marie Curie Momentum Research Transfer Network on Multidisciplinary Research and Training on Composite Materials Applications in Transport Modes. Contract number MRTN/CT/2005/019198).

References

1. Mouritz AP, Feih S, Kandare E, Mathys Z, Gibson AG, DesJardin PE, Case SW, Lattimer BY (2009) Review of fire structural modelling of polymer composites. Composites 40A(12):1800–1814
2. Gutierrez J, Parneix P, Bollero A, Hoyning B, McGeorge D, Gibson AG, Wright PNR (2005) Fire and materials conference. San Francisco, USA, 31 Jan–1 Feb:425–438

3. Gutierrez J, Breuillard A, Corrignan P, Marquis D, Chivas C, Guillaume E, Pavageau M (2008) Use of fire safety engineering for the design of marine structures. Composites in Fire-5, Newcastle, 10–11 July
4. Greene E (1993) Fire performance of composite materials for naval applications. US Navy Contract N61533-91-C-0017, Structural Composites Inc., Melbourne FL USA. www.marinecomposites.com
5. Murrell J, Briggs P (2008) Developments in the fire testing and certification of composites used in railway and marine applications. Composites in Fire-5, Newcastle, 10–11 July
6. CEN/TS 45545—Fire protection on railway vehicles—Part 2: Requirements for fire behaviour of materials and components
7. Mouritz AP (2008) Review of smoke toxicity of aerospace composites. Composites in Fire-5, Newcastle, 10–11 July
8. Dodd DC, Hall CTM, Pollard J, Snell MA (1994) Burnthrough resistance of fuselages: initial findings. CAA Paper 94002, Civil Aviation Authority, London
9. Marker TR (1999) Full-scale test evaluation of aircraft fuel fire burnthrough resistance improvements. DOT/FAA/AR-98/52, Office of Aviation Research, Washington, DC 20591
10. Babrauskas V (1982) Development of the cone calorimeter: a bench scale heat release rate apparatus based on oxygen consumption (NBSIR 82-2611), USA, National Bureau of Standards
11. Babrauskas V, Peacock RD (1992) Heat release rate: the single most important variable in fire hazard. Fire Saf J 18:255–272
12. Huggett C (1980) Estimation of rate of heat release by means of oxygen consumption measurements. Fire Mater 4:61–65
13. ISO 5660-1: 2002 Reaction to fire—heat release, smoke production and mass loss rate (cone calorimeter method)
14. Gibson AG, Hume J (1995) Fire performance of composite panels for large marine structures. Plast Rub Compos 23:175–183
15. Bamford CH, Crank J, Malan DH (1946) Proc Camb Phil Soc 42:166–182
16. Kung H-C (1972) Combust Flame 18:185–195
17. Kansa EJ, Perlee HE, Chaiken RF (1977) Combust Flame 29:311–324
18. Henderson JB, Weibelt JA, Tant MR (1985) J Compos Mater 19:579–595
19. Henderson JB, Wiecek TE (1987) J Compos Mater 21:373–393
20. Griffiths CA, Nemes JA, Stonesifer FR, Chang CI (1986) J Compos Mater 20:216–235
21. Milke JA, Vizzini AJ (1991) J Compos Technol Res 13:141–151
22. Sorathia U, Beck C, Dapp T (1993) J Fire Sci 11:255–270
23. Gibson AG, Wu Y-S, Chandler HW, Wilcox JAD, Bettess P (1995) Rev l'Inst Franc Petrol 50(1):69–74
24. Sorathia U, Lyon R, Gann R, Gritzo L (1996) SAMPE J 32:8–15
25. Looyeh MRE, Bettess P, Gibson AG (1997) Int J Numer Methods Heat Fluid Flow 7(6):609–625
26. Dodds N, Gibson AG, Dewhurst D, Davies JM (2000) Composites 31A:689–702
27. Pering GA, Farrell PV, Springer GS (1981) Degradation of tensile and shear properties of composites exposed to fire or high temperature. In: Springer GS (ed) Environmental Effects on Composite Materials. Technomic Publishing, New York
28. Massot JJ (1994) Glass reinforced plastics heavy load flooring for offshore platforms. In Composite Materials in the Offshore Industry, Rueil-Malmaison, France, 3–4 November, Institut Français du Pétrole. 9
29. Dao M, Asaro RJ (1999) A study on failure prediction and design criteria for fiber composites under fire degradation. Composites 30A:123–131
30. Mouritz AP, Mathys Z (1999) Post-fire mechanical properties of marine polymer composites. Compos Struct 47:643–653
31. Mouritz AP, Mathys Z (2001) Post-fire mechanical properties of glass-reinforced polyester composites. Compos Sci Technol 61:475–490

32. Gardiner CP, Mouritz AP, Mathys Z, Townsend CR (2002) Tensile and compressive properties of GRP composites with local heat damage. Appl Compos Mater 9(6):353–367
33. Gibson AG, Wright PNH, Wu Y-S, Mouritz AP, Mathys Z, Gardiner CP (2003) Modelling residual mechanical properties of polymer composites after fire. Plast Rub Compos 32(2): 81–90
34. Lua J, O'Brien JO (2003) Fire simulation for woven fabric composites with temperature and mass dependent thermal-mechanical properties. Composites in Fire-3, University of Newcastle upon Tyne, 9–10 Sept
35. Seggewiss PGB (2003) Properties of fire-damaged polymer matrix composites. Composites in Fire-3, University of Newcastle upon Tyne, 9–10 Sept
36. Gibson AG, Wu Y-S, Evans JT, Mouritz AP (2006) Laminate theory analysis of composites under load in fire. J Compos Mater 40:639–658
37. Gibson AG, Wright PNH, Wu Y-S, Mouritz AP, Mathys Z, Gardiner CP (2004) The integrity of polymer composites during and after fire. J Compos Mater 38:1283–1308
38. Liu L, Holmes JW, Kardomateas GA, Birman V (2005) Compressive response of composites under combined fire and compressive loading. Composites in Fire-4, Newcastle-upon-Tyne, 15–16 Sept
39. Zhou A, Keller T (2005) Structural response of FRP elements under combined thermal and mechanical loading: experiments and analysis. Composites in Fire-4, Newcastle-upon-Tyne, 15–16 Sept
40. Lattimer BY (2005) Using small samples to get large-scale results. Composites in Fire-4, Newcastle-upon-Tyne, 15–16 Sept
41. Keller T, Tracy C, Zhou A (2006) Structural response of liquid-cooled GFRP slabs subjected to fire—Parts I and II. Composites 37A(9):1286–1308
42. Mouritz AP, Feih S, Mathys Z, Gibson AG (2006) Mechanical property degradation of naval composite materials in fire. In: Couchman L, Mouritz AP (eds) Modeling of naval composite structures in fire. Acclaim Printing, Melbourne
43. Bausano JV, Lesko JJ, Case SW (2006) Composite lifetime during combined compressive loading and one-sided simulated fire exposure. Composites 37A:1092–1100
44. Key CT, Lua J (2006) Constituent based analysis of composite materials subjected to fire conditions. Composites 37A:1005–1014
45. Liu L, Kardomateas GA, Birman V, Holmes JW, Simitses GJ (2006) Thermal buckling of a heat-exposed, axially restrained composite column. Composites 37A:972–980
46. Luo C, Xie W, DesJardin PE (2006) Fluid-structure simulations of composite materials response for fire environments. In: Couchman L, Mouritz AP (eds) Modeling of naval composite structures in fire. Acclaim Printing, Melbourne
47. Lattimer BY, Ouellette J (2006) Properties of composite materials for thermal analysis involving fires. Composites 37A:1068–1081
48. Birman V, Kardomateas GA, Simitses GJ, Li R (2006) Response of a sandwich panel subjected to fire or elevated temperature on one of the surfaces. Composites 37A:981–988
49. Feih S, Mathys Z, Gibson AG, Mouritz AP (2007) Modelling the tension and compression strengths of polymer laminates in fire. Compos Sci Technol 67:551–564
50. Feih S, Mouritz AP, Mathys Z, Gibson AG (2007) Tensile strength modelling of glass fiber-polymer laminates in fire. J Compos Mater 41(19):2387–2410
51. Easby RC, Feih S, Konstantis C, La Delfa G, Urso Miano V, Elmughrabi AE, Mouritz AP, Gibson AG (2007) Failure model for phenolic and polyester pultrusions under load in fire. Plast Rub Compos 36(9):379–388
52. Bai Y, Vallée T, Keller T (2008) Modeling of thermal responses for FRP composites under elevated and high temperatures. Compos Sci Technol 68(1):47–56
53. Bai Y, Keller T (2008) Modeling of stiffness of FRP composites under elevated and high temperatures. Compos Sci Technol 68(15–16):3099–3106
54. Browne TNA (2006) A model for the structural integrity of composite laminates in fire. Ph.D. thesis, University of Newcastle

55. Easby RC (2006) Fire behavior of pultruded composites. Ph.D. thesis, University of Newcastle
56. Agarwal BD, Broutman LJ (1990) Analysis and performance of fiber Composites. Wiley, New York
57. Eckold G (1994) Design and manufacture of composite structures. Woodhead Publishing Ltd, Cambridge
58. Jones RM (1974) Mechanics of composite materials. Scripta Book Company, Washington
59. Boeing Specification Support Standard (1986) Advanced Composite Compression Tests, BSS 7260
60. Budiansky B, Fleck NA (1993) J Mech Phys Solids 41:183–211
61. Kulcarni AP, Gibson RF (2003) Non-destructive characterisation of effects of temperature and moisture on elastic moduli of vinyl ester resin and E-glass/vinyl ester resin composite. American society of composites, 18th Annual technical conference. Florida, 19–22 Oct
62. Mahieux CA, Reifsnider KL (2001) Property modeling across transition temperatures in polymer matrix composites: Part 1: Tensile properties. Polymer 42(7):3281–3290
63. Mahieux CA, Reifsnider KL (2002) Property modeling across transition temperatures in polymers: application to thermoplastic systems. J Mater Sci 37:911–920
64. Feih S, Manatpon K, Mathys Z, Gibson AG, Mouritz AP (2008) Strength degradation of glass fibers at high temperatures. J Mater Sci 44(2):392–400
65. Gupta PK (1988) Glass fibers for composite materials. In: Bunsell AR (ed) Fiber reinforcements for composite materials. Elsevier, New York
66. Gibson AG, Wright PNH, Wu Y-S (2004) A small-scale, low cost technique for fire resistance of composites. SAMPE conference, Long Beach, California, 16–20 May
67. Urso Miano V, Gibson AG (2009) Fire model for fibre reinforced plastic composites using apparent thermal diffusivity (ATD). Plast Rub Compos 38(2–4):367–373
68. Florio J, Henderson JB, Test FL, Hariharan R (1991) A study of the effects of the assumption of local thermal equilibrium on the overall thermally-induced response of a decomposing glass-filled polymer composites. Int J Heat Mass Transf 34:135–147
69. Boyd SE, Lesko JJ, Case SW, Bausano JV (2005) The viscoelastic/viscoplastic characterisation of glass-vinyl ester composites under fire conditions. Composites in Fire-4, University of Newcastle upon Tyne, 15–16 Sept